BODY FAT AND PHYSICAL FITNESS

BODY FAT AND PHYSICAL FITNESS

BODY COMPOSITION AND LIPID METABOLISM IN DIFFERENT REGIMES OF PHYSICAL ACTIVITY

JANA PAŘÍZKOVÁ, M. D.
Research Institute, Faculty of Physical Education
Charles University, Prague

1977

MARTINUS NIJHOFF B. V. / MEDICAL DIVISION
THE HAGUE

ISBN 90.247.1925.9

This book is published with the arrangement of
AVICENUM, Czechoslovak Medical Press, Prague

Printed in Czechoslovakia

Contents

Introduction

Man develops during phylogenesis and ontogenesis as an active creature and his most striking external manifestations include physical activity. From this ensue efforts to investigate the human organism with regard to its functional diagnosis mainly during activity, in relation to the level of that physical activity.

The amount and qualitative aspect of physical activity is subject to some laws associated with the developmental stage, type of higher nervous activity, health, nutritional status, external environment incl. social position, profession, hobbies, etc.; thus it is also one of the important ecological factors. During the period before the onset of technical civilization physical fitness and performance were essential prerequisites for survival and successful existence. At present and from the aspect of the perspective development of our civilization the importance of physical fitness is pushed into the background; nevertheless adequate physical activity level is even today an important prerequisite for normal function of the organism as a whole.

A serious shortcoming is that so far we possess only very few data not only on the total volume but also on the structure and temporal distribution of physical activity in micro- and macrocycles in different individuals by age, sex, occupation, etc. in different population groups, although it is one of the basic characteristics of the individual (obviously this is to some extent due to methodical difficulties associated with accurate and long-term investigations of these parameters in human subjects under quite normal conditions). Moreover, these properties are closely related to a number of other characteristics of the organism; in this connection we must emphasize in particular the caloric intake of the individual and his balance which is closely dependant on the physical activity as one of the most important components responsible for the above basal energy expenditure. Every man is according to Widdowson (1962) a "*nutritional individuality*" resulting from a number of factors. In addition to *certain dietary habits* and *preferences* there is in particular the aspect of *overall caloric intake* which may differ considerably (i.e. be more than treble) even in quite homogeneous groups. *Similar differences exist also in the total volume of physical activity.* As revealed e.g. by investigations of Soviet authors (Slonim and Smirnov 1972, Gapon 1972) the difference in the physical activity of Novosibirsk citizens in groups of equal age, occupation, sex, living conditions, etc. was sevenfold or greater (range 3,500–25,000 steps per day assessed by means of a pedometer or heart beat totalizer). Although there were certain day-to-day differences in physical activity, when measured for a prolonged period the *physical activity settled at a level typical for a given individual.* In quite homogeneous groups of Sprague Dawley rats Collier (1971b) proved individual differences which were as high as tenfold. Investigations of children (Ledovskaya 1972) revealed a *greater similarity of the physical activity of monozygotic than dizygotic twins* which suggests a *certain constitutional and hereditary basis.* Sklad (1972) also found *closer agreement in the structure of physical activity in monozygotic than dizygotic twins.* It is obvious that in the sphere of physical activity the individual also displays a certain *"motor individuality"*; this pertains to the *total volume of activity, its structure, distribution in time,* etc.

Activity levels can differ from the earliest periods of growth; Mack and Kleinhenz (1974) found strong inverse correlations between growth in weight and both activity level and growth in length suggesting that rapid development *of unique body configurations consistent with possible later obesity begin to emerge in the earliest weeks of life* (Rose and Mayer 1968). From this it ensues that the definition of physical activity based on accurate measurements is not only *one of the important characteristics of the organism* but promotes in addition the *understanding of the nature of "nutritional individuality"* (e.g. why with the same caloric intake some subjects deposit excessive fat while others do not) etc. and also some *other properties of the organism from the physiological and possibly also the pathological aspect.*

Views on the part played by physical activity regime under conditions of the present way of life still differ considerably. Although correct views of its importance and usefulness predominate, occasionally very extreme views are also encountered which vary between refusal to pay any attention to physical activity to the assumption that physical exercise can help to resolve all possible problems which vex humanity. This position can be explained by the fact that it is not always possible to present overall conclusive evidence on the importance of optimal physical activity regime or vice versa. This results in particular from the *variability of the human organism as regards the degree of spontaneous individual physical activity and its need* (so far we only know that it may vary within an extremely wide range), which is further *modified by a vast number of other factors which act on the organism during ontogenesis.* The same degree of physical activity thus represents a different stimulus in individual cases, in subjects of different age, with a different case-record, with different motivation and interest and generally different personal characteristics. *The problem of the optimum amount of physical activity for the individual, i.e. the total volume and structure with regard to his genotype and phenotype has not been resolved;* different recommendations are based on empirism and partial studies pertaining only to some aspects.

The majority of work on the influence of physical exercise is based on comparisons of individuals who decide to take up more intensive exercise (and adhere to it for some prolonged time) with those who are relatively inactive. An analysis of causes is lacking. Therefore we cannot rule out in these individuals a certain degree of *primary difference, either manifest or latent which leads to a different interest in exercise and which may be of various origin. These differences then can act as a feedback in particular in children and young persons*—initial success makes the individual persevere in sports or other activities, and conversely failure makes him detest exercise and leads to the preference of other interests. The problem is thus to differentiate inborn prerequisities (functional, morphological, psychological, etc.) from adaptational consequences to different physical activity and their mutual relationship in individual instances and thus to provide more convincing evidence on the action of different levels of physical activity. An exact trial in the normal human population is so far practically impossible. (It would be difficult to find groups of healthy normal subjects with the same constitution and genetic background, nutrition, living conditions, etc. and maintain them on a constant regime of physical activity or inactivity.)

Another aspect is that *under equal conditions increased physical activity exerts a differentiated action as regards different systems, organs, tissues, etc.* In some instances consequences of adaptation are manifested very clearly; in others the effect is manifested indirectly, it is mediated; and finally in some it is not manifested at all. If its action is inadequate the effect of a certain physical activity may also be negative which may apply in particular to subjects with poor physical disposition or weakened individuals (about 5–10% of the population according to WHO) or even with latent minor malformations (e.g. of the vascular system, etc., which may be manifested adversely only after an extreme load). Much depends also on the selected indicators and aspects. So far very few indicators are investigated most of them being directly associated with physical activity and muscular work.

Functional diagnosis attempts to classify the organism from different aspects, the latter include *morphological, vegetative, motor, biochemical etc. aspects.* The somatic characteristic is one of the substantial components of this diagnosis. The morphological shaping of the organism is the result of constitutional factors as well as factors of the external environment which play a part during ontogenetic development (e.g. health record, environmental hygiene, nutrition, regime of physical activity, etc.). The resulting condition ensuing from the action of these and other factors is, however, the basis which can influence and in some instances co-determine the functional capacity of the organism. *The functional diagnosis must be conceived dynamically, i.e. as defining the functional state of the organism which results from a certain previous development, and on this basis we may establish the prognosis of responses of the organism under conditions of a different physical load.*

Functional diagnosis has proved to be of basic importance, especially during growth when evaluating the level of development from a complex point of view. In recent decades the *secular trend of acceleration of growth* manifests (Morant 1950, Tanner 1962, 1973; Trotter and Gleser 1951, Karsaycvskaya 1964 etc.) mainly in industrially developed countries characterized inter alia by decreasing level of physical activity in everyday life. There are few data about changes of different parts of the organism, or different body components, organs, tissues etc. and in connection with that, of resulting changes of functional state of the organism. There is already some evidence that *these changes are not always positive and desirable from the point of view of functional capacity* (and thus also as regards *health prognosis and longevity) without further interventions* in hygiene, way of life, nutrition etc. and last but not least—also in regime of physical activity.

Among the wide range of morphological indicators there has been for a long time a desire to define one which is closely related to vegetative, motor, biochemical and other processes in the organism. Based on some functional studies, changes of body composition are in the foreground as being one of the most striking and regularly encountered consequences of adaptation to a different level of physical activity. *In this context we understand by body composition the assessment of relative and absolute lean body mass (LBM) comprising all tissues with the exception of depot fat which is the second main component* (Keys and Brožek 1953).

LBM is as compared with the total body weight more closely related with a number of physiological variables such as oxygen consumption under basal conditions and during different loads, cardiac output, vital capacity, respiratory volume, renal clearance, peformance etc. (Keys and Brožek 1953; Behnke et al. 1966; Buskirk and Taylor 1957; Zhdanova and Pařízková 1962; Pařízková and Šprynarová 1970; Malina 1975; Kitagawa et al. 1974; Fidanza 1975 etc.). As a result of different factors which act during ontogenesis on the development of body composition great individual differences are found in this respect even among subjects of similar age, height and body weight. Measurement of lean body mass and fat renders thus possible the evaluation of an important morphological and functional characteristic of the organism; moreover *lean body mass serves as one of basic reference standards* in addition to body weight, body surface etc. which do not always prove to be satisfactory especially from the point of view of energy metabolism (Holliday et al. 1967; Schmit-Nielsen 1970 etc.) during ontogeny.—Arshavsky (1972) established the role of skeletal muscles as one of the main factors which determine individual development and thus the whole process of evolution, and designated, in contrast to the energy rule of body surface, the "energy rule of the activity of skeletal muscles" (which represent the main part of lean body mass and which are *in vivo* hardly measurable).

In connection with the problem of body composition we may specify the problems in several spheres: they comprise above all *changes during ontogenesis* which *differ in the two sexes* and are very *typical in different stages of the life cycle. These developmental changes of LBM and fat are associated with the energy balance and level of the energy turnover* which itself undergoes marked changes during ontogenesis and thus is one of the main determining factors responsible for variations of body composition. All factors which influence this equilibrium—in particular *diet and muscular work*—are therefore *reflected in a significant way in the body composition and may modify its developmental trend.* At the same time they are factors by which we may interfere intentionally with the development of body composition and influence it in a desired direction.

We therefore paid attention to changes in LBM and fat throughout ontogenesis starting with earliest childhood up to old age. *As regards the influence of energy turnover we concentrated our attention on the component pertaining to energy output, represented by physical activity and muscular work* and secondarily the *corresponding caloric intake.* The spontaneous amount of physical activity which displays very wide individual differences can be reflected, no doubt, in functional, metabolic, morphological and other properties of the organism. So far we have no definite idea on these relationships as adequate data on physical activity during prolonged periods are lacking. During the so-called *critical periods,* e.g. early childhood (Seefeldt 1975) or the pubertal period, *it is obviously possible to produce by a different regime of physical activity a more marked actual effect or interfere with "programming" of subsequent development and influence late sequelae.* A more profound approach to these problems is only in its initial stages: experimental results assembled in recent years indicate that even the *action of some factors during pregnancy* (in particular the last stage) may be of fundamental importance in this respect.

Energy metabolism is closely related with general metabolism which affects the biochemical processess at a cellular level. The regulatory mechanisms which control these processes are the links in the chain of changes which in their final stage lead inter alia to more visible changes in body composition. Investigations of some *factors which are responsible for changes in lean body mass and fat in different age groups or during different periods of adaptation to a various intensity of physical activity (e.g. regulation of caloric intake, the level of metabolic activity of tissues, in particular adipose and muscular tissue) and finally the part played by body composition in some induced pathological situations* provided in some instances a basic solution for the elucidation of results obtained in cross-sectional and long-term investigations of LBM and fat in human subjects.

To study the above problems very varied methodical approaches were needed. Cross-sectional and longitudinal investigations of LBM and fat in human subjects and in turn their effect on energy metabolism, functional capacity, biochemical indicators etc. during loads, starting during the growth period and ending in old age were supplemented in various stages of research by studies on *experimental models using laboratory animals* to make more detailed analysis at a tissue level possible.

As we have worked in the human part of our studies only with healthy subjects who participate in our examinations on a voluntary basis, procedures were used causing as little inconvenience as possible, to enable us to keep in touch with the subjects for a number of years. This approach naturally restricted our examination methods (which cannot be compared with the opportunities of clinical research) in particular when working with children.

In attempting a more detailed analysis of processes and mechanisms which change body composition under the influence of the regime of physical activity during ontogenesis we tried to combine the results of methodical programmes and procedures which at first sight may seem incompatible. The sum of submitted results of experimental work therefore did not lead in all instances to a consequential solution of the problems but rather brought forth new problems. It was our desire to elucidate briefly, on the basis of actual results, the importance and impact of the assessment of body composition (used in the Physical Education Research Institute since 1957) and which has become in recent years an integral part of the functional diagnosis not only in research into physical fitness (e.g. in clinics of sports medicine, in research of physical fitness as part of the International Biological Programme IBP, etc.) but also in clinical research, human biology, physiology and pathophysiology of nutrition and other disciplines.

When summarizing the results we considered two possibilities: to list in a logical sequence individual data and their interpretation to resolve different problems consecutively. This would imply alternation of experimental studies in laboratory animals with observations obtained in human subjects. The second approach was to concentrate studies in experimental animals into a special section preceding or followed by studies in humans. The laborious experiment required for the second alternative made us finally return to the first. Nothing prevents the reader from reading chapters containing results obtained in laboratory animals (I, IV, VI, VII, XII) and those pertaining to human subjects (chapters II, III, V, VIII, IX, X, XI) separately. The intention and desire of the author was, however, to follow up the work as it developed in the course of recent years.—Statistical evaluation of the results using common methods (Fisher 1950) was accomplished in collaboration with Z. Roth (Prague) to whom we are greatly indebted for his collaboration.

I. Body composition and metabolic activity of tissues during ontogenesis

1. Ratio of lean body mass and fat in relation to energy turnover

Comparison of the young and adult organism revealed the tendency to enhanced deposition of body fat with advancing age in mammals. This ensues not only from the altered calorie balance but in particular from the different level of energy turnover during ontogenesis. *The young growing organism* ingests a substantially *larger amount of food per body weight unit* than the full grown or old organism. The *basal metabolic rate during growth is at least double* that of the full grown organism (Richet 1889, Rubner 1916, Brody 1945, Holliday et al. 1967) and it declines still further in old age. In addition to energy needed for growth there are from the aspect of caloric requirements changes in the trend of spontaneous physical activity, i.e. muscular work which determines the energy output above the basal metabolic rate. *Spontaneous physical activity is highest in the early stages of ontogenesis and declines in later life.* This was assessed fairly accurately in experimental animals (e.g. Smith and Dugal 1965, Collier 1971a, b) as well as in man (Ledovskaya 1972, Gapon 1972).

Confrontation of all these data pertaining to different constituents of the energy turnover indicates that *in early stages of ontogenesis the level of energy intake and output per unit of weight and time is highest followed by a significant decline during subsequent stages of life* (Fig. 1). With the decline of physical activity we may assume in advanced age also a more readily upset balance between calorie intake and output.

One of the manifestations of general changes of the energy turnover during ontogenesis is also different intensity of metabolic activity (characterized e.g. by $Q\,O_2$) of various tissues (Kleiber and Rogers 1961, Davies 1961 etc.). *The increased metabolic activity reflecting the general higher energy turnover obviously prevents in the young growing organism excessive deposition of fat* which is manifested from the morphological aspect by a typical body composition—*a high ratio of lean,*

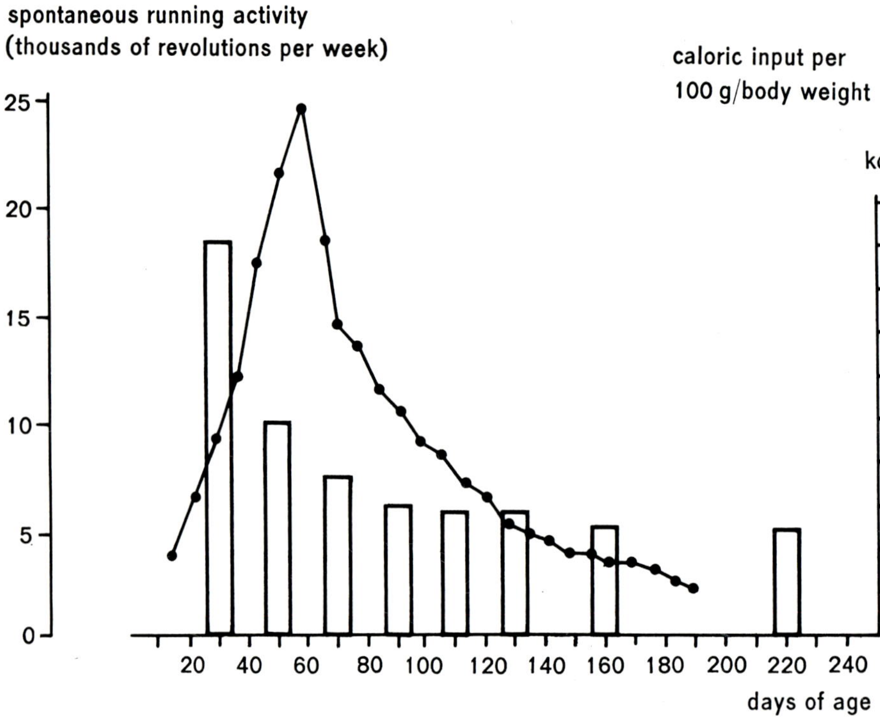

Fig. 1. Changes in spontaneous physical activity and caloric intake in male rats during ontogeny (full points, full line – running activity, i. e. thousands rotations of the drum per week, ordinate – left side; white columns – caloric intake per 100 g body weight and one day, right side). Abscissa – age in days (Smith and Dugal 1965, Pařízková 1968g).

fat-free body mass (LBM) despite increased lipogenesis (Benjamin et al. 1961, Gellhorn et al. 1962). During ageing the ratio of LBM declines. This trend is apparent on an *ad libitum* dietary intake in different animal species. Fig. 2 indicates changes in the body fat ratio and body weight in male and female rats (Wistar strain) assessed by the extraction method.

The total body fat of rats (*Rattus norvegicus laboratorius*, strain Wistar) was estimated by weighing the chloroform extract of the organism saponified by a mixture of 30% KOH in 50% alcohol (Keys et al. 1959, Pařízková and Staňková 1964). Fat-free body mass (which is comparable but not identical with lean body mass estimated in human subjects by densitometry — Behnke et al. 1942) was evaluated as the difference between weight (g) and absolute amount of fat (g).

The percentage of fat was lowest in young animals, males and females. The calculation of variation coefficients revealed a great variability of body fat values although the experimental animals were from equally sized litters (eight pups per mother weaned always by the 30th–32nd day) and lived under similar conditions (Larsen mixture *ad libitum*, size of boxes cca 30 × 45 × 28 cm).

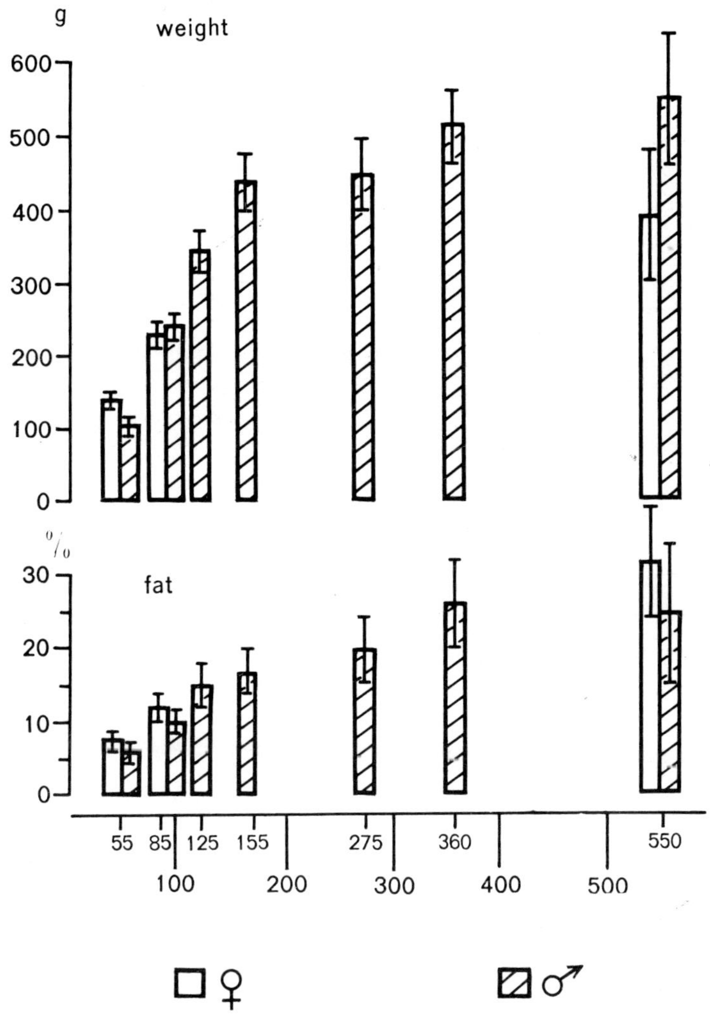

Fig. 2. Changes of weight (g – upper part) and percentage of body fat (% – lower part) in male and female rats during ontogenesis (x̄ ± SD). Abscissa – age in days (Pařízková 1968g).

The results of body fat ratio measurements under these conditions, also under this set-up, are in keeping with the trends of ontogenetic changes in the energy turnover (Fig. 1) (Pařízková 1968f,g, Smith and Dugal 1965). *The considerable individual variability of body fat* in rats of similar age may be associated among others factors with the above-mentioned *variability in spontaneous physical activity* (Collier 1971; Ledovskaya 1972; Gapon 1972; Slonim and Smirnov 1972). When comparing shorter periods of time, the physical activity of an organism varies considerably; in longer time periods the differences are, however, compensated and settled down on a typical individual value which may cause also a different metabolic stereotype.

With the development of body fat various factors may interfere in the earliest stage of ontogenesis, in particular *nutritional factors* (Widdowson and McCance 1975; Widdowson and Kennedy 1962). Kennedy and Mitra (1963) demonstrated that by rearing experimental animals in different sized litters the development of body weight and body fat at a later age can be influenced. Our experiments confirmed this finding (Faltová and Pařízková 1970); male rats fed in groups of three per nest had at the age of nine weeks a significantly higher body fat ratio and body weight than animals fed in litters of 14, although after weaning (30th day) they lived under equal conditions and on the same diet (*see* Fig. 91). Knittle and Hirsch (1968) described in rats fed in small litters a different development of fat cells and altered metabolic activity in the epididymal fat of rats.

Investigation in groups of male rats fed a high-fat diet during the period between the 18–30th day indicates a more rapid growth and higher body fat ratio as adults (230 days) than in control rats. Animals fed a high-fat diet during early ontogenesis displayed, as compared with controls, during a certain period (cca between the 50th and 80th day) a *different self-selection of food,* i.e. they *spontaneously ingested significantly more fat* which led to a *higher calorie intake during a certain critical period.* This obviously contributed to the development of a different metabolic stereotype and thus also to a more potent somatic development and greater development of body fat during a period when both groups had the same regime, i.e. after the 30th day (Pařízková 1961b).

Developmental stimuli act obviously most markedly in the earliest stages of ontogenesis (Kennedy and Mitra 1963); the possibility, however, cannot be ruled out that the *development of adipose tissue* is influenced even earlier (Brook 1972), i.e. *during the last stage of pregnancy.* These early consequences are modified by factors acting later, obviously, however, during subsequent life a *certain tendency towards a readier or more limited deposition of fat persists* even when the conditions—diet, activity etc. are the same (Lemonnier et al. 1973 etc.).

2. Composition of lean body mass

The development of lean body mass (LBM) depends both on genetic factors (in humans especially during growth) (Gaidash and Savostyanova 1975) as height and body build (Wolański 1970), and environmental stimuli (nutrition, physical activity etc.). E.g. the number of fibres in skeletal muscles, which represent the main part of LBM is settled already during the 4–5th month of embryonic life (Åstrand 1972b) similarly as the ratio of white and red muscle fibres. Later changes in the absolute amount of LBM take place thus within a certain range determined genetically even when LBM and the depot fat ratio vary widely due to ontogenetical stages, environmental factors etc.—LBM itself changes as regards composition during onto-

TABLE 1.
Mean values ($\bar{x} \pm$ SD) of body weight, percentage of body fat and relative weights (mg/100 g weight or fat-free mass-FFM) of internal organs and skeletal muscles (Pařízková 1968g)

Age (days)		50		160		440		550	
n		16		14		11		10	
Weight	$\bar{x}$	102.2		316.4		448.7		545.3	
(g)	SD	11.1		20.5		36.4		87.8	
Fat (%)	$\bar{x}$	5.8		7.9		16.9		24.7	
	SD	0.9		2.1		4.4		9.8	
Relat. weights		mg/100g weight	mg/100g FFM	mg/100g weight	mg/100g FFM	mg/100g weight	mg/100g FFM	mg/100g weight	mg/100g FFM
Heart	$\bar{x}$	351.9	375.5	257.1	279.6	238.0	307.7	218.0	293.0
	SD	35.2	36.0	22.9	21.1	25.6	25.9	31.0	31.0
Liver	$\bar{x}$	3581.6	3826.4	2316.0	2593.0	2956.4	3834.2	2948.0	3959.0
	SD	288.5	313.4	202.8	211.0	199.9	333.0	327.0	523.0
Spleen	$\bar{x}$	558.2	605.5	293.1	319.1	181.5	235.2	170.0	231.0
	SD	162.6	173.2	32.9	32.9	7.1	36.0	31.0	44.0
Adrenals	$\bar{x}$	24.3	26.4	13.6	14.8	9.7	12.5	9.9	13.2
	SD	3.5	3.7	8.9	2.2	1.2	1.4	1.9	1.7
Soleus	$\bar{x}$	40.8	43.5	36.0	39.1	28.4	36.7	29.6	39.9
muscle	SD	5.8	5.7	1.7	1.7	2.9	2.8	4.1	6.4
Tibialis	$\bar{x}$	178.9	191.1	170.2	186.1	136.8	176.4	130.0	174.0
muscle	SD	11.1	12.0	9.6	10.2	15.6	12.5	31.0	10.0

genesis: the ratio of LBM formed by internal organs, muscles, skeleton (which under normal conditions is a very constant part of LBM) (Trotter 1956) differs during growth and in old age. During growth, i.e. period of high energy turnover internal organs account for a significantly higher ratio than in adult life and old age. These *metabolically highly active organs* do not increase proportionately during growth and maturation as other parts of the body. It has been already described that the weights of *liver, heart, spleen* and *adrenals* in early stages of ontogenesis are higher in relation to the total body weight than later (Holliday et al. 1967). This is not due to altered relations of LBM and body fat at different age periods but applies also in relation to lean body mass of the organism (Table 1) (Pařízková 1968g). The above organs *form the highest proportion of LBM during the period of growth and this ratio declines during ageing*. From this ensues that *not only the ratio of the main components of lean body mass and fat but also their composition changes during ontogenesis, in keeping with the general level of energy turnover.*

According to Lesser et al. (1970) the increase of lean body mass in the laboratory rat (Sprague-Dawley) proceeds up to the age of 500 days. After this period neither the lean body mass nor the water and potassium content undergo any changes. The size of the metabolically most active organs remains also the same.

Analysis of individual organs or muscles also revealed changes as regards percentage of organ fat.

Fat was extracted from the tissues crushed with sea sand, using a mixture of chloroform-methanol at a ratio of 3 : 1 and after evaporation it was assessed gravimetrically.

The increase of fat was most marked in the soleus muscle (Table 2). *In the heart the percentage of fat increased only slightly,* and in the tibialis muscle it did not change. Comparison of the percentage of fat in the liver and kidneys of growing and full grown rats did not reveal any marked difference.—An enhanced lipid synthesis in the heart can be demonstrated e.g. in oxygen deficiency (Harris and Gloster 1972).

TABLE 2.
Mean percentage of fat ($\bar{x} \pm$ SD) in heart and skeletal muscles of male rats of different age

Age (days)	85		125		360		440		550	
n	12		7		7		11		10	
	$\bar{x}$	SD	$\bar{x}$	SD	$\bar{x}$	SD	$\bar{x}$	SD	$\bar{x}$	SD
Heart	2.7	0.3	2.8	0.5	2.8	0.5	2.8	0.2	3.1	0.4
Soleus muscle	3.4	0.9	2.7	0.6	3.7	0.8	7.4	1.6	8.3	2.6
Tibialis muscle	2.0	0.9	1.9	0.4	2.6	0.5	1.9	0.2	2.0	1.0

3. Composition and metabolic activity of adipose tissue

Adipose tissue of growing laboratory rats is more cellular and contains more deoxyribonucleic acids (DNA), i.e. the fat cells are smaller than in adult age (Jelínková and Myslivečková 1965). Also in human ontogenesis fat cells not only increase in number but also their size increases with age from childhood to adult age (Hirsch and Knittle 1970). Between the size of fat cells and the blood supply of adipose tissue there is a significant negative relationship (Di Girolamo et al. 1975) which has a significant effect on the metabolic activity of tissue. Significant negative relationships were ascertained between blood flow in the adipose tissue on the one hand, and body weight, the degree of overweight and mean skinfold thickness of women on the other hand, and a positive relationship between the release of free fatty acids (FFA) into the medium after adrenalin, and blood flow in the adipose tissue. Muscular work enhanced blood flow in subcutaneous adipose tissue by 64 % (Rath 1971).—Catecholamines which are synthetized to a greater extent in a young organism especially during early periods of growth (as indicated e.g. by greater activity of tyrosine hydroxylase in the adrenals, as related to body weight—Kvetňanský et al., in press) enhance the blood flow through adipose tissue (Mjös and

Akre 1971). Lipogenesis in the growing organism is more intense (Benjamin et al. 1961; Gellhorn et al. 1962), but Altschuler et al. (1962) and others (Jelínková and Myslivečková 1965 etc.) demonstrated that adipose tissue of young rats of small size and low weight releases after the same stimulus, i.e. the addition of the same relative amount of adrenalin into the incubation medium, a significantly higher amount of FFA than adipose tissue of large older rats. In our experiments we obtained in relation to weight and in particular in relation to the accurate age of the experimental animals similar results (Fig. 3).

The epididymal adipose tissue was incubated in Krebs-Ringer phosphate buffer with addition of 3 % human albumin at a temperature of 37 °C, pH 7.4, for a period of 60, 100 and 210 min. FFA were titrated according to Dole (1956).

Spontaneous FFA release was very marked in rats aged 85 days (i.e. before the stage of exponential growth was terminated). At the age of 360 days FFA were not released spontaneously after 60 – 120 min. After addition of adrenalin into the medium (2 or 4 μg per 100 mg tissue/1 ml medium) the amount of released FFA was again graded by age—it was highest in the youngest rats and lowest in the oldest. From this ensues that *adipose tissue of the young growing organism is able, if necessary, as e.g. during muscular work when increased amount of catecholamines are released into the blood stream* (Spitzer and McElroy 1961) *to liberate in response to the same stimulus larger amounts of FFA* (and obviously also other lipid meta-

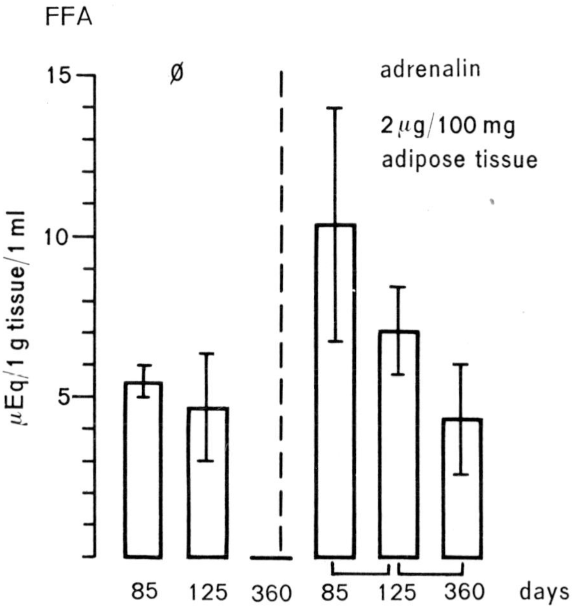

Fig. 3. Release of free (non-esterified) fatty acids (FFA, in μEq/ml/1 g – ordinate) from epididymal adipose tissue *in vitro* in male rats of different age (left – spontaneous release; right – released free fatty acids after addition of 2 μg adrenalin per 100 mg of adipose tissue; x̄ ± SD). Abscissa – days in days. └──┘ means statistical significance of differences (at least $p < 0.05$) (Pařízková and Staňková 1967, Pařízková 1968e,g).

bolites e.g. glycerol—Havel and Carlsson 1963) from the same volume of adipose tissue which serves as energy substrate. *In the early stage of ontogenesis thus adipose tissue not only accounts for a lower proportion of the body weight but it also differs markedly from the aspect of metabolic activity* (Pařízková 1968f.g., 1971b, Pařízková and Staňková 1967). A decrease of lipolytic activity in adipose tissue with ageing was found further e.g. by Macho and Kolena (1975). Lipid mobilizing hormones (ACTH, noradrenalin) lowered the concentration of cyclic 3,5-AMP in the adipose tissue, and also an impaired stimulation of lipolytic activity was found in old rats. A smaller release of glycerol and FFA by cAMP was observed in old animals where obviously a lower lipolytic activity per volume of tissue and lipid mass was available, spontaneously and after hormone stimulation. Therefore the accumulation of lipids in fat depots is facilitated in older animals.

4. Lipid metabolism in muscular tissue

In conjunction with the above properties of adipose tissue of young growing male rats certain corresponding metabolic differences were also found in muscular tissue. The lipoprotein lipase (LPL) (Biale et al. 1956) activity was investigated using Cherkes and Gordon's method (1957) which on perfusion of the heart with heparin correlates significantly with the increased uptake and oxidation of fatty acids (Crass and Meng 1966). The higher activity of LPL is also found concurrently with a raised activity of beta-oxidative enzymes (Pette 1966).

Specimens of heart and skeletal muscle (m. tibialis anterior and m. soleus), cca 100 mg per 1 ml medium, were incubated under constant shaking in Krebs-Ringer phosphate buffer, pH 7.4, containing 5 units heparin per 1 ml medium. After 1 hour incubation 1 ml medium was added to 1 ml substrate (8 parts 10 % albumin, 1 part human plasma, 1 part Ediol — 5 % at pH 8.7). 0.5 ml of this mixture was withdrawn for estimation of FFA (according to Dole 1956) and the remainder was incubated for another hour. Then FFA were again estimated and the LPL activity was expressed as the amount of released FFA (Cherkes and Gordon 1957).

In 50-day-old male rats the LPL activity in skeletal muscle was significantly higher than in 160-day-old rats. The LPL activity in the heart did not change with advancing age (Fig. 4). These results seem to provide indirect evidence of an *increased ability of the growing skeletal muscle to utilize fatty acids as a source of energy which is in keeping with findings of an increased capacity of young adipose tissue to release fatty acids* (Pařízková and Koutecký 1968; Pařízková and Staňková 1964ab, 1967). This increased ability is also suggested by findings of Beatty and Bocek (1970) on the increased uptake of palmitate-^{14}C by muscle fibres from the extremities of the monkey *Maccaca mulata in vitro:* the uptake of palmitate-^{14}C was significantly higher in muscle fibres of foetuses and newborn monkeys than in adults.

The above data obtained in experimental animals revealed that changes in body composition during ontogenesis, i.e. in particular an increase of the body fat ratio reflecting obvious changes in the general level of energy turnover, are based on

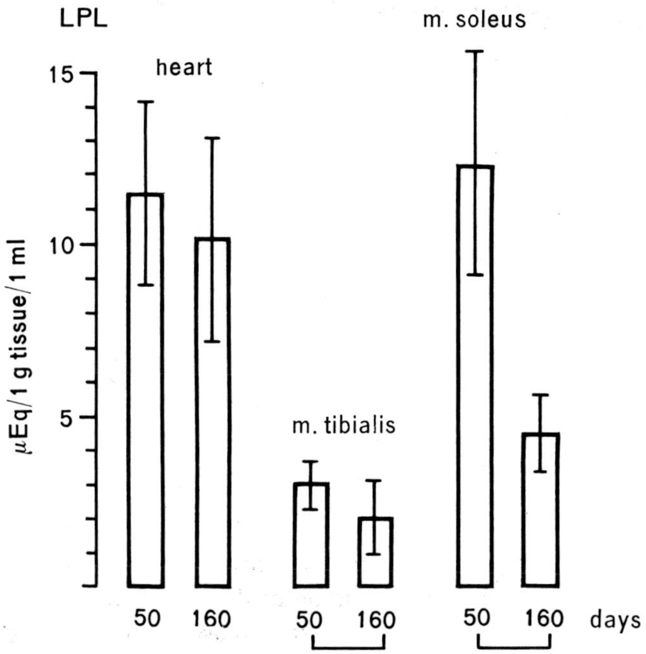

Fig. 4. Activity of lipoprotein lipase (LPL) in the heart, tibialis and soleus muscles in male rats of different age (abscissa – days). Expressed as μEq of free fatty acids / 1 g tissue / 1 ml medium: $\bar{x} \pm SD$ (Pařízková and Koutecký 1968).

marked changes of fat metabolism in adipose as well as muscular tissue. The total body fat ratio may therefore under normal conditions serve as an approximate indicator of the level of energy turnover and thus also as an indirect indicator of the level of lipid metabolism in the above tissues.

II. Lean body mass and depot fat during ontogenesis in humans

In the ontogenesis of man somatic changes are limited not only to the growth period. The main somatic indicators such as height increase up to 18 to 20 years, some other signs may, however, change up to the end of the third decade. Data on our Czechoslovak population assembled at Spartakiades (mass gymnastic displays) e.g. in 1965 indicate that on average the body-weight increases with advancing age (Fetter et al. 1967). The increase of body-weight is even more marked when evaluated in relation to height: values of relative body-weight (calculated on the basis of data assembled by Fetter et al. 1967), using Broca's index, rise between 18 and 64 years in men from 91.7 to 107, in women from 93.8 to 115.2. This all leads to the question of *how body composition changes during ontogenesis and whether these changes only correspond to the increase in body-weight or whether (e.g. in advanced age) they can be manifested even in the absence of changes in body-weight.*

Least data were obtainable so far on quantitative changes of lean body mass and fat in children and adolescents where till recently only data on subcutaneous fat measured by means of different calipers or by X-rays were available (Reynolds 1950, Garn 1956, Brožek and Keys 1951, Tanner 1962, etc.). Some measurements of body composition made in children using old methods (Boyd 1923, Zook 1938) are not comparable with densitometric (Pařízková 1959b, 1961a,c, 1962a, Novak 1963, Hunt and Heald 1963) or ^{40}K measurements (Forbes and Amirhakimi 1970, Novak 1973, Novak et al. 1970, Mann et al. 1974 etc.). The growth rate and magnitude of weight increment changes markedly during development ("growing up" and "filling down") which is manifested as periods of robustness and slenderness (Hampton et al. 1966). Knowledge of the development of body composition of normal healthy children was thus the first essential task (Pařízková 1957, 1959a,b).

A very important and so far not completely resolved problem in the evaluation of child development are criteria of optimal and adequate growth. Physiological and clinical studies done in recent years indicate that the orientation using only growth grids and nomograms, based on values of height and weight of children from industrially developed countries, is not always satisfactory. The question therefore still remains for the future of what is optimal in a given category from the aspect of somatic growth (Blažek 1971). *Attainment of ever increasing values of body-weight and height are not always an advantage,* particularly if these data are not concurrently confronted with other developmental parameters incl. body composition and functional indicators. On these problems ontogenetic investigations were focused where *for the first time in the child population the development of the relative and absolute amount of LBM was evaluated by the densitometric method* (Pařízková 1959b, 1961a, 1962a). Another aspect were investigations of the development of subcutaneous fat.

1. Changes of subcutaneous fat during ontogenesis

The development of subcutaneous fat in children immediately after birth and at an early and preschool age we could investigate only by assessing skinfold thickness by means of a caliper; other methods available for us were not feasible in these age groups.

We used a Best's caliper (1954) (Plate 1) modified for our needs (Pařízková 1957, 1960a,c, Motyčka 1966). The caliper exerts a constant pressure on the measured skinfold and transmits it on contact terminals (3 mm in diameter, circular shape) by means of a spring calibrated for a constant pressure of 200 g (i.e. cca 28 g/mm^2). The skinfold is lifted between the thumb and index finger, the terminals of the caliper are applied about 1 cm from the fingers flat in relation to the body surface. The axis of the caliper is normal to the axis of the skinfold (Plate 1). The reading is taken when the calibration marks of the caliper coincide. We made measurements at ten sites of the body surface (Allen et al. 1956): (1) on the cheek, below the temple (skinfold horizontally, on the line connecting the tragus and nostrils); (2) on the chin below the hyoid bone with the head slightly lifted (direction of the skinfold vertical, the skin of the neck must not be stretched); (3) on the chest in the anterior axillary fold (thorax I — oblique along the borderline of the m. pectoralis major); (4) on the posterior surface of the m. triceps (vertical direction, half-way on the line connecting the acromion and olecranon); (5) on the back beneath the lower angle of the scapula (oblique along the ribs – subscapular); (6) on the chest above the 10th rib at the point of intersection with the anterior axillary line (direction of skinfold along ribs; thorax II); (7) on the abdomen (on the line connecting the navel — and spina ilica ventralis, a quarter of the distance, more closely to the navel); (8) on the hip above the crista ossis ilii, also at the point of intersection with the prolonged anterior axillary line (direction of the skinfold along the edge the ilium – suprailiac); (9) on the thigh above the knee (cca 4–5 cm above the patella, direction of the skinfold vertical, leg slightly bent, supported lightly on tip of foot); (10) on the calf about 5 cm beneath the popliteal fossa (direction of skinfold vertical, leg also slightly bent). Later also (11) the skinfold above the m. biceps measured on the arm in a supine position with the elbow slightly bent was added (direction of skinfold along axis of arm). All measurements were taken on the right side of the body (Pařízková 1959a, 1961a,c). In later studies skinfolds 4, 5, 8, 10, 11 were measured by Harpender caliper (*see* Plate 3) on both sides of the body (Tanner 1962, Weiner and Laurie 1969).

To evaluate the ontogenetic trend of changes in body composition, not influenced by an elevated or reduced body weight, we selected for our experimental groups only comparable subjects. In children and youths several growth grids were used for orientation so that according to all the mean height and weights corresponded

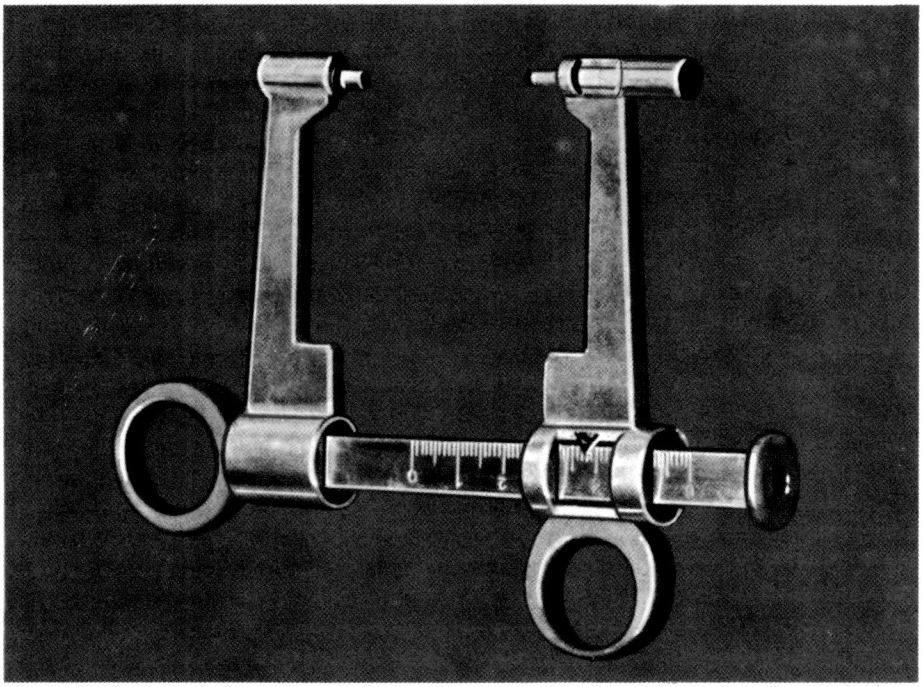

Plate 1. Caliper after Best (1954) modified by Pařízková (1957, 1959) and Motyčka (1966).

to normal (Kapalín 1967, Tanner et al. 1966, Wetzel 1942). In adults we evaluated the relative weight according to Broca's index (ideal weight = height in cm – 100 cm; relative weight = $\frac{\text{actual wt.} \times 100}{\text{ideal wt.}}$). At the same time as a check we confronted the basic somatic characteristics with standard values for the Czech population measured in Spartakiades (Fetter et al. 1967; Suchý 1971). The selected age groups did not thus correspond to the mean Czechoslovak population but rather to optimum values (Hejda and Hátle 1960).

The skinfold thickness in newborn infants was measured during the first two days after birth (4 – 48 hours) in the maternity home. Already during this period a tendency of greater subcutaneous fat deposition in girls was apparent (Fig. 5). *The skinfold on the hip was significantly greater in girls* (n = 23) than in boys (n = 25), *the sexual difference in the amount of body fat is thus apparent immediately after birth* (Pařízková 1963a). The body-weight and height of boys was as a rule also somewhat greater (3,450 ± 477 g; 50.9 ± 2.7 cm) than in girls (3,287 ± 439 g; 50.2 ± 1 cm). The sexual differences in subcutaneous fat persisted also during the normal drop of weight after birth between the 3rd – 5th day of life (Fig. 5). Data indicate a marked difference in subcutaneous body fat by sex as well as interindividual differences, although all the infants were born in term from healthy mothers.

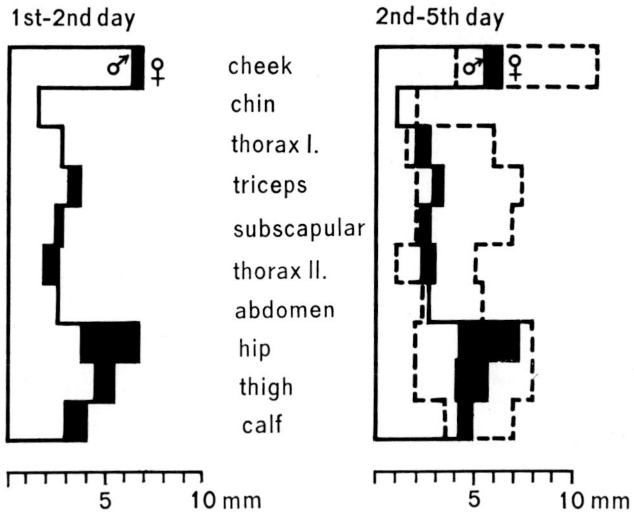

Fig. 5. Mean skinfold thickness (mm – measured by means of modified Best caliper (1954) (Pařízková 1962a) in newborns. Left: white area – values for boys, white and black areas – values for girls. Right: dtto; interrupted line more to the left side – values for children born before term, interrupted line on the right side – values for children born in term from diabetic, metabolically decompensated mothers (i. e. with hyperglycaemia) (Pařízková 1963a).

Further observations revealed possible factors which influence during intrauterine life the layer of subcutaneous body fat: *children from mothers with metabolically uncompensated diabetes had a significantly increased amount of body fat* (Pařízková 1963a) and a higher body-weight (n = 16; Fig. 5). Evidence was provided that in mothers with metabolically compensated diabetes without a raised blood sugar level the weight of newborns was increased only slightly (Přibylová and Znamenáček 1971) and obviously there was no increase of adipose tissue. The body-weight of newborns from diabetic mothers correlates with the blood sugar level in cord blood—the higher the blood sugar level, the higher the birth-weight of the infants (Hoet 1971) and obviously also the subcutaneous fat (Fee and Well 1963). It seems thus that the *fluctuations in blood sugar level of mothers, in particular during the last months of pregnancy* (when in humans adipose tissue is already developing and increasing—Adolf and Hegeness 1971) can exert a considerable effect on insulin and growth hormone levels in the foetus and thus also on the development of adipose tissue cellularity and thus influence later development of body fatness.

On the other hand, *premature infants have a significantly smaller skinfold thickness* (Fig. 5—Pařízková 1963a). Brans et al. (1974) also showed the effect of gestational age on the amount of subcutaneous fat in newborns, which correlated positively with birth weight.

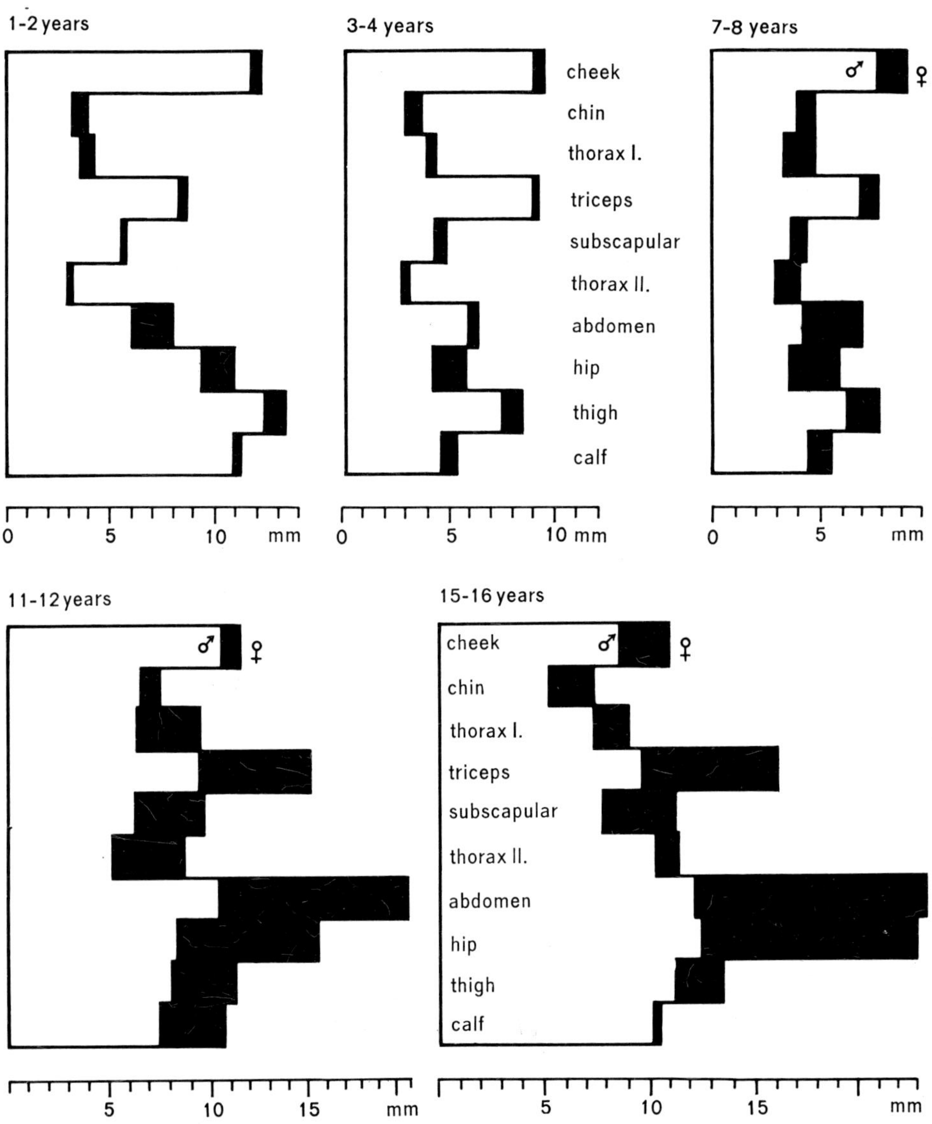

Fig. 6a. Mean values of skinfold thicknesses in children and adolescents (Pařízková 1959a, b, 1962b, 1963a).

The investigation of 1460 subjects of both sexes revealed a *steady increase of skinfold thickness throughout life.* During growth and development also the sexual differences increase (Fig. 6a); *boys and girls differ relatively most at the peak of puberty* (Pařízková 1959a, 1960a,c) when in boys a reduction of subcutaneous fat occurs (Table 3). *During adult and old age, when subcutaneous fat increases in both sexes the*

TABLE 3.
Mean skinfold thicknesses ($\bar{x} \pm SD$) in children and adolescents from 1 to 16 years of age, measured by modified Best's caliper (1954) (Pařízková 1957, 1959, 1963a)

Age (years)		1	SD	2	SD	3	SD	4	SD	5	SD	6	SD	7	SD	8	SD	9	SD	10	SD
1—2	♂	11.9	2.9	3.3	0.9	4.0	0.9	8.3	1.6	5.6	1.8	3.0	0.3	6.0	2.2	9.5	3.2	12.5	1.8	11.1	2.6
	♀	12.2	2.6	4.0	2.1	3.7	2.0	8.6	2.8	5.8	2.9	3.2	1.5	8.0	4.5	11.1	4.2	13.4	3.4	11.0	3.0
2—3	♂	11.8	2.4	3.8	1.0	3.3	1.5	9.0	2.8	5.5	1.8	2.9	1.6	5.0	1.5	5.6	3.0	10.1	2.9	8.7	2.6
	♀	10.6	2.0	3.2	1.1	3.5	0.9	8.6	2.3	5.4	1.3	3.2	0.9	6.9	2.8	7.6	3.8	11.5	2.4	7.8	2.2
3—4	♂	9.5	1.2	3.7	1.3	4.3	2.2	9.2	2.1	4.5	1.3	2.9	1.3	6.0	3.1	4.4	2.4	7.7	2.1	5.4	1.8
	♀	9.1	2.0	3.1	1.2	4.0	2.1	9.3	2.5	4.7	1.3	3.1	1.2	6.3	2.4	5.8	2.2	8.6	2.5	4.9	2.2
4—5	♂	8.3	3.0	2.9	1.1	2.8	1.2	7.4	1.9	3.7	1.1	2.5	0.7	4.4	2.3	2.9	1.6	5.7	2.0	3.6	1.5
	♀	9.0	2.4	3.0	1.5	3.8	1.6	10.0	2.5	5.1	2.0	3.3	1.6	7.2	4.1	5.7	4.1	8.3	2.8	4.9	1.9
5—6	♂	8.7	2.7	3.5	1.4	3.1	1.3	8.2	2.4	4.0	1.1	3.0	1.2	5.4	3.3	4.0	2.7	5.4	1.8	3.8	1.7
	♀	7.5	2.2	3.0	1.4	3.2	1.4	8.5	2.6	4.1	1.4	2.8	1.3	5.6	3.2	4.4	2.4	6.5	2.2	4.2	1.9
6—7	♂	7.9	1.6	3.0	0.9	2.3	0.6	5.8	1.4	3.4	0.8	2.4	0.7	3.8	2.4	2.9	0.9	5.4	1.0	3.0	0.8
	♀	8.0	1.9	3.2	1.3	3.0	1.5	6.9	3.7	3.8	1.9	3.0	1.2	5.2	3.3	4.7	2.9	5.8	2.6	4.0	1.8
7—8	♂	8.5	1.6	4.3	1.4	3.5	1.3	7.1	2.2	3.9	1.7	3.0	1.7	4.4	0.7	3.7	1.4	6.5	1.9	4.6	1.8
	♀	9.3	1.4	4.8	1.4	4.8	2.2	7.9	3.1	4.4	2.1	4.1	4.3	7.2	1.1	5.9	4.0	7.8	2.6	5.5	2.7
8—9	♂	8.1	1.9	4.5	2.4	4.1	2.2	7.5	3.0	4.0	2.8	3.9	3.1	6.3	2.6	5.4	4.2	6.6	2.6	5.3	2.6
	♀	9.8	2.0	5.5	1.9	5.3	1.8	9.8	2.9	5.7	2.5	4.4	3.6	7.8	2.9	8.3	6.1	8.9	2.9	5.5	3.0
9—10	♂	8.8	1.7	4.9	1.4	4.3	1.7	8.0	2.2	4.7	1.4	3.8	2.9	6.0	1.1	4.6	1.8	6.7	1.8	5.1	2.2
	♀	8.7	1.7	5.9	2.0	6.4	1.8	9.8	2.6	6.0	2.1	5.1	3.8	10.5	2.5	9.3	4.9	8.5	3.0	6.7	2.4
10—11	♂	9.6	3.2	5.2	1.7	5.1	1.8	8.8	2.9	5.5	2.1	4.7	3.5	7.9	2.5	6.4	4.2	8.0	2.7	6.2	2.4
	♀	10.9	2.9	6.2	2.3	6.7	3.9	10.7	3.4	7.2	3.2	5.8	4.5	13.3	2.9	11.1	8.2	9.2	3.5	8.0	3.0
11—12	♂	10.8	2.2	6.7	2.3	6.5	3.1	9.6	2.4	6.2	2.6	5.3	3.9	10.6	2.8	8.4	5.8	8.2	3.2	7.5	2.8
	♀	11.6	3.3	7.6	3.0	9.6	4.5	14.9	4.5	9.8	5.5	8.6	5.5	19.6	3.9	15.2	8.9	11.2	3.7	10.7	3.6
12—13	♂	11.2	2.8	7.0	2.8	7.0	4.1	9.9	3.9	6.5	3.5	6.2	4.3	12.4	3.9	10.3	7.6	9.5	2.4	7.8	3.2
	♀	11.0	2.8	6.9	2.5	8.7	4.6	12.4	4.9	8.6	3.7	8.2	4.5	17.8	3.5	15.3	7.8	11.1	3.4	10.3	3.4
13—14	♂	9.4	3.6	6.1	3.0	6.2	4.3	9.0	3.8	6.6	3.7	6.4	4.3	11.5	3.5	9.7	7.1	9.2	3.4	7.7	3.8
	♀	11.4	3.1	6.6	2.2	7.3	3.3	11.9	3.2	10.8	5.1	10.4	5.4	21.0	4.4	18.4	9.6	12.1	3.2	11.4	3.9
14—15	♂	8.8	2.1	5.5	1.5	6.7	3.3	11.5	3.2	6.9	2.6	6.7	5.6	11.6	3.7	9.1	4.8	9.6	3.7	8.2	4.5
	♀	11.2	2.9	7.1	2.2	9.4	3.5	14.8	4.0	12.0	5.8	11.0	7.7	22.6	4.6	23.0	9.4	13.2	3.4	11.3	3.2
15—16	♂	8.5	2.3	5.1	1.7	7.3	3.9	9.6	3.6	7.9	2.6	10.3	4.3	12.6	4.3	12.6	4.3	11.3	4.2	10.1	4.2
	♀	10.8	2.7	7.3	2.4	8.9	4.2	16.0	4.2	11.1	3.3	11.3	8.0	23.1	4.2	22.9	8.9	13.4	2.0	10.5	3.9

(1 — cheek, 2 — chin, 3 — chest I, 4 — triceps, 5 — subscapular, 6 — chest II, 7 — abdomen, 8 — hip (suprailiac), 9 — thigh, 10 — calf)

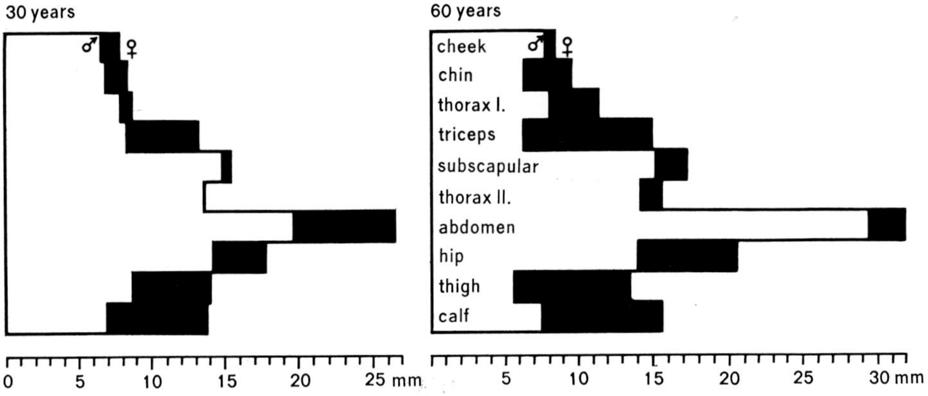

Fig. 6b. Mean values of skinfold thicknesses in adult and aged men and women (Pařízková 1962b).

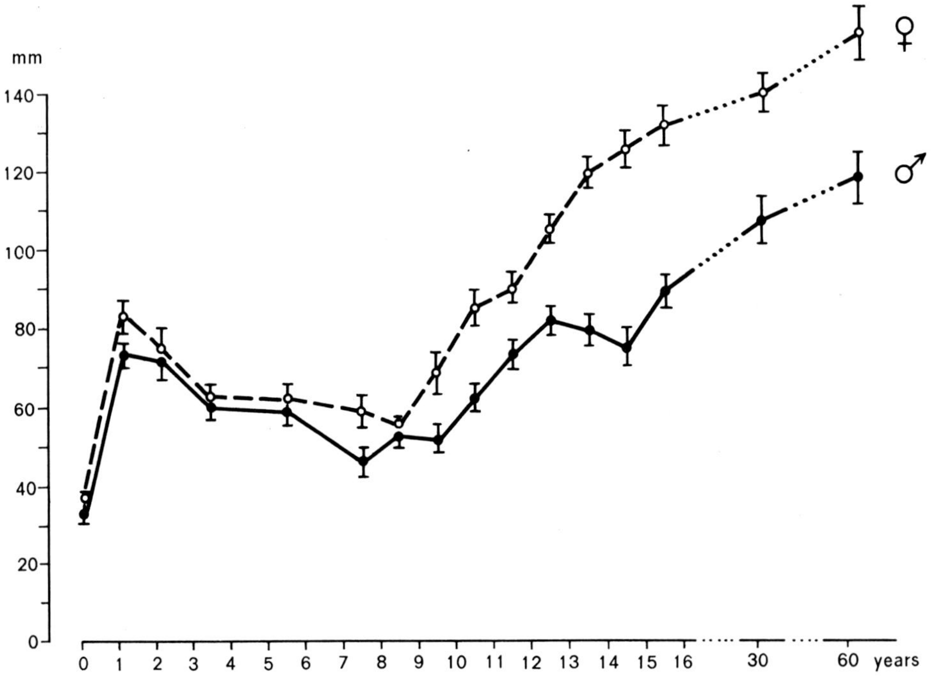

Fig. 7. The development of mean values ($\bar{x} \pm$ SE) of the sum of ten skinfolds (see Fig. 5) in males and females. Abscissa – age in years, ordinate – sum of ten skinfolds in mm (♂ n = 715, ♀ n = 745) (Pařízková 1959b, 1960a, c).

TABLE 4.
Mean skinfold thicknesses ($\bar{x} \pm SD$) on arm (triceps — I) and back (subscap. — II) in men and women in Czech regions and Slovakia (measured by modified Best's caliper) (Pařízková and Kreipl 1971)

			Bohemia and Moravia				Slovakia				
		Age (years)	18—25	26—35	36—45	46—55	18—25	26—35	36—45	46—55	Total
Women	I	n	182	194	226	176	44	54	72	39	987
		$\bar{x}$	14.6	16.0	18.3	18.7	15.5	15.6	18.4	18.3	17.0
		SD	5.9	6.9	7.6	8.0	6.3	5.9	8.5	7.3	7.3
	II	$\bar{x}$	13.2	15.9	18.8	19.1	12.6	15.5	17.7	19.4	16.7
		SD	6.5	7.5	8.9	8.3	7.3	6.3	8.9	8.9	8.2
Men	I	n	153	173	214	149	33	40	58	48	868
		$\bar{x}$	8.9	9.5	9.4	9.4	10.4	10.1	11.1	10.7	9.6
		SD	5.3	4.8	4.7	5.0	6.2	6.0	5.6	9.6	5.3
	II	$\bar{x}$	10.3	12.0	13.5	14.6	10.4	12.5	13.0	12.5	12.6
		SD	5.6	4.9	5.6	7.4	5.2	6.6	5.8	7.2	6.1

sexual difference is still maintained at a significant level (Pařízková 1963a, 1968g, 1971b) (Fig. 6b).—The development of the sum of all ten skinfolds expresses the general changes of subcutaneous fat during ontogenesis—the rise up to the age of one, a drop up to 7–8 years with a subsequent systematic increase of skinfold thicknesses with the exception of a temporary decline in boys during puberty (Fig. 7). The skinfold thickness is related in a significant way to somatotypes according to Wetzel (1942) (Pařízková 1962a).

During ageing also the relative distribution of subcutaneous fat changes. While *in the youngest children the maximum of subcutaneous fat is deposited on the extremities and the minumum on the trunk* (Fig. 5, 6a), *in adults and in particular in elderly people the reverse is true* (Fig. 6b; Pařízková 1963a, 1971b). In some subjects the amount of body fat on the trunk increases simultaneously with a diminution of fat on the extremities.

The above measurements were made on a sample of the Prague population selected according to the described criteria. Ontogenetic changes in adults and elderly people were tested also on a nation-wide representative random sample.

The selected men (n = 868) and women (n = 987) were part of a sample of 13,000 subjects investigated in the research programme "Investigation of the physical activity of the population of Czechoslovakia". As regards body composition only skinfold thicknesses on the arm above the triceps and on the back beneath the lower angle of the scapula (subscapular) were investigated. The data from Czech and Slovak regions were evaluated separately.

As apparent from Table 4, in women the values of the skinfold thickness increased on the arm as well as on the back; in men only on the back. In women an increase was observed in the Czech as well as Slovak regions. In Slovak regions this increase was not observed in men, while it was significant in the men from Czech regions. This difference, however, may be due to a greater ratio of manual workers in the sample of the oldest age group in Slovakia (which is still less industrialized). On the whole, however, the results of these measurements were in keeping with the trend of changes which were found in a smaller sample of the Prague population (with the above mentioned exception in Slovak men), i.e. with advancing age in normal subjects increasing amounts of subcutaneous body fat were deposited even when the body-weight remained within a normal range (Pařízková and Kreipl 1971).

2. Ontogenetic changes of the total body fat and lean body mass ratio

The application of the densitometric method rendered also the quantitative evaluation of the main body constituents (Bashkirov 1958) during development possible starting with children of early school age. Men were examined up to the age of 80 and above, women between 50–60 years (Pařízková 1962a, 1963a, 1971b, Pařízková and Eiselt 1966) in subgroups comprising always 15–18 subjects.

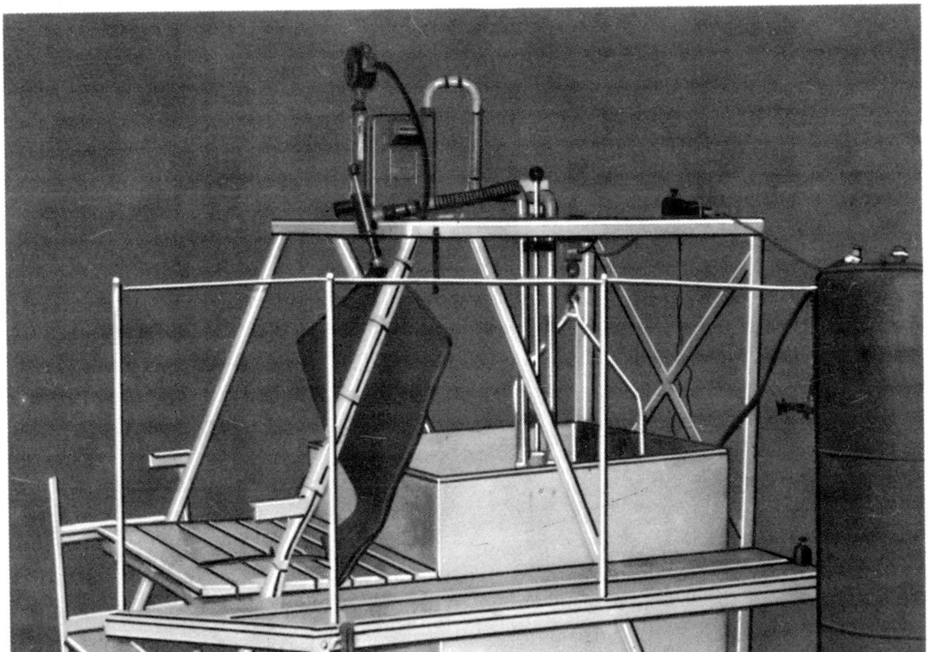

Plate 2. Apparatus for assessement of body density, i. e. hydrostatic weight with open circuit for measurement of the air in the lungs and respiratory passages (modification after Keys and Brožek 1953, Brožek et al. 1953, Pařízková 1959b, 1961a, c).

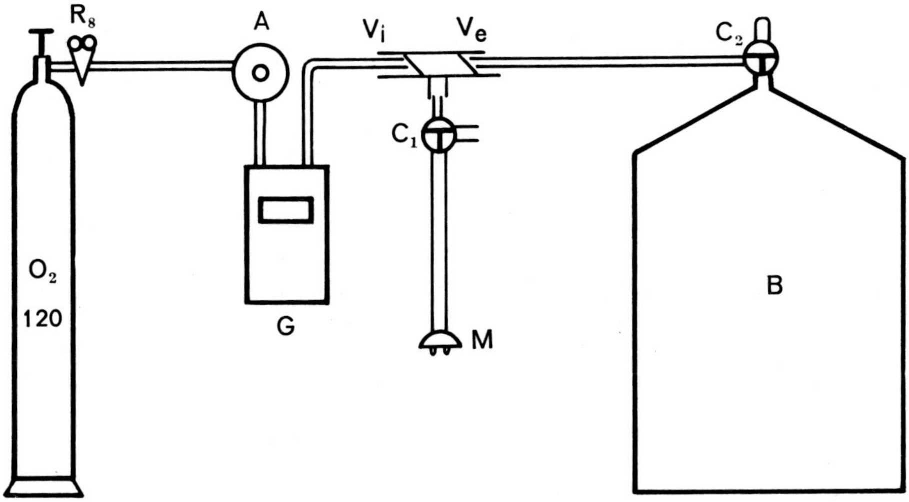

Fig. 8. Scheme of the open circuit apparature (nitrogen dilution method) for measuring the volume of the air in the lungs and respiratory passages. O_2 120 Atm. = oxygen cylinder, R = pressure regulator from 120 to 8 Atm.; A = automatic valve from breathing set; G = gas meter; $C_{1,2}$ = change-over cocks; M = mouthpiece, $V_{i,e}$ = ventiles dividing inspiration and expiration; B = Douglas bag (Cournand et al. 1940; Navrátil et al. 1958; Pařízková 1959, 1961a).

The body density was assessed by hydrostatic weighing (Plate 2) based on Archimedes principle with the simultaneous estimation of the volume of air in the lungs and respiratory passages (Brožek et al. 1953, 1963, Keys and Brožek 1953, Pařízková 1959b, 1961a,b). To assess the volume of air in the lungs we used the nitrogen dilution method, as described by Navrátil et al. (1958) (Fig. 8) which is based on the older method of Cournand et al. (1940). The expired gases are analyzed by means of an interferometer. The above method was further modified for examination under water (Pařízková 1959b, 1960c, 1961c, 1962a, 1963a etc.).

The density was calculated according to Brožek's formula (Brožek et al. 1963):

$$\text{density} = \frac{wt_a \times 0.996}{wt_a - wt_w - VALR \times 0.996}$$

(wt_a = weight in normal atmosphere, wt_w = weight under water, VALR = volume of air in lungs and respiratory passages, 0.996 = specific density of water at 37 °C in which measurements are made).

$$\%\ \text{fat} = \left(\frac{4.201}{\text{density}} - 3.813\right) \times 100 \qquad \text{(Keys and Brožek 1953)}$$

% LBM = 100 — % fat. kg fat = % fat × body weight : 100
kg LBM = % LBM × body weight : 100.

During repeated measurements the values differed on average only by 0.5 %. In the course of the day (morning, afternoon, etc.) the density values did not vary significantly (Pařízková 1959b). — Other methods used for evaluation of body composition, e.g. assessment of total body water by means of D_2O or T_2O were not used in healthy children in view of difficulties associated with the method. Indirect assessment from the basal oxygen consumption or urinary creatinine excretion is too inaccurate (Cheek 1968), e.g.

when urine is collected for eight hours the variation coefficients of the results is 18.5, during 72 hours 6.9 (Viteri et al. 1971). The method of assessment of body composition most frequently used recently, i.e. assessment of ^{40}K by means of whole-body counters (Anderson and Langham 1959, Forbes 1964, 1975, Kirton and Pearson 1963, Novak 1972, etc.) was not available for us. This method uses for the calculation of LBM a theoretical formula based on analysis of mEq K^+/kg LBM from adult subjects (Forbes and Hursh 1963); when used for smaller children and adolescents, this method, though expensive, does not always give very reliable results as regards absolute amounts of both fat and LBM (Forbes and Amirhakimi 1970) (see footnote on page 51).

Comparison of individuals with a normal mean body weight displays a considerable variation of body composition during life (Fig. 9). *The highest ratio of LBM was found in men aged cca 20 years* (Pařízková 1962a, 1963a, 1968c, 1971a; Pařízková et al. 1960). *Already in early school age there is a significant difference in the body composition of boys and girls* which diminishes temporarily during the prepubertal period (Pařízková 1959b, 1961a). *Starting with the third decade the ratio of LBM declines and depot fat increases, even when the body-weight remains relatively constant* (Pařízková 1963a, 1968c, 1971b). *The sexual difference remains still significant.* The diminution of LBM in the organism during ageing was confirmed also by assessment of ^{40}K by means of whole body counters (Anderson and Langham 1959, Allen et al. 1960, Novak 1972 etc.). With the finding of a diminution of LBM in old age agrees also the finding of a decline of the basal metabolic rate in relation to body-weight in old people (Behnke 1956), similarly as the finding of an increased amount of subcutaneous body fat (Pařízková and Eiselt 1962, 1966).

The period of the maximum ratio of LBM corresponds also to the period of the highest absolute values of aerobic capacity assessed as the maximum oxygen consumption (Åstrand and Rodahl 1970). At the age of about 20 years 1 kg LBM of an average man with normal weight carries the smallest amount of fat; this is of great importance for the economy of work performance, in particular work where the whole body-weight is shifted. The drop of LBM and increase in fat deposition during ageing runs parallel with the decline of aerobic capacity of the organism (Robinson 1936, Åstrand 1972a etc.), reduced oxygen saturation of blood, reduced oxygen tension in tissues etc. (Sirotinin 1972, Davies 1972).

Comparison of ratios of LBM, fat and skinfold thicknesses is difficult with data from Czechoslovak authors or workers from other countries who do not use an identical procedure. Values in adolescents do not differ markedly (Novak 1963, 1966, Hunt and Heald 1963). In adults the results are in keeping with those of Consolazio et al. (1966) which were assembled in soldiers, i.e. a selected population group. As a rule, in older age groups a higher body fat ratio was found. This is, however, due to a different method of selection of experimental subjects (men and women with *average body-weight* were examined; during advanced age the latter increases in the majority of developed industrialized countries—Brožek and Keys 1951, Brožek et al. 1953, Young et al. 1963, Petrásek et al. 1965, in press, Krzywicki and Vhinn 1967, Mašek 1970, Durnin and Womersley 1974, Novak 1972 etc.). As mentioned before, we selected in all age groups subjects who were *comparable as to their relative*

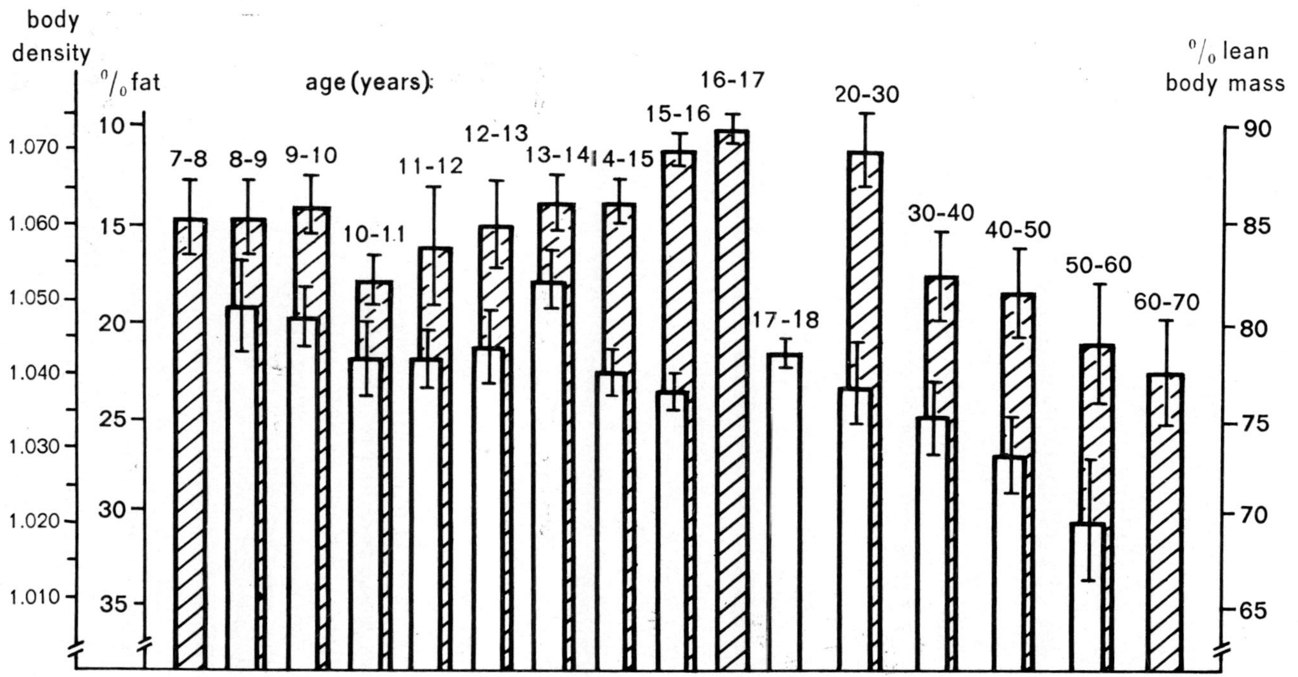

Fig. 9. Changes in body density, i. e. percentage of depot fat (ordinate left) and lean body mass (right) in males and females of comparable relative weight (i. e. approximately 100%) in various age categories during growth and ageing ($\bar{x} \pm SE$, ♂ n = 253, ♀ n = 218) (Pařízková 1959b, 1961a, 1963a).

weight. This enabled us to evaluate purely *ontogenetic changes in body composition without interference of other factors;* higher values of absolute and relative weight influence body composition even at a very young age. Without selection of experimental subjects from the above aspects it would not be possible to differentiate in cross-sectional studies ontogenetic differences from the influence of weight changes and other possible factors (Pařízková 1963a, 1965, 1968c).

3. Relationship of total and subcutaneous fat during ontogenesis

As apparent from previous data *changes of total and subcutaneous fat are in mutual agreement with certain age-dependent differences*. These relations were tested by correlation analysis. *They were all highly significant* and it was thus possible to derive *regression lines and to prepare nomograms where the ratio of body fat can be obtained from the skinfold thickness—individual skinfolds, the sum of skinfolds or selected combinations of skinfolds.*

For analysis of these relations the investigated groups were divided into boys (n = 66) and girls (n = 57) from 7–12 years and boys (n = 54) and girls (n = 62) aged 13–16 years. Adults were divided into males (n = 100) and females (n = 97) aged 17–49 years and finally men aged 50–65 years and 66–80 years (n = 170). We included in the experimental groups not only healthy people with normal weight (Fig. 9), but also underweight or overweight, i.e. the entire range of population. The correlations were close and highly significant particularly in adolescent and adult individuals. The correlation coefficients r were higher in boys than girls (Tables 5, 6) and in older boys as compared with younger ones. In the younger age groups (9–12 years) the order of correlation coefficients was almost the same in boys and girls. After the age of 13 the order differed. *The closest relations were proved for the sum of all ten skinfolds* which also had *the lowest variation coefficient $V\bar{x}$ during repeated, i.e. tenfold measurements of the same subjects* (Pařízková 1961c, 1962a). The regression equations (Table 7) and nomograms (Figs. 10a,b) were calculated and worked out for the mentioned groups of younger and older boys and girls and also for groups of adult and older men (Pařízková et al. 1960, Pařízková and Eiselt 1962, 1966) and finally for women of the given age groups (Pařízková 1962a).

When comparing the shape of regression lines with similar regressions derived e.g. for the Taiwan male and female population (Allen et al. 1956), we did not reveal significant differences (Pařízková et al. 1960). *The relationship of total and subcutaneous fat is thus obviously very similar or even identical in ethnically very different groups* with different morphological characteristics. The practical implication of this finding is that it is possible to apply the above equations for the evaluation of the total body fat ratio from skinfolds in other populations than our own (if the same procedure and caliper are used).

TABLE 5.
Correlation coefficients (r) of the relationship between body density and percentage of body fat resp., and skinfold thickness during growth and development (measured by Best's caliper 1954) (Pařízková 1961c, 1962b)

	Boys		Girls	
Age (years)	9—12	13—16	9—12	13—16
Cheek	0.816	0.895	0.554	0.543
Chin	0.917	0.917	0.741	0.689
Thorax I	0.873	0.894	0.775	0.792
Triceps	0.846	0.931	0.736	0.744
Subscapular	0.878	0.892	0.804	0.803
Thorax II	0.737	0.840	0.798	0.760
Abdomen	0.886	0.864	0.755	0.767
Suprailiac	0.860	0.858	0.748	0.755
Thigh	0.868	0.853	0.580	0.698
Calf	0.814	0.839	0.724	0.734
Triceps, subscapular	0.885	0.950	0.807	0.824
Sum of ten skinfolds	0.897	0.916	0.811	0.833

TABLE 6.
Correlation coefficients (r) of the relationship between body density and percentage of body fat resp., and skinfold thicknesses in adults (measured by modified Best's caliper 1954) (Pařízková 1961c, 1962b)

	Men			Women
	17—45	50—65	65—79	17—45
Cheek	0.733	0.527	(0.243)	0.724
Chin	0.805	0.465	0.443	0.809
Thorax I	0.845	0.590	0.431	0.875
Triceps	0.624	0.603	0.639	0.896
Subscapular	0.850	0.514	0.628	0.872
Thorax II	0.901	0.760	0.474	0.853
Abdomen	0.878	0.750	0.461	0.895
Suprailiac	0.862	0.730	(0.377)	0.829
Thigh	0.763	0.575	(0.369)	0.855
Calf	0.715	0.678	0.486	0.804
Subscapular + thorax II	0.876	—	—	Triceps + thorax II 0.898
Sum of ten skinfolds	0.898	0.788	0.559	0.929

Values in parentheses are not significant

TABLE 7.
Regression equations of the relationship between the sum of ten skinfolds (x — measured by Best's caliper 1954) and percentage of body fat (y) (Pařízková 1961c, 1962b)

	Age	Equation (y =	s
Boys	9—12	2.660x — 3.134	3.7
Girls	9—12	2.399x — 2.457	3.8
Boys + girls	9—12	2.594x — 2.947	3.7
Boys and girls	13—16	2.982x — 4.046	3.5
Men	17—45	22.32x — 29.00	2.4
	50—65	22.20x — 25.35	
	65—79	18.77x — 17.03	
	50—79	13.99x — 7.85	4.7
Women	17—45	39.572x — 61.25	3.3

x = sum of ten skinfolds, log

Regression lines for the relationship of total body fat assessed by densitometry and from skinfolds in children could not be compared, as so far these equations do not exist for other child populations. In 1967 similar equations were derived for adolescents (12.7 – 15.7) and adults by Durnin and Rahaman (1967) who used for confrontation with densitometric values the measurements of four skinfolds by means of a Harpenden caliper (Edwards et al. 1955). For this caliper a similar equation was derived also for boys and girls aged 7.5 to 18 years by Forbes and Amirhakimi (1970) who, however, assessed the body fat ratio indirectly by estimating ^{40}K using a whole-body counter (the authors themselves consider, however, the estimation of body fat by densitometry more reliable). The same procedure was used by Burmeister and Fromberg (1970) in German children.

The regression lines for individual groups were further tested mutually to evaluate whether they were in agreement or not. Statistical analysis of differences between different regression lines revealed differences between boys aged 9 – 12 years and boys aged 13 – 16 years; the same applies to girls. No significant differences were proved, however, between groups of younger boys and girls and older boys and girls. *It was thus possible to derive the same regression equations for combined groups of both younger and older boys and girls together* (Table 7). The body fat ratios for boys and girls are given in Table 8 where from the sum of ten skinfolds the percentage of body fat is obtained. In these tables common values for boys and girls are given only in the older group where the equations were identical (only $\underline{s}$ was higher in girls aged 13 – 16 years). In the younger group even in the absence of a significant difference there was a certain distinction (Fig. 10a); therefore the percentage of body fat are given separately for boys and girls.

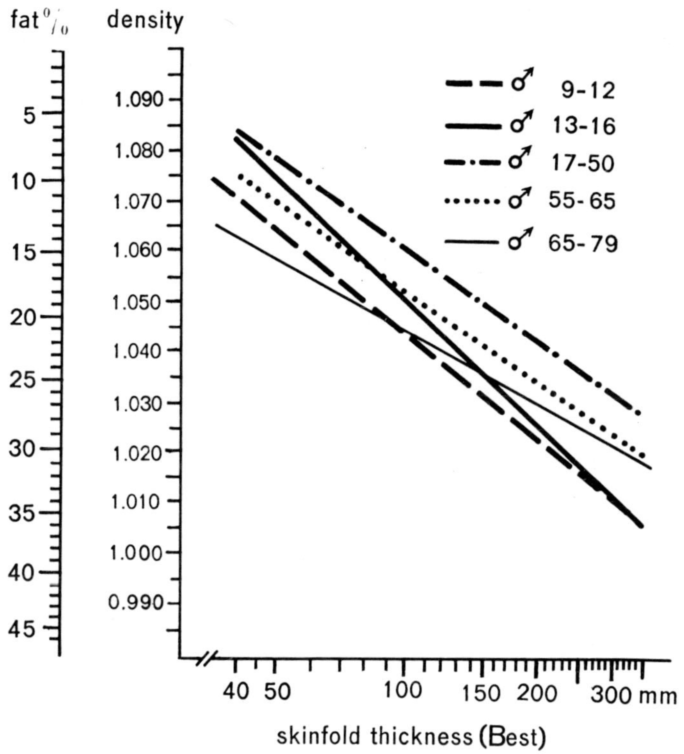

Fig. 10a. Nomogram for the evaluation of percentage of body fat from the sum of ten skinfolds (abscissa = sum of ten skinfolds in mm, ordinate = % body fat, or body density in males of different age for the measurements by modified Best caliper (1954; Pařízková 1957, 1959a,b, 1961c, 1962a etc.).

There is a relatively great difference in the regression lines between younger and older girls and boys (Figs. 10a,b) and thus also the percentage of body fat differs even when the sum of skinfolds is the same (Table 8). This becomes apparent particularly when we compare children who are of not very different age but belong into different age groups. The course of regression lines was therefore tested in another group of children, average age 10–12 years, which should be an intermediary group. The shape of regression lines in boys (mean age 10.55) was practically the same as in the age group 8–12 years, in somewhat older girls (mean age 11.55) it was the same as in adolescent girls. *During the period of prepubertal growth acceleration and during the onset of clinical puberty a marked sudden change in the ratio of total and subcutaneous body fat obviously occurs* but not at the identical age in all children. This change was proved also in a quite different group investigated several years later (Pařízková and Roth 1972).

In adult age the shape of regression lines by sex differed significantly; in both instances these lines differed from those obtained for younger age groups and in elderly men (Pařízková 1962a). Between the two groups of elderly men there was no

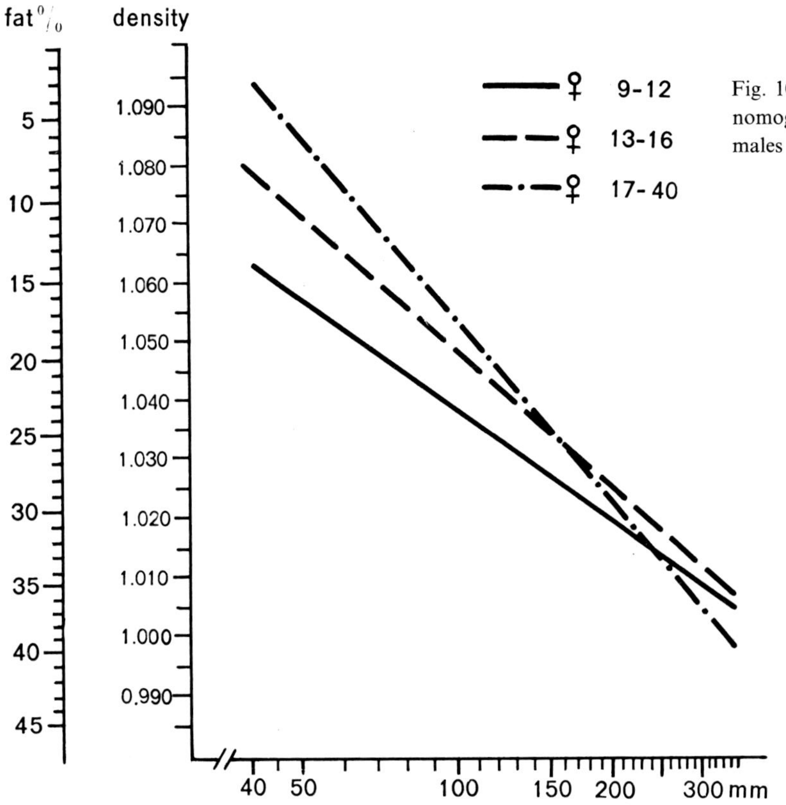

Fig. 10 b. The same nomogram for females of different age.

significant difference in the regression lines for the relationship between total and subcutaneous body fat. Therefore for men aged 50–80 years a single regression equation was calculated to estimate the percentage of body fat from ten skinfolds (Table 7). The percentage of body fat from the sum of ten skinfolds can be obtained from Table 9. The same table gives also values for adult men and women.

The differences between groups were manifested not only in the regression equations derived for total body fat based on measurements of all ten skinfolds but also in regression equations for individual skinfolds (Pařízková 1962a, 1971b), which can be used for the calculation of the percentage of body fat. The median error of estimation is, however, in that case somewhat higher than when the logarithm of the sum of all ten skinfolds is substituted (Pařízková, unpublished data).—From our data (i.e. percentage of fat from densitometry, four selected skinfolds) Möhr derived another regression equations (1969) which have been used in his subsequent research in German Democratic Republic.

We derived also *equations for two skinfolds which are recommended most frequently for the evaluation of adiposity—the skinfold on the arm above the triceps and on the*

TABLE 8.
Table for calculation of percentage of body fat from the sum of ten skinfolds measured by modified Best's caliper (1954) in youth (Pařízková 1961c)

mm	9—12	years	13—16	mm	9—12	years	13—16	mm	9—12	years	13—16
	♂	♀	♂ + ♀		♂	♀	♂ + ♀		♂	♀	♂ + ♀
30	8.4	11.3	4.1	73	18.2	20.2	15.1	116	23.6	25.0	21.1
31	8.7	11.7	4.6	74	18.4	20.3	15.3	117	23.7	25.1	21.2
32	9.0	12.0	5.0	75	18.5	20.5	15.5	118	23.8	25.2	21.3
33	9.4	12.3	5.3	76	18.7	20.6	15.6	119	23.9	25.3	21.5
34	9.7	12.6	5.7	77	18.8	20.7	15.8	120	24.0	25.9	21.7
35	10.0	12.8	6.0	78	18.9	20.9	16.0	125	24.5	25.7	22.1
36	10.4	13.1	6.4	79	19.0	21.0	16.1	130	24.9	26.1	22.2
37	10.7	13.4	6.7	80	19.3	21.0	16.3	135	25.4	26.5	23.1
38	10.9	13.7	7.0	81	19.4	21.2	16.5	140	25.8	26.9	23.6
39	11.2	13.9	7.3	82	19.6	21.4	16.6	145	26.2	27.3	24.0
40	11.5	14.2	7.7	83	19.7	21.5	16.8	150	26.6	27.6	24.5
41	11.8	14.3	8.0	84	19.8	21.6	16.9	155	27.0	28.0	24.9
42	12.0	14.4	8.3	85	19.9	21.7	17.1	160	27.4	28.3	25.3
43	12.3	14.6	8.5	86	20.1	21.7	17.2	165	27.7	28.7	25.7
44	12.6	14.9	8.8	87	20.2	21.9	17.4	170	28.1	29.0	26.1
45	12.8	15.0	9.1	88	20.4	22.1	17.5	175	28.5	29.3	26.5
46	13.1	15.3	9.4	89	20.5	22.2	17.7	180	28.8	29.6	26.9
47	13.3	15.7	9.6	90	20.6	22.3	17.8	185	29.1	29.9	27.3
48	13.5	16.0	9.9	91	20.8	22.4	18.0	190	29.4	30.1	27.6
49	13.7	16.2	10.1	92	20.9	22.6	18.1	195	29.6	30.4	28.0
50	14.0	16.4	10.4	93	21.0	22.7	18.2	200	30.1	30.7	28.3
51	14.2	16.6	10.6	94	21.1	22.8	18.4	205	30.4	31.0	28.7
52	14.4	16.8	10.9	95	21.3	22.9	18.5	210	30.6	31.2	28.9
53	14.5	17.0	11.1	96	21.4	23.0	18.6	215	30.9	31.5	29.3
54	14.8	17.1	11.4	97	21.5	23.1	18.7	220	31.2	31.7	29.6
55	15.0	17.3	11.6	98	21.6	23.2	18.8	225	31.5	32.0	29.9
56	15.2	17.5	11.8	99	21.7	23.3	18.9	230	31.7	32.2	30.2
57	15.4	17.7	12.0	100	21.9	23.4	19.1	235	32.0	32.4	30.3
58	15.6	17.9	12.2	101	22.0	23.5	19.3	240	32.3	32.7	30.8
59	15.8	18.0	12.4	102	22.1	23.6	19.4	245	32.5	32.9	31.1
60	16.0	18.2	12.7	103	22.2	23.7	19.5	250	32.8	33.1	31.4
61	16.2	18.4	12.9	104	22.3	23.8	19.7	255	33.0	33.3	31.0
62	16.4	18.5	13.1	105	22.4	23.9	19.8	260	33.2	33.5	31.9
63	16.6	18.7	13.3	106	22.5	24.0	19.9	270	33.5	33.9	32.4
64	16.7	18.9	13.5	107	22.6	24.1	20.0	280	33.7	34.3	32.9
65	16.9	19.0	13.7	108	22.7	24.2	20.2	290	33.9	34.7	33.3
66	17.1	19.2	13.9	109	22.8	24.3	20.3	300	34.2	35.1	33.9
67	17.3	19.3	14.0	110	22.9	24.4	20.4	310	35.4	35.5	34.4
68	17.4	19.5	14.2	111	23.1	24.5	20.5	320	35.8	35.8	34.8
69	17.6	19.6	14.4	112	23.2	24.6	20.6	330	36.2	36.1	35.2
70	17.6	19.8	14.6	113	23.3	24.7	20.8	340	36.6	36.4	35.6
71	17.9	19.9	14.8	114	23.4	24.8	20.9	350	36.9	36.8	36.1
72	18.1	20.0	15.0	115	23.5	24.9	21.0	360	37.3	37.1	36.4

TABLE 9.

Table for calculation of percentage of body fat from sum of ten skinfolds measured by modified Best's caliper (1954) in men and women (Pařízková 1962b, 1973b)

mm	17—50 years ♂	17—50 years ♀	50—80 ♂
30	1.5	—	12.8
31	1.9	—	13.0
32	2.3	—	13.2
33	2.7	—	13.4
34	3.1	—	13.6
35	3.5	—	13.7
36	3.8	0.4	13.9
37	4.1	0.8	14.1
38	4.5	1.3	14.2
39	4.8	1.7	14.4
40	5.1	2.1	14.6
41	5.4	2.6	14.7
42	5.7	3.0	14.8
43	6.0	3.4	15.0
44	6.3	3.8	15.1
45	6.6	4.2	15.3
46	6.9	4.5	15.4
47	7.2	4.9	15.5
48	7.4	5.3	15.7
49	7.7	5.6	15.8
50	7.9	6.0	15.9
51	8.2	6.3	16.0
52	8.4	6.6	16.1
53	8.7	7.0	16.3
54	8.9	7.3	16.4
55	9.1	7.6	16.5
56	9.4	7.9	16.6
57	9.6	8.2	16.7
58	9.8	8.5	16.8
59	10.0	9.8	16.9
60	10.2	9.1	17.0
61	10.4	9.4	17.1
62	10.6	9.7	17.2
63	10.8	9.9	17.3
64	11.0	10.2	17.4
65	11.2	10.5	17.5
66	11.4	10.7	17.6
67	11.6	11.0	17.7
68	11.8	11.2	17.8
69	12.0	11.5	17.9
70	12.2	11.8	17.9
71	12.3	12.0	18.0
72	12.5	12.2	18.1
73	12.7	12.5	18.2
74	12.9	12.7	18.3
75	13.0	12.9	18.4
76	13.2	13.1	18.5
77	13.4	13.4	18.5
78	13.5	13.6	18.6
79	13.7	13.8	18.7
80	13.8	14.0	18.8
81	14.0	14.2	18.8
82	14.2	14.5	18.9
83	14.3	14.7	19.0
84	14.5	14.9	19.1
85	14.6	15.1	19.1
86	14.8	15.3	19.2
87	14.9	15.5	19.3
88	15.0	15.7	19.3
89	15.2	15.9	19.4
90	15.3	16.1	19.5
91	15.5	16.3	19.5
92	15.6	16.4	19.6
93	15.7	16.6	19.7
94	15.9	16.8	19.7
95	16.0	17.0	19.8
96	16.1	17.2	19.9
97	16.3	17.3	19.9
98	16.4	17.5	20.0
99	16.5	17.7	20.1
100	16.6	17.9	20.1
101	16.8	18.1	20.2
102	16.9	18.2	20.2
103	17.0	18.4	20.3
104	17.1	18.6	20.4
105	17.3	18.7	20.4
106	17.4	18.9	20.5
107	17.5	19.0	20.5
108	17.6	19.2	20.6
109	17.7	19.4	20.6
110	17.9	19.5	20.7
111	18.0	19.7	20.7
112	18.1	19.8	20.8
113	18.2	20.0	20.9
114	18.3	20.1	20.9
115	18.4	20.3	21.0
116	18.5	20.4	21.0
117	18.6	20.6	21.1
118	18.7	20.7	21.1
119	18.8	20.9	21.2
120	18.9	21.0	21.2
125	19.9	21.7	21.5
130	20.0	22.4	21.7
135	20.4	23.0	21.9
140	20.9	23.7	22.2
145	21.3	24.3	22.4
150	21.8	24.9	22.6
155	22.2	25.4	22.8
160	22.6	26.0	23.0
165	23.0	26.5	23.1
170	23.3	27.0	23.3
175	23.7	27.5	23.5
180	24.0	28.0	23.7
185	24.4	28.5	23.8
190	24.7	28.9	24.0
195	25.1	29.4	24.2
200	25.4	29.8	24.3
205	25.7	30.2	24.5
210	26.0	30.6	24.6
215	26.3	31.0	24.8
220	26.6	31.4	24.9
225	26.9	31.8	25.0
230	27.1	32.2	25.2
235	27.4	32.6	25.3
240	27.7	32.9	25.4
245	27.9	33.3	25.5
250	28.2	33.6	25.7
260	28.7	34.3	25.9
270	29.1	35.0	26.2
280	29.6	35.6	26.4
290	30.2	36.2	26.6
300	30.5	36.8	26.8
310	30.9	37.3	27.0
320	31.3	37.8	27.2
330	31.7	38.4	27.4
340	32.0	38.9	27.6
350	32.4	39.4	27.7
360	32.5	39.9	27.9

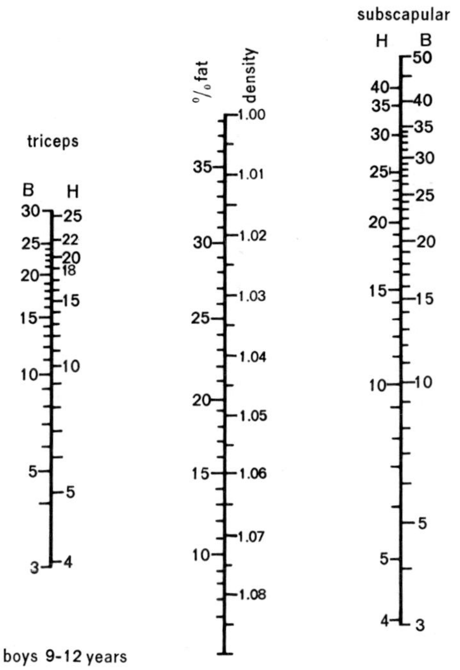

Fig. 11. Nomogram for the evaluation of percentage of body fat (or density – middle scale) from two skinfolds: triceps – left; subscapular – right; external sides of both extreme scales = values for modified Best caliper (B), internal sides of extreme scales (H) = values for Harpenden caliper (and Lange's caliper resp.). The value of the percentage of body fat is read on the middle axis, on the cross-section point of the line connecting particular values on the scales for triceps and subscapular skinfolds. This nomogram refers to the boys 9–12 years old (Pařízková 1961c).

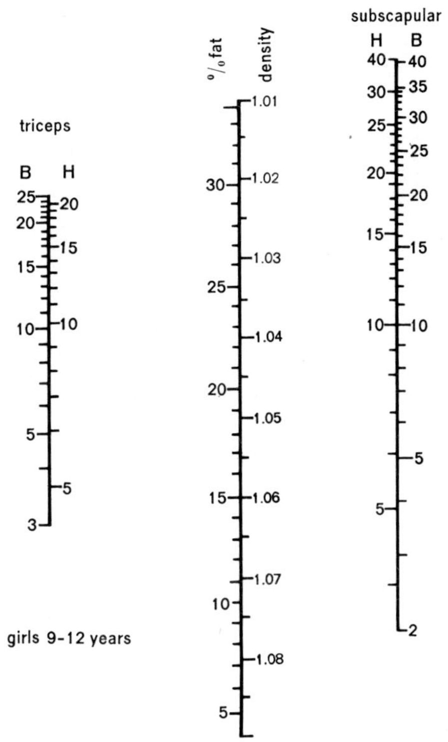

Fig. 12. Nomogram for the evaluation of percentage of body fat (or density – middle scale) from two skinfolds: triceps – left, subscapular – right, measured by Best or Harpenden (and Lange's caliper resp.). For explanation see Fig. 11. This nomogram refers to girls 9–12 years old (Pařízková 1961c, 1962b).

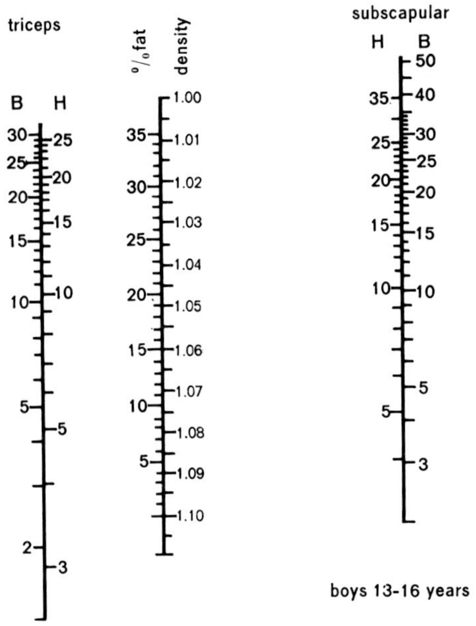

Fig. 13. Nomogram for the evaluation of percentage of body fat (or body density – middle scale) from two skinfolds: triceps – left, subscapular – right, measured by Best or Harpenden, (and Lange's caliper resp.). For explanation see Fig. 11. This nomogram refers to boys 13–16 years old (Pařízková 1961c, 1962b).

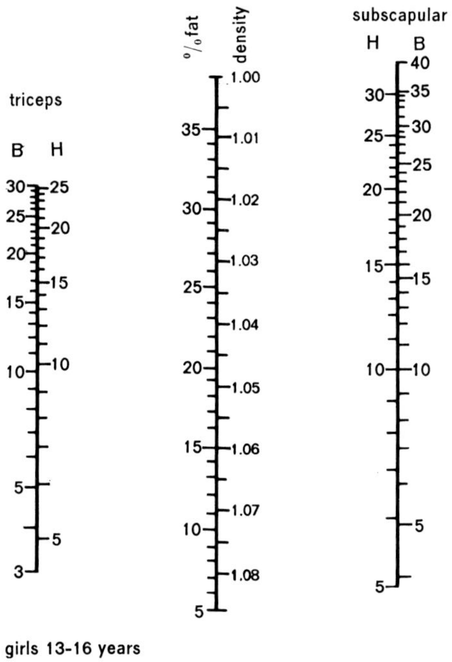

Fig. 14. Nomogram for the evaluation of percentage of body fat (or body density – middle scale) from two skinfolds: triceps – left, subscapular – right, measured by Best or Harpenden, (and Lange's caliper resp.). For explanation see Fig. 11. This nomogram refers to girls 13–16 years old (Pařízková 1961c, 1962b).

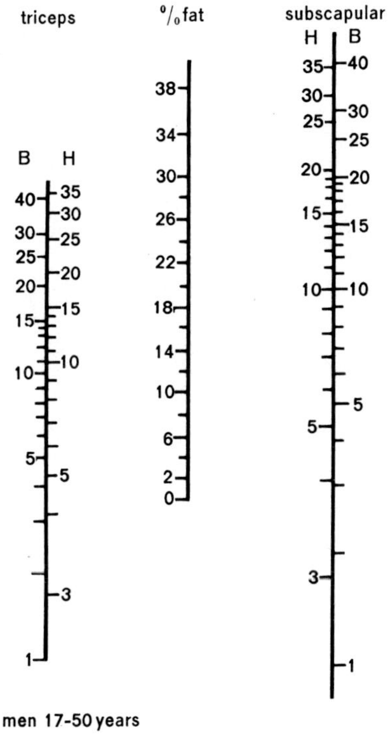

Fig. 15. Nomogram for the evaluation of percentage of body fat (or body density – middle scale) from two skinfolds: triceps – left, subscapular – right, measured by Best or Harpenden (and Lange's caliper resp.). For explanation see Fig. 11. This nomogram refers to men 17–50 years old (Pařízková et al. 1960, 1962b).

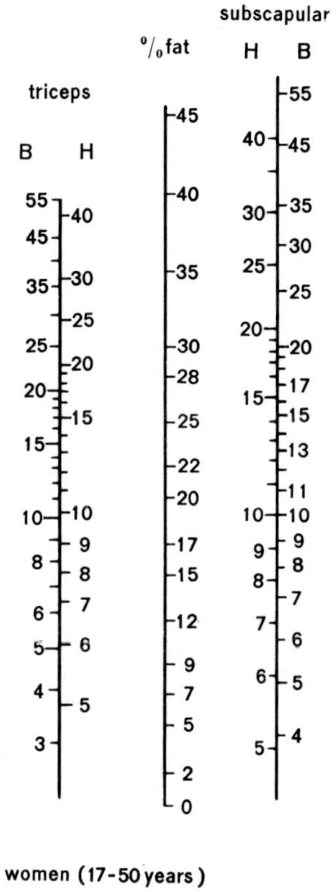

Fig. 16. Nomogram for the evaluation of percentage of body fat (or body density – middle scale) from two skinfolds: triceps – left, subscapular – right, measured by Best or Harpenden (and Lange's caliper resp.). For explanation see Fig. 11. This nomogram refers to women 17–50 years old (Pařízková 1962b).

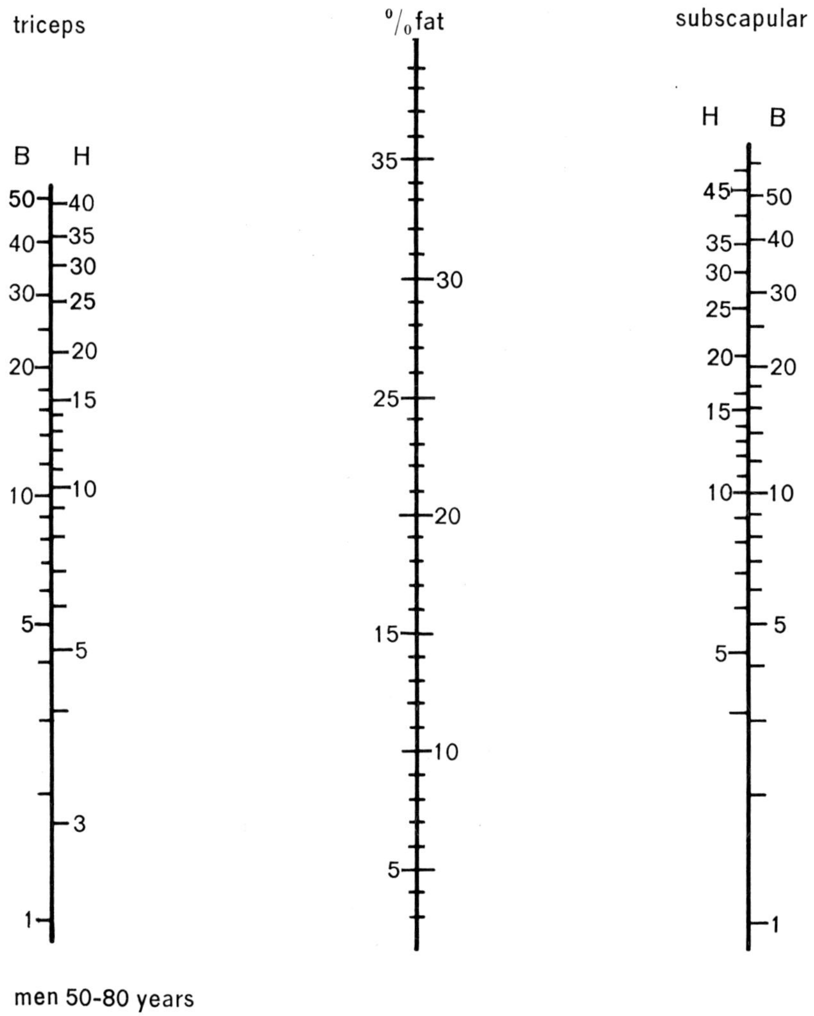

Fig. 17. Nomogram for the evaluation of percentage of body fat (or body density – middle scale) from two skinfolds: triceps – left, subscapular – right, measured by Best or Harpenden (and Lange's caliper resp.) For explanation see Fig. 11. This nomogram refers to men 50–80 years old (Pařízková and Eiselt 1962, 1966).

back beneath the scapula (i.e. subscapular). Scales for both *Best* and *Harpenden caliper* values (Pařízková and Goldstein 1970) are given. Nomograms which give readings of the percentage of body fat for these two skinfolds measured by both calipers (resp. also by *Lange's caliper* as its measurements do not differ from the Harpenden one) (Sloan and Shapiro 1972) for different categories by age and sex are presented in Figs. 11–17.

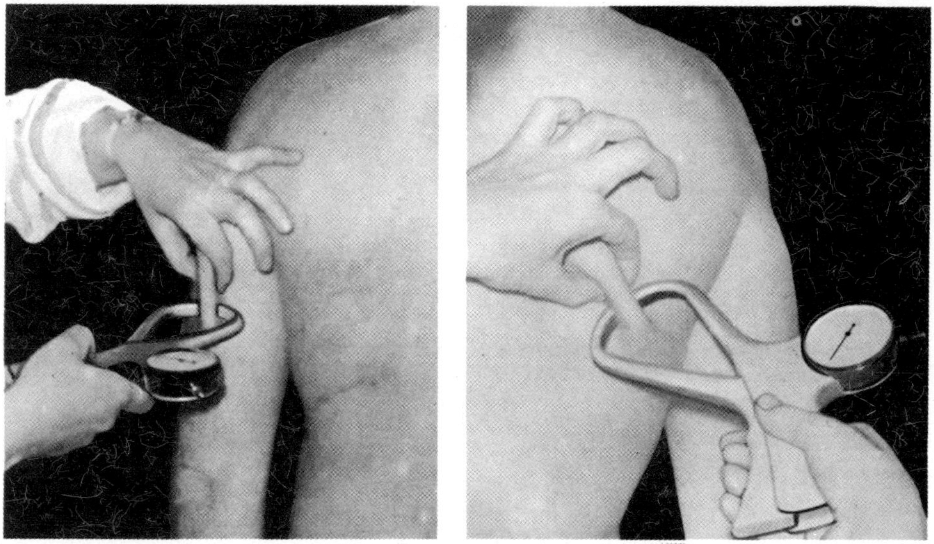

Plate 3. Measurement of the skinfold over triceps and subscapular region using Holtain caliper (modified Harpenden, i. e. Tanner-Whitehouse caliper; fa Siber Hegner, Zurich).

4. Results of comparison of skinfolds measured by means of different calipers

One of the most frequently used calipers is the Harpenden caliper (Edwards et al. 1955). This caliper has, however, quite different characteristics; it has larger (12 × × 6 mm) contact areas of an oblong shape and the pressure exerted per 1 mm^2 is 10 g (Plate 3a,b). This pressure was adopted in 1959 as a uniform value for the assessment of skinfold thickness. It is thus not possible to compare data obtained by different calipers (Rehs et al. 1975). Harpenden calipers, however, were not available commercially in the Czechoslovak market until 1973, are more expensive and more difficult to manufacture; in view of their original use (measurements of the thickness of leather) it is sometimes difficult to use them in infants and very young children. Many authors have used it, however, for measurement in large numbers of youth and adults in all parts of the world. The possibility of comparing our values and those assessed by means of a Harpenden caliper was therefore desirable. This is why we *analyzed the differences between values obtained by the two calipers (i.e. our modified Best caliper and the Harpenden caliper)*.

We measured the skinfold thickness on the arm above the triceps, on the back below the scapula (subscapular), the supracristal skinfold on the hip, on the leg and finally on the arm above the biceps muscle in 863 subjects aged 6–70 years of

TABLE 10.
Prediction equations for converting skinfold thicknesses assessed by modified Best's caliper (x) in corresponding values assessed by a Harpenden caliper (y; all data in mm) (Pařízková and Goldstein 1970)

Skinfolds	Biceps	Triceps	Subscapular	Suprailiac
Males (6—70 years)	y = 1.43 + 0.75x	y = 1.51 + 0.81x	y = 1.42 + 0.85x	y = 0.92 + 0.82x
s	(0.71)	(0.89)	(0.87)	(1.14)
Females (6—70 years)	y = 2.02 + 0.70x	y = 2.13 + 0.77x	y = 1.80 + 0.32x	y = 1.26 + 0.75x
s	(0.80)	(0.94)	(0.89)	(1.40)

y = skinfold in mm as measured by a Harpenden caliper
x = skinfold in mm as measured by a Best caliper
s = estimated standard deviations of prediction

TABLE 11.
Correlation coefficients (r) and regression equations (±s) of relationship between skinfold thicknesses assessed by a Harpenden caliper in boys and girls aged 8—12 years (n = 71; y = percentage of fat) (Pařízková and Roth 1972)

		r	Regression equation (y =	s
Boys	I	0.849	32.914x — 21.973	4.93
	II	0.863	29.344x — 27.410	4.70
	III	0.862	30.768x — 39.409	4.72
Girls	I	0.871	39.032x — 30.084	5.02
	II	0.886	39.024x — 43.435	4.73
	III	0.904	40.384x — 59.439	4.37
Boys + girls	I	0.859	35.567x — 25.330	4.94
	II	0.868	32.689x — 33.108	4.79
	III	0.875	33.910x — 46.669	4.66

(y = % fat; I x = log 2 skinfolds (triceps and subscapular)
II x = log 5 skinfolds (I + suprailiac + calf + biceps)
III x = log 11 skinfolds (II + cheek + chin + chest I, II + abdomen + thigh)

both sexes. Certain *constant differences were revealed between the two calipers* which were *expressed by means of linear regressions.* These regressions were calculated for individual skinfolds and for all age groups combined (there were no age-conditioned differences), separately for the two sexes. These equations (Table 10) *render it possible to calculate from values obtained by our caliper corresponding values for the Harpenden caliper* and thus also *to compare results obtained in different populations by means of these different calipers* (Pařízková and Goldstein 1970).

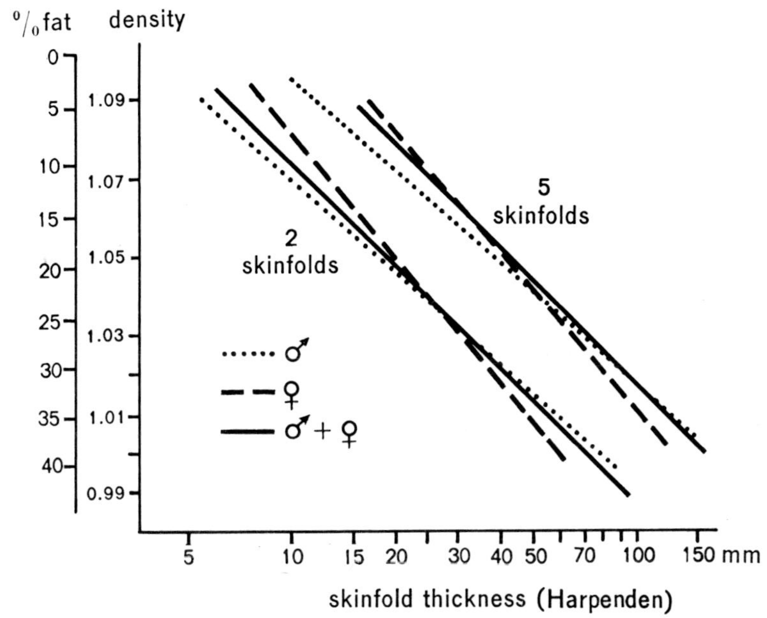

Fig. 18. Nomogram for the evaluation of the percentage of body fat (or body density – ordinate) from the sum of two (triceps and subscapular – left) or five (triceps, subscapular, suprailiac, calf, biceps – right; abscissa, mm) in boys (......) and girls (------) and together (——— ♂ + ♀) at the age of 8–13 years (Harpenden caliper, Pařízková and Roth 1972).

In subsequent investigations of body composition and subcutaneous fat since 1966 we used both calipers concurrently. This made it possible to compare both methods of skinfold measurement and *to derive regression equations for the relationship between total body fat and skinfolds* assessed by the Harpenden caliper on the arm above the triceps and biceps and beneath the scapula, on the hip (suprailiac skinfold) and leg (calf skinfold). Fig. 18 shows shape of the regression lines for boys and girls aged 8–13 years (n = 71) from which a reading of the percentage of body fat can be obtained. Individual equations are given in Table 11. For adolescents Durnin's and Rahaman's (1967) equation can be used. When comparing individual sites, *skinfolds over the triceps were regularly smaller on the right side,* and *those over the biceps on the left side of the body, in both boys and girls.* The differences were statistically significant. In *boys the suprailiac skinfold on the right side was significantly greater than on the left side;* there was *no difference in girls* of this age group, i.e. 8.5–12.9 years. There were also no differences in the values of subscapular and calf skinfolds measured on the right and left sides (Pařízková and Roth 1972).

In the same way measurements were made in young men aged 17–40 years (n = 101). In that case linear regression equations proved most suitable (Table 12)

TABLE 12.
Correlation coefficients (r) and regression equations ($\pm$s) for the relationships between percentage of fat (y) and skinfolds (individual x_1–x_5—A) and in sums (B) assessed by means of a Harpenden caliper in men (n = 101; Pařízková and Bůžková 1971)

	R	Regression equation (y =	s
A	0.430	$y_1 = 4.019 + 0.894x_1$	1.44
	0.563	$y_1 = 2.333 + 0.998x_2$	1.43
	0.673	$y_1 = 4.069 + 0.819x_3$	1.54
	0.592	$y_1 = 2.618 + 2.410x_4$	0.92
	0.489	$y_1 = 2.743 + 1.327x_5$	1.21
B	0.571	$y_1 = 9.729 + 0.630x_6$	1.80
	0.653	$y_1 = 1.187 + 0.398x_7$	2.23
	0.659	$y_1 = 0.969 + 0.338x_8$	2.35
	0.665	$y_1 = 0.174 + 0.317x_9$	2.49

y = % fat
x_1 = skinfold over triceps
x_2 = subscapular
x_3 = suprailiac
x_4 = skinfold over biceps
x_5 = calf skinfold

$x_6 = x_1 + x_2$
$x_7 = x_1 + x_2 + x_3$
$x_8 = x_1 + x_2 + x_3 + x_4$
$x_9 = x_1 + x_2 + x_3 + x_4 + x_5$

(Pařízková and Bůžková 1971). The nomogram which makes it possible to take a reading of the percentage of fat from two, three to five skinfolds is given in Fig. 19. The percentage of body fat cannot be derived so far from skinfolds measured by the Harpenden caliper in the older population.

Body fat can be calculated from the values of skinfold thicknesses also using older *formulas of Matiegka* (1933).

$D_{(fat)} = d \,.\, S \,.\, k_3$ ($d = \frac{1}{2} \cdot \frac{d_1 + d_2 + \ldots d_6}{6}$; d = skinfold thickness — d_1 = over biceps, d_2 = volar side of the forearm, d_3 = above quadriceps femoris muscle, d_4 = calf, d_5 = chest, half-way distance between the nipple and navel, d_6 = abdomen, half-way between the navel and spina ilica ventralis, S = body surface, $k_3 = 0.13$.

LBM can be calculated by means of another formula of Matiegka (1933) LBM = M + O + R. $M_{(musculature)} = r^2 \,.\, L \,.\, k_3$ ($r = \frac{r_1 + r_2 + \ldots r_4}{4}$; r_{1-4} = radiuses calculated from the circumference of the arm, forearm, thig and calf, after substraction of the thickness of the subcutaneous fat and skin. L = length of the body in m . $k_3 = 6.5$). $O_{(skeleton)} = o^2 \,.\, L \,.\, k_1$. ($o = \frac{o_1 + o_2 \ldots o_4}{4}$; o_{1-4} = breadth measures of humeral and femoral condyles, and the breadths of the wrist and ankle . $k_1 = 1.2$) R = rest.

Between the values of LBM and depot fat resp. calculated by means of mentioned formulas of Matiegka and the values of LBM and depot fat ascertained by densitometry high positive correlations were shown, proving thus the reliability of the

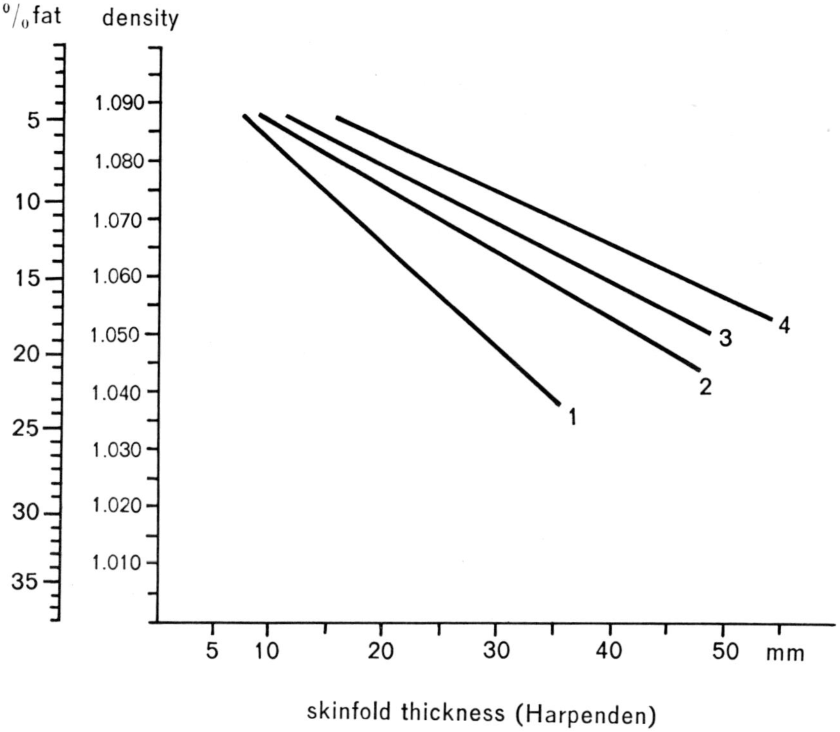

Fig. 19. Nomogram for the evaluation of the percentage of body fat (or body density – ordinate) from two (1 = triceps + subscapular), three = 1 + suprailiac), four (3 = 2 + calf) and five (4 = 3 + biceps) skinfolds (abscissa, mm) in men from 17 to 50 years (for Harpenden caliper – Pařízková and Bůžková 1971).

above-mentioned formulas. In groups of athletes e.g. the correlation coefficients (r) ranged from 0.75 to 0.98 (Malkovská, in press).

The above results indicate that the *ratio of LBM and total depot fat,* similar as the *amount and distribution of subcutaneous fat, has a marked ontogenetic trend which differs in the two sexes and is variable throughout life.* Assessment of body constituents by means of densitometry in the laboratory or indirectly by measurement of skinfolds by means of different calipers not only *extends the morphological characteristics of the individual* (Nagamine et al. 1974) but can also *serve as an indirect indicator of the energy turnover and calorie balance in the organism.* The use of calipers is simple and therefore suited for field work. Evaluation of body composition by means of the above equations or nomograms will be useful in particular *in functional studies* where the calculations of LBM *serves together with body weight as a reference standard.*

*) Differences in lean, fat-free, essential, active etc. body mass and methods of their measurement were analyzed in detail elsewhere (Pařízková 1959b, 1962a).

III. Changes in the maximum level of metabolic activity of lean body mass during ontogenesis

When evaluating changes of body composition in different age groups, it is essential to consider not only the ontogenetic aspect from the morphological point of view, i.e. the relative and absolute amount of LBM in relation to depot fat but also the *aspect of the level of their metabolic activity characterized e.g. by oxygen consumption under different conditions* (von Döbeln 1956, Buskirk a. Taylor 1957). Behnke (1956) described changes in the oxygen consumption in relation to LBM under basal conditions at rest: his observations were made in adult and elderly subjects. *The basal oxygen consumption in relation to LBM declined significantly during ageing:* the author explained this finding by changes in the composition of LBM (relative diminution of internal organs which under basal conditions have the highest oxygen consumption; in that case muscles consume cca 25% of oxygen, although as regards weight they form the largest constituent of LBM, and also by changes in the internal structure of tissues the sum of which is LBM (sclerotization, increased ratio of fibrous tissue, enhanced deposition of minerals, lipofuscin, etc.). Another aspect in this connection is the *maximum level of aerobic processes during ontogenesis related to LBM*. Aerobic capacity declines with ageing (Robinson 1936, Åstrand and Rodahl 1970, Hollman 1963, Davies 1972 etc.). Here in particular an important part is played by muscular tissue where the intensity of metabolic processes increases most markedly during a maximal load. This maximal metabolic level in relation to LBM has not been compared so far for a wide age range.

1. Changes of the relationship of aerobic capacity and lean body mass during ontogenesis

Data on body composition from youngest to the oldest age groups were used for this purpose (Pařízková 1959b, 1961a,c, 1962a, 1971b, etc.; Pařízková and Eiselt 1966,

1968) as well as data on the maximum oxygen consumption (Šprynarová 1966, Pařízková and Šprynarová 1968, 1970, Macková 1968, Eiselt and Pařízková 1975).

The maximal oxygen consumption was measured on a treadmill in a horizontal position. Every examination was started by assessment of the oxygen consumption during a 10 minute run at a standard rate of 6.5 km/min. After 10 min. rest the oxygen consumption was measured during a graded work-load, i.e. the rate of the treadmill was increased every minute by 0.5 km. The examined subjects ran till they reached the point of subjective exhaustion. The oxygen consumption was assessed continuously using low resistence valves with tubes 3 cm in diameter. The inspired air passed through a gasometer: the minute ventilation volume was recorded on a kymograph. For analysis of the inspired air a modified Bőhlau metabolimeter was used which recorded the decrease of oxygen in the expired air every 20 s. For the calculation of oxygen consumption the minute volume of inspired air was used with correction for STPD multiplied with the average percentage of oxygen decrement per minute. As indicator of the aerobic capacity the highest recorded value of oxygen consumption during the graded load was taken. The pulse rate was recorded electrocardiographically (Šprynarová 1966, 1974).
In old men the aerobic capacity was investigated on a bicycle ergometer under a somewhat different set-up. After 5 min adaptation to the mask and 5 min assessment of values at rest the oxygen consumption was measured during a 50 W load for a period of 3 min; then while the rate of pedalling was unaltered (70/min), the resistance was increased every minute till the sensation of subjective exhaustion was reached (in old age this criterion, however, need not always equal the maximum possible performance). The subsequent measurement was done in the same way as above (Eiselt 1968, Fischer et al. 1965). When using a veloergometer we must foresee during the maximum load oxygen values by 5—8 % lower (Åstrand and Rodahl 1970, Hermansen and Saltin 1969). A total of 156 men were examined divided into eight age groups starting with the mean age of 10.8 to 73.7 years. For the experimental groups we selected healthy subjects from the normal population who were not engaged systematically in any sports activities. As to adults we selected only subjects with a sedentary occupation. As so far has not been possible to examine the aerobic capacity of a sufficient number of women the comparison of ontogenetic changes of the maximum level of aerobic capacity of LBM was made only in men.

The highest absolute body weight figures were recorded at the age of 35.4 years; although we selected in all age groups subjects with normal range of height and weight, the relative body weight (related to height according to Broca's index) rose steadily from the youngest to the oldest age group. The percentage of LBM reached the highest levels between 18 – 25 years. In the fourth decade the ratio of LBM was significantly reduced and declined further with advancing age.

The absolute values of the aerobic capacity were highest at the age of 18.0 years, however, the values at the age of 14.2 (Šprynarová 1966, 1974) were not significantly lower, similarly as in the other groups, up to the fourth decade (Macková 1968). The same applied to values of maximal ventilation. Only in the seventh and eighth decade the values of the maximum pulse rate were very low; in the remaining groups they reached the appropriate level of 187 – 202/min. The oxygen pulse was lowest in the youngest and oldest age groups; between 14.2 – 35.4 years it remained at the same level. From the fifth decade onwards the values of oxygen pulse declined (Pařízková et al. 1972b).

The highest values of maximal oxygen consumption in relation to LBM were recorded at the age of about 15 years (Fig. 20). In the youngest boys and men aged 18 – 35 years these values did not differ significantly. In the fifth decade the values of the maximal

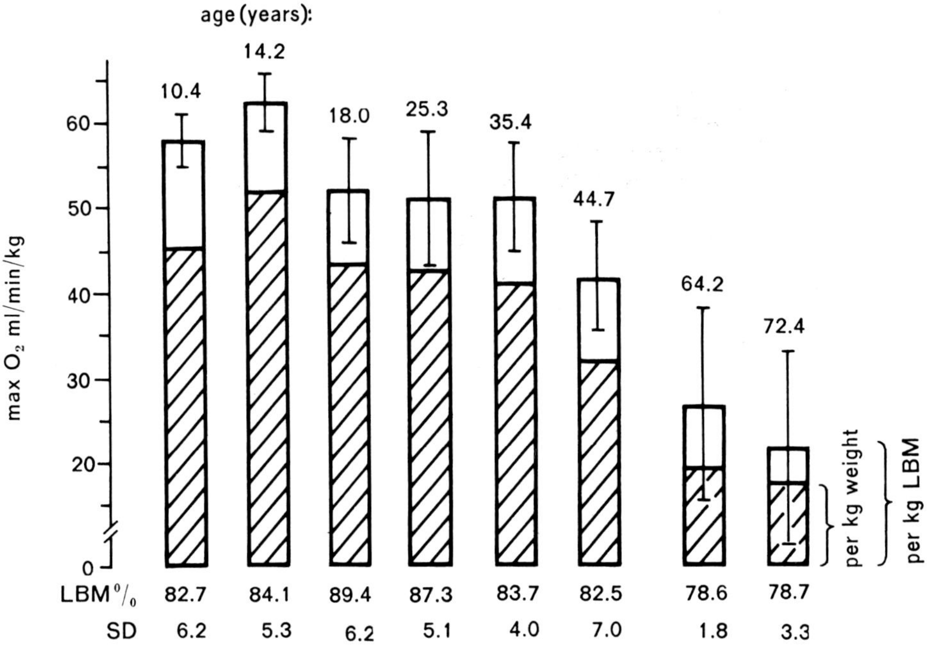

Fig. 20. Changes in maximal oxygen uptake as related to total body weight and lean body mass during ontogeny in men. Abscissa – age in years; ordinate – ml max. O_2/min/kg ($\bar{x} \pm$ SD) (Pařízková et al. 1972b).

oxygen consumption in relation to LBM declined significantly. At that age a break in the aerobic capacity occurs, although body weight, absolute values of lean body mass, maximal ventilation and pulse rate did not differ significantly from values assessed in the fourth and third decade (Macková 1968). Here we may consider the possibility of a reduced capacity of tissues, in particular muscles, to reach the maximum level of aerobic processes. In previous investigations in old men a significant correlation was found between the oxygen pulse and maximal oxygen consumption related to LBM. Also in the above age groups (Fig. 20) along with a decline of the maximal oxygen consumption in relation to LBM in the 5th decade a significant drop of oxygen pulse values was found. The reduced efficiency of the transport capacity for oxygen to working tissues is together with the lower oxygen utilization from ventilated air one of the most important links in the chain of causes leading to a lower level of aerobic processes of LBM under conditions of a maximum load (Pařízková et al. 1972b).

The peak of aerobic capacity of LBM is thus attained by the end of puberty, i.e. before the period when somatic development is completed and the highest ratio

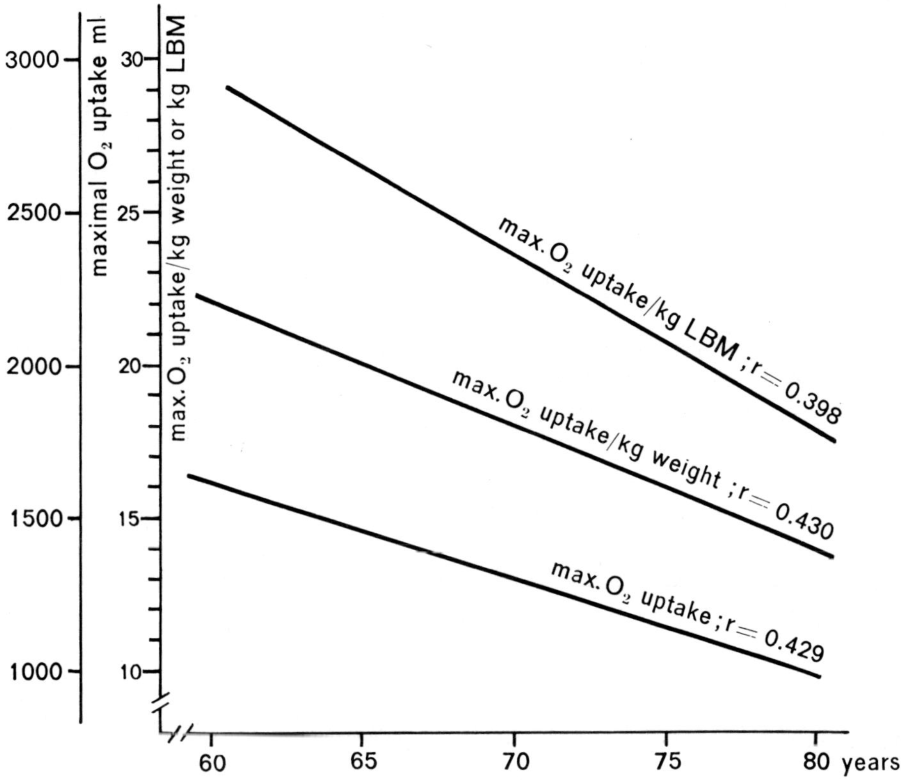

Fig. 21. Relationship between age and maximal O_2 uptake (ml/min) in absolute values (lowest line, ordinate – left side) as well as related to body weight (middle line, ordinate – right side – ml O_2/min/kg weight) or to lean body mass (ml O_2/min/kg LBM – line above) in men 60–80 years old (abscissa – years) (Fischer et al. 1965; Pařízková 1963a).

of LBM and highest maximum oxygen consumption is reached. The same applies to aerobic capacity related to total body weight (Fig. 20).

Fig. 21 shows in greater detail the declining trend of the aerobic capacity in relation to LBM, to body weight recorded in man from 60–80 years: *the drop of the maximum oxygen consumption applied to absolute as well as relative values in relation to body weight and LBM* (Fig. 21). The relationship with age in these two decades is significant and can be expressed by regression equations (Fischer et al. 1965, Pařízková 1963a).

2. Changes of the capillary network in skeletal muscle in relation to body composition and aerobic capacity

The previous findings indicate that functional precedes morphological involution (Figs. 20, 21). As a significant correlation has been proved between the maximum oxygen pulse and maximal oxygen consumption in relation to LBM, it may be assumed that there also exists a significant relationship between the reduction of the transport capacity of the circulation and the reduction of the maximal metabolic activity of LBM. *The reduced capacity of the circulation may be in this respect one of the most important limiting factors of the maximal metabolic level of tissues, similar to the maximum performance and aerobic capacity in old age.* In this connection also the problem of adequate supply of tissues with oxygen and other necessary substances comes to the fore and depends e.g. on the density of capillaries in relation to the number of muscle fibres in particular in large skeletal muscles. We compared therefore this indicator in the quadriceps femoris muscle along with body composition and the maximal oxygen consumption in young men (students at the Faculty of Physical Education) and old men with an average, physical activity and with a sedentary occupation.

Comparison of somatic characteristics revealed a greater height and weight in young men; the same relative weight and the same Quetelet index indicated a similar proportionality and constitution within the range of normal values in both age groups (Fig. 22). LBM was also greater in young men—in relative as well as absolute values. Comparison of the body composition of these groups of young and old men with results obtained in larger previously investigated groups of the normal population (Pařízková 1963a, 1971b, Pařízková and Eiselt 1966) did not differ significantly. The circumferences of the extremities were also greater in young men.

The maximal oxygen consumption measured during a graded load on a bicycle ergometer in absolute amounts as well as in relation to body weight and LBM was, in keeping with previous results, higher in young men (Fig. 22). As compared with physical education students in other countries our values were lower (Bottin et al. 1968) and thus more comparable to values of untrained subjects. E.g. in untrained normal men of similar age during a maximum load values of cca 50 ml/kg body weight were obtained (however when running on a treadmill—Hermansen and Wachtlová 1971). Values assessed in old men were also in keeping with former findings (Eiselt 1968, Eiselt and Pařízková 1971, 1975) and did not differ markedly from data of other authors (Robinson 1936, Felder 1959, Hollman 1963, Luft 1973 etc.).

Along with somatic and functional results we analyzed differences in the muscle structure with regard to the number and size of muscle fibres in relation to the number of capillaries. These indicators were investigated in biopsy specimens of the quadriceps femoris muscle.

Specimens were collected by means of a biopsy needle from the lateral portion of the quadriceps femoris muscle using Bergstrøm's technique (1962). After fixation of the specimen with formalin (3 weeks) the

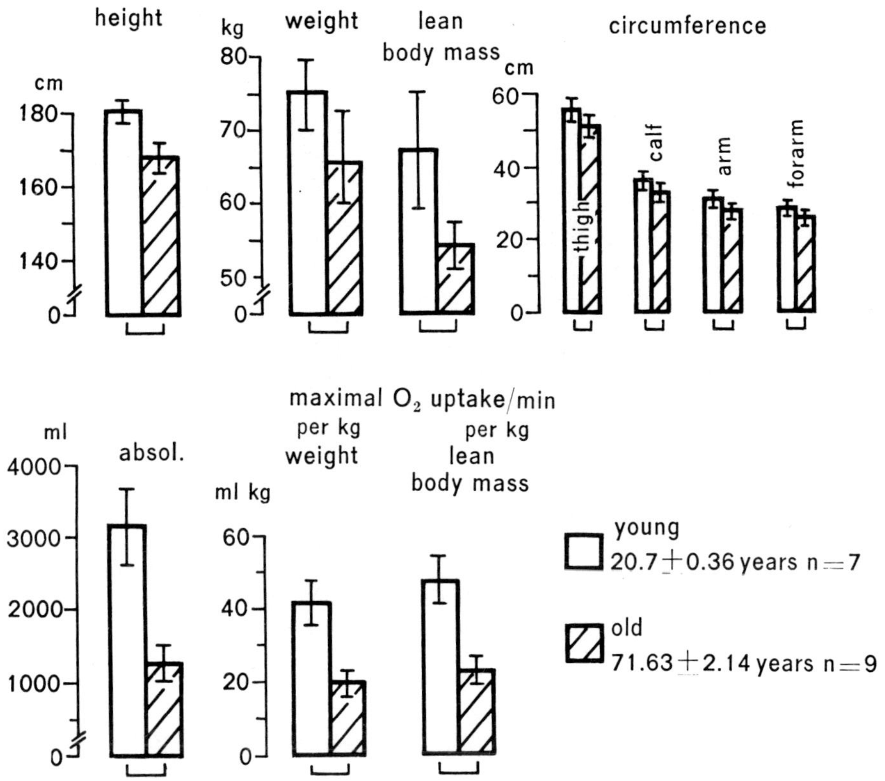

Fig. 22. Mean values of morphological (upper part – height, weight, lean body mass) and functional parameters (lower part – max. O_2 uptake in absolute values – ml O_2/min, and as related to weight and lean body mass – ml O_2/min/kg) in groups of young men (white) and old men (hatched columns). ($\bar{x} \pm$ SD: └──┘ means statistical significance of differences, p at least < 0.05) (Pařízková et al. 1971a).

microstructure of the muscle was visualized by means of the PAS reaction (Hecht 1958). The number of capillaries and muscle fibres from transverse section was calculated under the microscope using a vertical camera (Zeiss) from 20 fields in each specimen. The size of fields for all evaluations was 40,000 sq. μ. In addition to the absolute number of fibres and capillaries the ratio capillaries: fibres was evaluated as well as the diffusion distance (D/2) according to Krogh (1929).

The number of capillaries per sq.mm from biopsy muscle specimens displayed a great variability in both groups (young $V_{\bar{x}} = 36.7$, old $V_{\bar{x}} = 30.5$). Individual differences in this respect are thus considerable. There was no difference in capillarization between the group of young and old men. *The absolute number of muscle fibres per sq.mm was significantly lowest in young men, i.e. the fibres had the greatest diameter. The ratio capillaries: fibres was therefore more favourable, i.e. higher in young men where there was a greater number of capillaries in relation to the same*

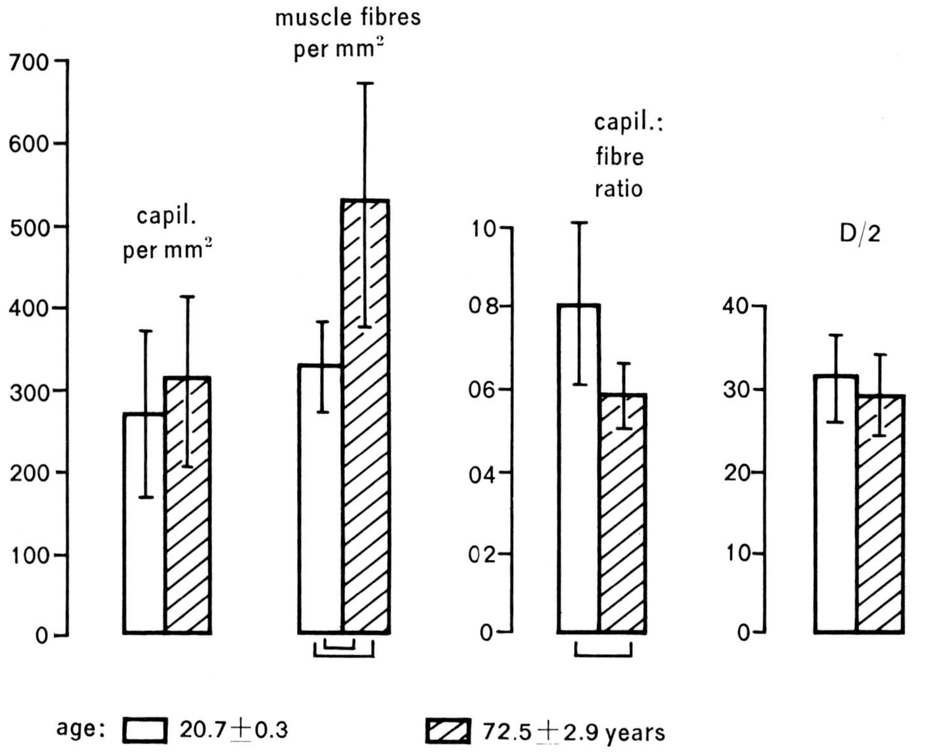

Fig. 23. Morphological structure of skeletal muscle (biopsy from quadriceps femoris muscle), i. e. number of capillaries/mm², number of muscle fibres/mm², fibre: capillary ratio, and diffusion distance in young and old men. (For explanation see Fig. 22) (Pařízková et al. 1971a).

number of fibres (Pařízková et al. 1971a). The diffusion distance, however, did not differ significantly (Fig. 23).

Data on the number of capillaries in young men are in agreement with data of Hermansen and Wachtlová (1971). The morphological structure of muscle from biopsy specimens in old men has not been described so far. A reduced cross section of fibres (i.e. a greater number of fibres per sq.mm) corresponds to general senile tendencies—a reduction of LBM, body weight and circumferences of extremities (Pařízková et al. 1971a).

Confrontation of results pertaining to the ratio capillaries: fibres and the maximum oxygen consumption display a certain parallelism in young men: *high values of aerobic capacity and a high maximum oxygen pulse are found in men with a higher ratio capillaries: fibres* on the quadriceps femoris muscle ($r = 0.850$; $r = 0.800$). These correlations were significant only in young men and not in men of more advanced age. A higher maximal oxygen consumption was also found in athletes who had moreover a higher capillary: fibre ratio in the same muscle; the reverse was true in untrained subjects (Hermansen and Wachtlová 1971). A higher aerobic capacity was thus usually found in individuals with a more favourable i.e. higher ratio of capillaries to muscle fibres. In younger age categories apparently the morphological structure of muscle plays a more important part in the functional aerobic capacity. In the eighth decade the position deteriorates; this applies to the aerobic capacity as well as muscle structure. In view of the unaltered diffusion distance and the absence of significant relations between the ratio capillaries: fibres in the muscle and indicators of aerobic capacity, these changes in muscle do not seem to be of primary importance for the reduction of the maximum oxygen consumption in old age. The poorer supply of muscle fibres is obviously has a minor impact, as compared with other senile changes in other parts of the circulation, i.e. in particular in the heart muscle and large vessels.

IV. Some consequences of adaptation to increased or restricted activity during ontogenesis

In the normal course of ontogenesis the level of the energy turnover changes markedly (i.e. the calorie intake as well as expenditure) which among others is also linked to the level of spontaneous physical activity. The great variability of physical activity depends on internal as well as external factors (Oliverau 1971). As has been mentioned before the differences in experimental animals (Collier 1971) as well as in man (Gapon 1972 etc.) may be as much as tenfold. Physical activity is also associated with the level of excitability of the central nervous system (CNS) which under various set-ups is also evaluated according to the level of physical activity. A high level of excitability of the CNS is tested in experimental animals, for instance in special boxes used to promote a greater exploratory activity i.e. increased movement of the animal (Lát 1963). Although there is a very wide range of interindividual variability it may be said that during growth the mean physical activity is high and during adult life and advanced age it declines. A very similar trend is also displayed by ontogenetic changes in the level of excitability of the CNS (Lát 1963).

The question thus arises what changes may take place in the organism when the level of physical activity is altered. This change can be induced by increasing or reducing physical activity; the change can be in line (e.g. increased activity during the growth period) *or at variance with the actual ontogenetic trend* (restriction of activity during the developmental period or conversely a great increase in activity in adult life or advanced age). All this applies to the average population. In extreme instances, however, induced changes of the regime of physical activity may (depending on individual properties) act as a stimulus of quite a different quality and importance.

A certain mean effect of altered physical activity can be evaluated according to a number of indicators. If the energy output is raised above a certain level, this also implies an altered caloric intake. Mayer (1968) demonstrated that changes in the caloric intake and body weight depend on the intensity as well as the duration of physical activity. After a small amount of exercise the caloric intake of rats does not increase (rather the reverse) and the body weight declines. In response to a medium load the caloric intake increases parallel with the energy output, and body weight does not change (the so-called range of proportional response). When the load is excessive and the caloric intake does not increase further the body weight declines; this condition implies overburdening.

When evaluating the response to physical activity in particular of a medium type, we cannot be satisfied with recording body weight only. Although the growth curves (in particular during the period of exponential growth) are a very sensitive indicator, we must also obtain information on body composition and the size of different organs and muscles. These changes may take place even when the body weight does not change significantly.

1. Growth curves and body composition during adaptation to different loads

Experiments in rats concerned with manifestations of adaptation to different types of physical loads were focused on the sequelae of increased physical activity as well as on those of marked restriction of activity. To increase the intensity of physical activity we used running on a treadmill driven by an electric motor (Plate 4). In some experiments we modified the physical activity in such a way as to prevent a negative effect on the body weight curve during the experiment as a whole (up to 360 days). In other trials we purposely used an intensity increased to such an extent that the growth curve remained retarded up to the completed stage of exponential growth as compared with the growth curve of controls: the duration and rate of activity on the treadmill were greater and supplemented moreover by a static load (hanging on a ladder). Adaptation to different physical loads began either very early, i.e. before weaning (18th – 19th day of life) or after weaning (30th – 32nd day), after puberty (50 – 55th day) or in adult life (160th day).

All these experiments concerned with the consequences of adaptation to different types of physical activity were conceived so that the *stimulus,* i.e. running on the treadmill (possibly supplemented by a static load), *was precisely defined,* and *tolerable for all animals included in the experiment.* By this means we tried *to eliminate the effect of selection.* When the load is too great, a certain proportion of the animals always drop out (this is usually not mentioned in papers of this type), because they cannot tolerate the load. Thus at the end of the experiment only those animals are examined who were able to endure and tolerate the load, and this may imply a certain primary difference. We tried to eliminate this in our experimental set-up.

The load on the treadmill (designed by Hyrš and Zelenka) with separate pathways (Plate 4) was uniform in all experiments, i.e. gradual, from a very low rate of 5—8 m/min for a few minutes up to the definite load continuing for as much as 3 hours per day at a rate of 18—20 m/min. The final load was attained usually after 30 – 40 days (Pařízková and Staňková 1964a, 1967, Pařízková et al. 1966a,b, Pařízková and Koutecký 1968 etc.). The run on the treadmill then represented a medium load depending on its

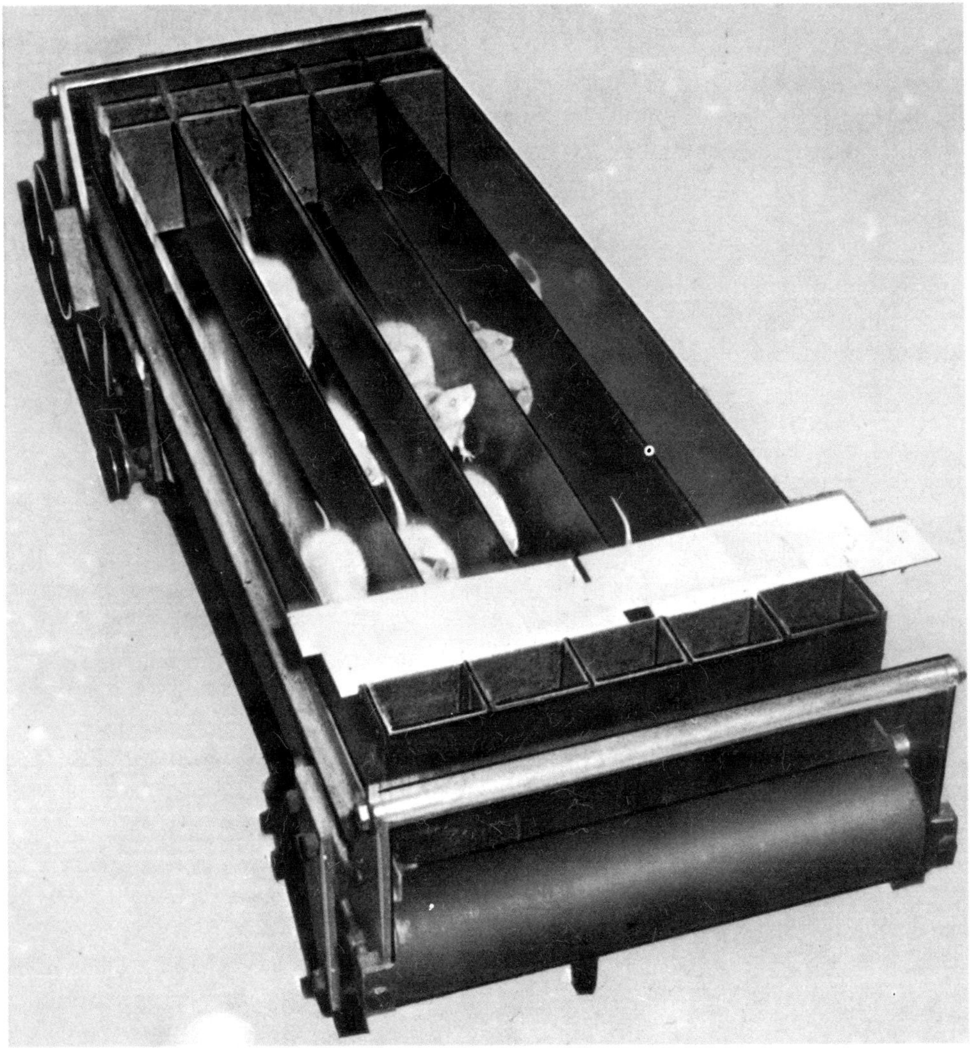

Plate 4. Motor-driven treadmill for exercising the rats (Hyrš and Zelenka 1971).

duration. In selected experiments in addition we used a static load, i.e. three hours hanging on vertical ladders made from wire splints and fixed in a vertical position from a horizontal board in such a way that the rat was unable to sit on top (Pařízková et al. 1972c, Pařízková and Lát 1973a etc.). Below the ladder the space was arranged in such a manner that if the rats fell from the ladder they could not escape. The run on the treadmill as well as hanging on the ladder was under constant supervision so that the animals could not be injured. In view of the variations of spontaneous motor activity during the oestrous cycle (Kennedy and Mitra 1963) we used only male rats in these experiments. All experimental animals were fed Larsen mixture *ad libitum*.

Restriction of activity was achieved by placing the animals after weaning (31st—32nd day) in small boxes

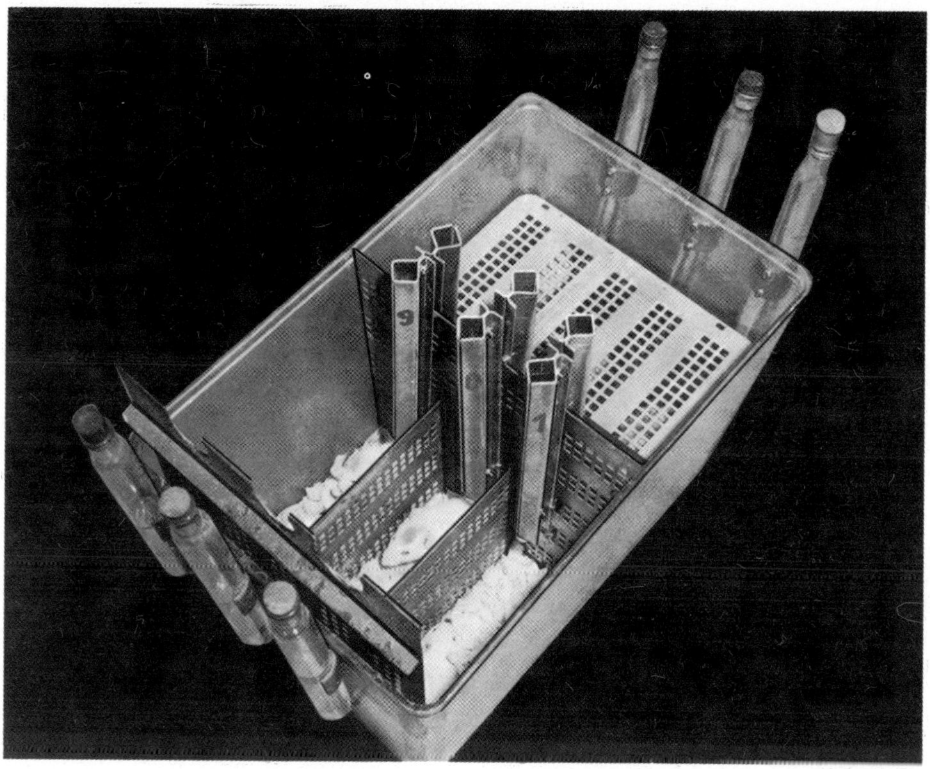

Plate 5. Cages with small compartments (8 × 12 × 20 cm) for the artificial restriction of physical activity of laboratory rats (Pařízková and Staňková 1964a,b; 1967).

20 × 12 × 8 cm (Plate 5) (Pařízková and Staňková 1964, 1967, Pařízková and Faltová 1969, 1970, etc.) the walls of which were made of perforated aluminium or wire netting (to reduce the strain of isolation and the absence of olfactory, thermal and other stimuli). Feeding pots were placed in the boxes which rendered it possible to record the amount of food and water ingested during different time intervals (Pařízková and Staňková 1964a, Pařízková and Poledne 1974a,b, etc.).
The controls lived in normal cages cca 30 × 45 × 28 cm. The results of both groups mentioned above were compared with findings obtained in controls (the question remains open, however, whether the regime of activity of controls shut up throughout life in a small cage represents for this type of rats — although "domesticated" in laboratory animal houses for more than a century — really normal, natural conditions. Laboratory rats — as has been mentioned before (Collier 1971a,b) display when they have the opportunity e.g. in boxes leading to a rotational wheel a great spontaneous physical activity. This fact is usually forgotten in experiments with this type of rat. Rats subjected to a certain load have obviously in this respect much more normal conditions).

Fig. 24 presents the growth curves from several series of experiments where animals adapted to running on the treadmill were followed up. 85-day-old animals ran for three hours a day at a rate of 20/min and 125-day-old animals for two hours a day

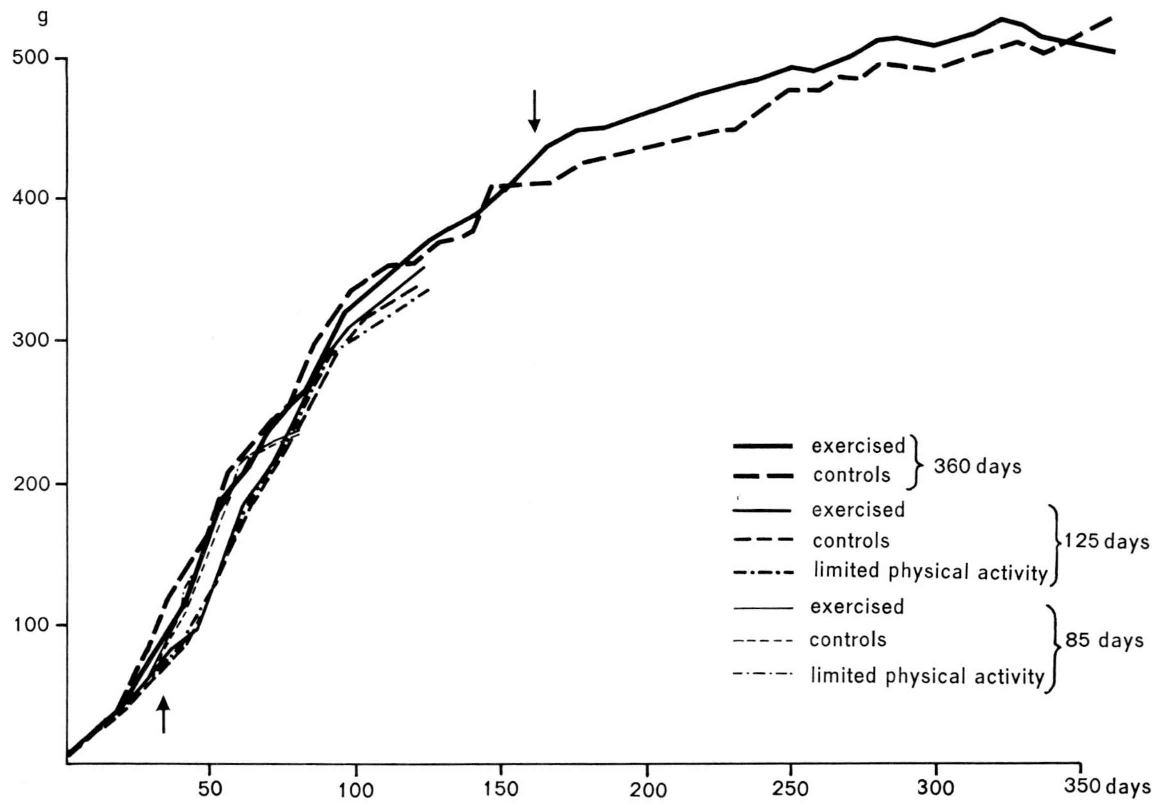

Fig. 24. Growth curves (g, weight – ordinate) of male rats adapted to different motor activity regime up to 85, 125 and 360 days of life (abscissa – age in days). Arrows indicate the beginning of daily exercise on a motor driven treadmill (30th day in the youngest, 160th day in the oldest group). (Pařízková and Staňková 1964a,b, 1967).

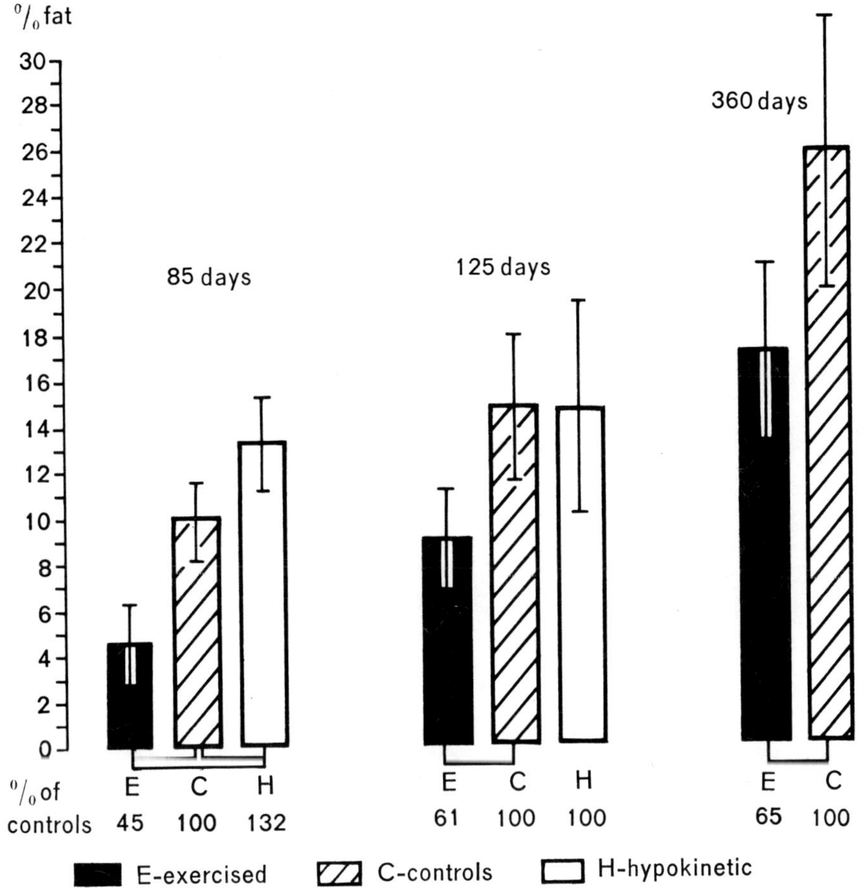

Fig. 25. Percentage of body fat ($\bar{x} \pm SD$) in male rats adapted to different motor activity regime (black – active, exercised; hatched – controls; white columns – hypokinetic animals (growth curves see Fig. 24) at the age of 85, 125 and 360 days (Pařízková and Staňková 1964a,b, 1967). ⎣___⎦ means statistical significance of difference, p at least < 0.05.

at the same rate. Both groups began to run after weaning. 360-day-old animals started to run only at the age of 150 days and were able to run only for one hour per day at the above rate. All groups of animals attained the possible maximum. When the rate was increased or the period of running prolonged, injuries occurred frequently and the number of experimental animals diminished; a situation we regarded as undesirable. When *this type of load was used, the growth curves were almost identical* (Fig. 24). The body composition differed, however, significantly—*the body fat ratio of the exercised animals was in all instances significantly lowest* (Pařízková 1966, 1969 etc.). In the youngest groups (85 days) the percentage of fat in the animals

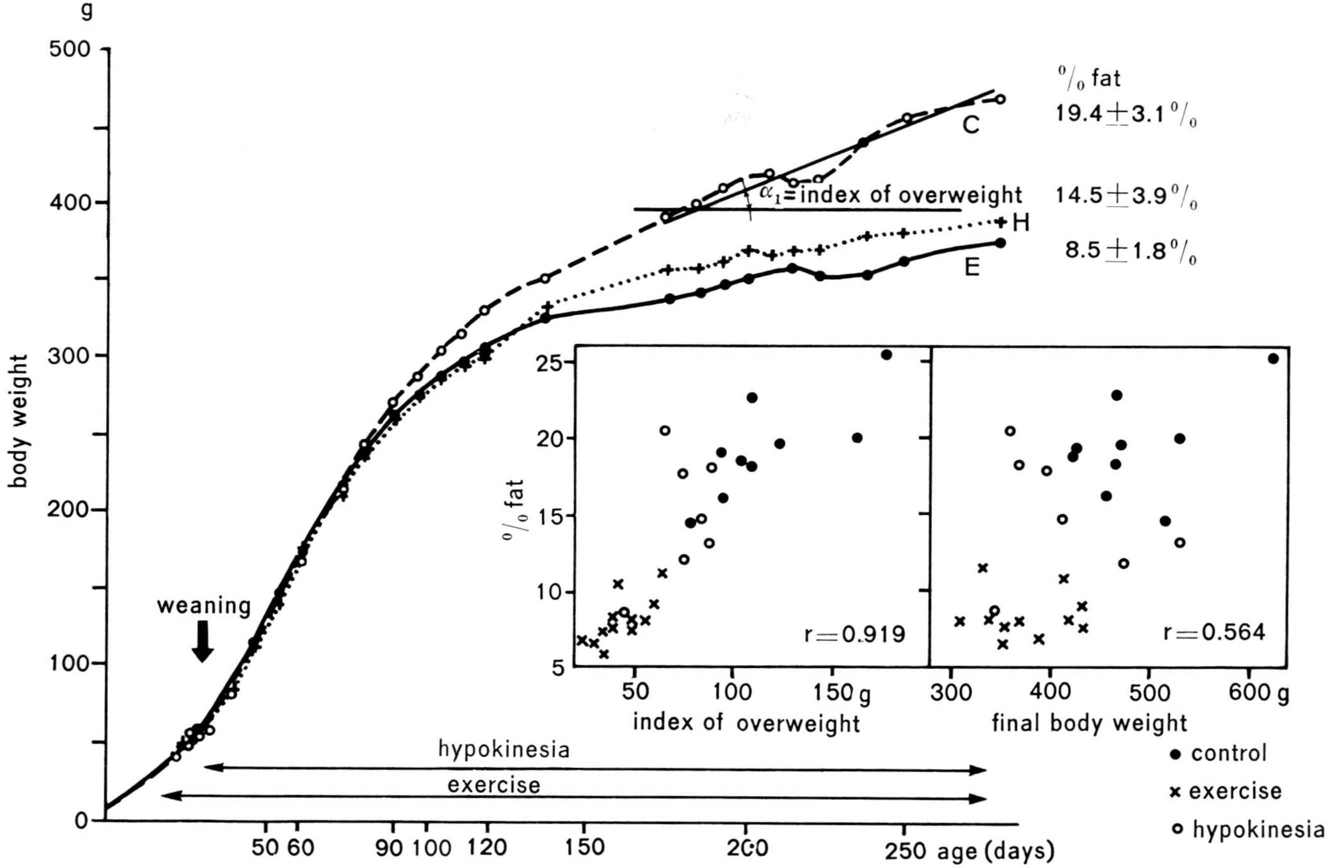
g
500
400
300
200
100
0
body weight
weaning
% fat
19.4 ± 3.1 %
14.5 ± 3.9 %
8.5 ± 1.8 %
C
H
E
α_1 = index of overweight
25
20
15
10
5
% fat
r = 0.919
r = 0.564
50
100
150 g
index of overweight
300
400
500
600 g
final body weight
● control
× exercise
○ hypokinesia
hypokinesia
exercise
50 60
90 100 120
150
200
250 age (days)

with restricted activity was higher than in controls. At the age of 125 days (i.e. full grown animals) restriction of activity was not manifested in this way. In the oldest group (360 days) we did not investigate the effect of restricted activity (Fig. 25).

As apparent from the results presented, the percentage of body fat in the running rats aged 125 days was the same as in 85-day-old controls. The same applies to the comparison of 360-day-old running and 125-day-old control animals. *The increased intensity of activity caused the body fat ratio to remain at a level corresponding to a younger age group. The reverse can be shown when comparing 85-day-old restricted and 125-day-old control animals.* Between these two groups there is again no difference (Fig. 25).—Changes in body composition were confirmed also by our later experiments with ^{131}I which revealed the greatest plasma volume in running animals (Pařízková and Poledne 1974a,b).

In this series of 125-day-old animals we did not find a difference between the absolute and relative weights of the adrenals with the exception of the 125-day-old animals (Pařízková and Staňková 1964a,b, 1967).

In the subsequent series of experiments where a *more intensive load was used* (i.e. three hours running and three hours hanging on a ladder) to which the animals were exposed from the 18th day of life, we showed *at the age of 285 days significant differences between weight curves* (Fig. 26). The controls had roughly from the 110th to 120th day a higher body weight and this discrepancy increased. The *"overweight index"* calculated from the slope of the linear line expressing weight increments after the stage of exponential growth (Fig. 26) was *in controls also significantly greater* than in the two remaining groups, i.e. running rats and those with restricted activity. The percentage of body fat was significantly highest in the controls (19.4 ± ± 3.1 %) than in exercised animals (8.5 ± 1.8 %) and in those with restricted activity (14.5 ± 3.9 %). The overweight index correlated significantly with the percentage of body fat (r = 0.919; index of overweight: final weight of animal = 0.564) (Pařízková and Lát 1973b).

In one trial we also checked the size of different organs in running animals (31st to 160th day of life) as compared with controls of similar age and still growing 50-day-old animals (also kept as controls). Table 13 shows that while the changes in body composition were as expected, *there was a smaller difference between 50-day and 160-day exercised animals* as regards the relative size of the liver, spleen and adrenals than between 50-day and 160-day old male controls. *The relative size of organs in relation to the total as well as lean body mass in the exercised animals persisted on a level closer to that found in young growing animals.* The differences were, however, not very marked as the load in this experiment acted only for a brief period. Relative

◀ Fig. 26. Growth curves of male rats adapted to different motor activity regime (E – active exercised male rats – 3 hours running on a motor-driven tread-mill + 3 hours of static work load – hanging on vertical ladders; C – controls; H – hypokinetic). Abscissa – age in days; ordinate – weight (g). Bottom right: correlation between the overweight index and percentage of fat (r = 0.919), and overweight index and final total body weight (r – 0.564) (Pařízková and Lát 1973b).

TABLE 13.
Mean values ($\bar{x} \pm$ SD) of total weight, body composition and relative weights of internal organs in young and full grown male rats (Pařízková et al. 1966a)

Groups		Young		Adult : Exercised		Controls	
Age (days)		50		160		160	
n		10		12		9	
		$\bar{x}$	SD	$\bar{x}$	SD	$\bar{x}$	SD
Weight (g)		102.2	11.1	306.1	43.8	316.4	20.5
Fat (%)		5.8	0.8	6.2	1.5	7.9	2.1
Fat-free body mass (g)		96.2	10.2	287.3	58.4	291.6	21.2
Liver:	weight (mg)	3659	468	8182	1319	7656	915
	mg/100 g weight	3581	288	2677	244	2416	202
	mg/100 g fat-free weight	3826	313	2859	83	2593	211
Spleen:	absol. weight (mg)	569	170	1056	233	929	115
	mg/100 g weight	558	162	345	64	293	32
	mg/100 g fat-free weight	605	173	369	69	319	33
Adrenals:	absol. weight (mg)	27.7	3.1	53.4	7.4	43.4	6.9
	mg/100 g weight	24.3	3.5	17.2	3.5	13.6	1.9
	mg/100 g fat-free weight	26.4	3.7	18.2	3.6	14.8	2.2

weights of organs were also investigated in a series of other experiments. Fig. 27 shows the results of investigations of 110-day-old animals with a different regime of physical activity (i.e. exercised for 3 hours on a treadmill at a speed of 18 – 20 m/min, controls and hypokinetic animals in small cages since weaning). The weight and percentage of fat were lowest in the exercised animals; the absolute weight of the heart did not differ but the relative heart weight was highest in the exercised. Both absolute and relative weights of the adrenals, soleus muscle and seminal vesicles were higher in the exercised as compared to the hypokinetic animals, and so were the relative weights. The tibialis muscle and the hypothalamus in the exercised animals compared with the controls and hypokinetic animals were highest only when related to total body weight (Pařízková 1974d, 1975—in press).

Greater relative weights of the heart, adrenals and skeletal muscles indicate morphological adaptation to an increased work load, i.e. adaptation of organs involved during increased motor activity. The finding of an increased weight of the seminal vesicles in the exercised animals seems to indicate that *adequate and natural stress,* which the organism is able to cope with, *can also have a stimulating effect on gonadotrophic function.* Excessive stress, on the other hand, has an inhibitory effect on this function as shown e.g. by Mikulaj et al. (1975). A positive effect of adequate stress on gonadotrophic function was also demonstrated in athletes by the same authors. Comparison of testosterone levels before and after a parachute jump and during 180 min of recovery phase revealed higher values in trained parachutists as compared to beginners of the same age. Adequate stress activating

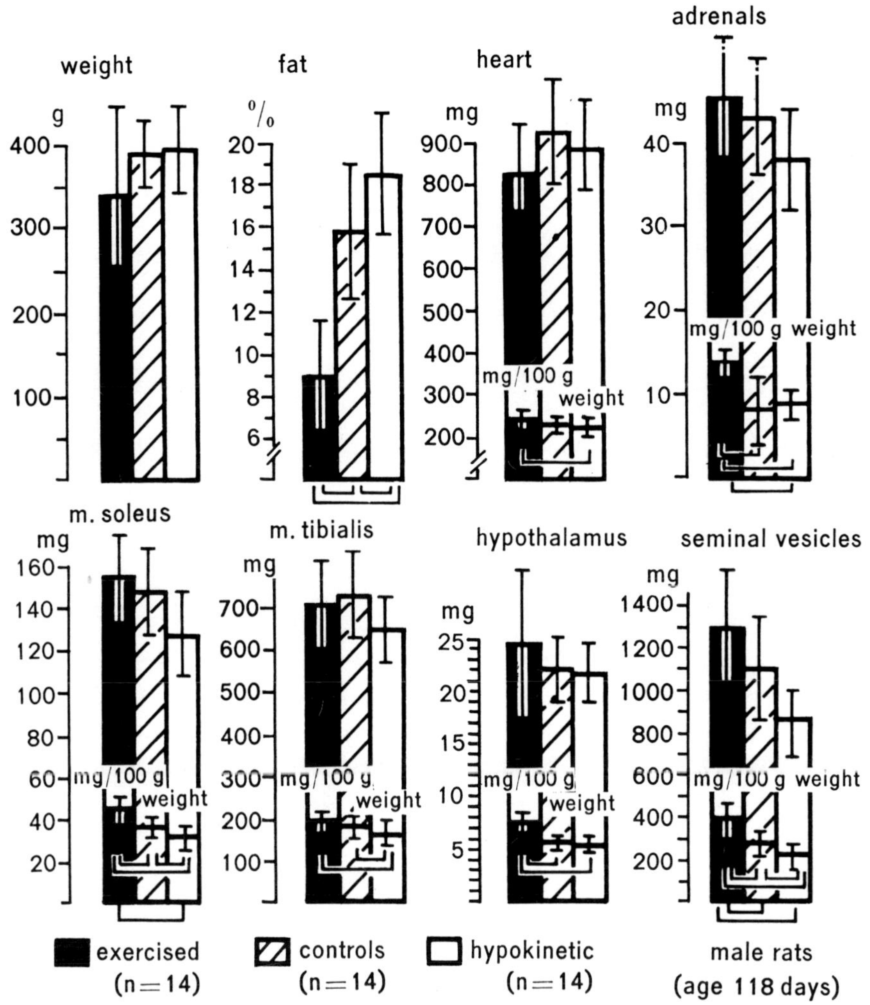

Fig. 27. Mean values ($\bar{x} \pm$ SD) of total body weight, percentage of fat and of absolute and relative values (mg; mg/100 g body weight) of weights of selected organs and muscles in male rats 110 days old with different physical activity regime (Pařízková 1974d).

the whole hypothalamo-hypophysary-adrenal axis seems also to have an impact on the weight of the hypothalamus (Fig. 27). Changes of the above organs were examined in a subsequent series of experiments (Pařízková and Poledne 1974b, 1975, Kvetňanský et al. 1975, Mikulaj et al. 1976).

Some authors (Erankö et al. 1962, Kenyon and Toressani 1963, Oscai et al. 1971 etc.) described in animals exposed to exercise (running, swimming, etc.) changes in the weight of the whole organism, heart, adrenals etc. The explanation of these differences is due to the type of load. In some of our experiments it was graded in

TABLE 14.
Mean values ($\bar{x} \pm SD$) of total weight, percentage of fat and relative weights of internal organs and skeletal muscles in wild *(Rattus norveg.)* and laboratory male rats *(Rattus norveg. labor.)* (Pařízková et al. 1972c).

	Wild rat		Laboratory rat			
			Exercised		Controls	
n	6		8		6	
	$\bar{x}$	SD	$\bar{x}$	SD	$\bar{x}$	SD
Weight (g)	249.0	11.2	235.6	26.7	258.3	21.4
Fat (%)	6.7	1.9	7.8	1.9	13.0	2.9
Heart mg/100 g weight	336.0	43.8	294.1	12.5	281.4	12.7
Adrenals mg/100 g	19.8	5.3	11.1	5.3	11.7	1.9
Tibialis muscle mg/100 g weight	161.0	28.0	201.5	28.0	168.0	15.8
Soleus muscle mg/100 g weight	38.0	6.9	37.1	3.7	34.6	3.6

such a manner as not to interfere with the growth curve or to affect it only after termination of the exponential growth by reducing the ratio of body fat but not by affecting the lean body mass. This type of load was used in our experiments as we were *interested in the sequelae of adaptation to an optimum and not an excessive load during growth and development,* and in subsequent stages of ontogenesis. A much more marked effect is exerted naturally by a load which the experimental animals are subjected suddenly without a preliminary stage of gradual adaptation to muscular work.

The most marked difference from the aspect of *effect of motor activity in phylogenesis was* assumed in *animals living wild in nature,* although in these animals the simultaneous effect of other factors such as irregular or inadequate food intake, stress etc. cannot be ruled out. We compared therefore the body composition and relative size of selected organs in wild rats *(Rattus norvegicus)* and laboratory rats *(Rattus norvegicus laboratorius)* adapted to exercise (running) and controls. For comparison animals of similar weight were selected (in wild rats supplied by the rodent control service the age was not known). The *percentage of body fat in wild rats was lower* but it *did not differ, however, significantly from the percentage of fat in laboratory rats adapted to daily running* (Table 14). The wild rats had the relatively largest heart and adrenals in relation to body weight. The relative weight of the m. soleus was the same and of the m. tibialis greater in the running laboratory rats. The *question arises whether wild living rats have systematically such a high physical activity as assumed* or, in particular as *compared with the domesticated type adapted to daily running (cca 2.5 km per day)* on a treadmill *throughout life.* In view of the nature of the differences it is also possible to consider the effect of *food shortage* (reduced percentage of fat) and the effect of *stress* threatened life in free nature (rapid flight). These differences would have to be tested in larger groups of wild rats where we would also have to know the exact age. This is not possible in wild rats supplied by the rodent control service.

It seems thus that *muscular work and physical activity act or do not act as an important stress, depending on the way in which and for how long the organism can become adapted to them.* The above results indicate that various characteristics of the organism such as the percentage of fat may be very markedly influenced without an increase in weight of the adrenals or without hypertrophy of the heart muscle. It is *important to enforce physical exercise and muscular work in particular during growth and development when there is interest in physical exercise* and when *it acts as an optimal biological stimulus.* The load can be relatively intensive and it can be started at a very early age (i.e. in rats before weaning); the organism must, however, get used to it gradually and individual needs must be taken into account.

2. Caloric intake and physical activity

Assessment of the oxygen consumption in rats during exercise on a treadmill with concomittant recording on an interferometer during a 1-hour run revealed that when the caloric expenditure for the whole day is calculated this run represents only an increase of 5–7% (Staňková and Jánský, unpublished data). This increase is relatively small but under living conditions of rats in cages it is significant. Next we also assessed the oxygen consumption in the course of 24 hours and evaluated separately the oxygen consumption during day and night (Table 15).

For the 24-hour oxygen consumption the closed circuit method described by Luštinec (1956) was used. The animals were placed in a small glass container and their activity was thus restricted. The oxygen consumption was determined according to the above author by the decline of the water column.

As apparent from Table 15, the *mean oxygen consumption per 24 hours was significantly raised in rats adapted for a prolonged period to a physical load with lower*

TABLE 15
Oxygen uptake (ml/1000 g/1 hour) in male rats 120 days old, with different physical activity regime (exercised, control, hypokinetic) (Petrásek, Pařízková and Poledne 1975)

		Day	Night	Mean	Body weight (g)
Exercised	$\bar{x}$	1136.6	1580.8	1358.7	371.2
	SD	112	128	117	15
Control	$\bar{x}$	816.6	1120.8	968.7	417.3
	SD	83	212.3	83	32
Hypokinetic	$\bar{x}$	1000.8	1191.6	1096.2	428.0
	SD	55	76	63	12

body weight. When calculated per body weight and body surface, the values of oxygen consumption were always highest in exercised animals. When the day- and night-oxygen consumption is differentiated, it is found that the increase in the exercised animals is manifested particularly during the night hours (7.p.m. – 7a.m.). This can be explained by the fact that in rodents the night is the period of greatest activity. In exercised animals this activity during the night is, obviously, due to long-term adaptation to the daily run, even greater than in controls and hypokinetic animals. – The slight increase in animals adapted to restricted activity may be due to the fact that the space in which the oxygen consumption is measured is somewhat greater than the space in which the hypokinetic animals are usually kept. This may cause their somewhat greater physical activity and thus a slightly higher oxygen consumption than in controls. The difference was, however, not significant (Petrásek et al. 1975).

Next we checked the long-term caloric intake in other groups of rats running for 1 hour for a period of 110 days. The *food intake in relation to body weight declined with advancing age* (Fig. 28) and there were *considerable variations from day to day.* The *mean amount of Larsen mixture in g per day throughout the experiment was significantly higher in rats running for 1 hour per day* (Fig. 28), compared with controls and with another group of animals which after 70 days at the age of 180 days discontinued regular running (Pařízková 1966). The increase of caloric intake in the running animals expressed as a percentage of the values obtained in controls roughly met the increased energy output corresponding to the assessed values of oxygen consumption. This means that in rats the *regulation of caloric intake in relation to output is fairly reliable.* (It must, however, be taken into account that in this regulation in rats fed Larsen mixture and exposed to different regimes of activity only the quantitative aspect plays a part and not others such as different gustatory stimuli, etc.).

Between the groups of rats mentioned (Fig. 28) there were no differences in the weight curves; there was, however, a *significant difference in the percentage of fat which was lowest in running rats with the highest caloric intake,* as in previous experiments (see Figs. 24, 25). *A higher level of energy turnover in running animals follows from this, while the resulting equilibrium is the same as in controls. This condition induces a situation resembling that in younger growing animals.*

Adapted animals differ also as regards their *response to a load. The oxygen consumption measured within two minutes immediately after a 20-min run on a treadmill was in animals adapted to this load significantly lower* than in non-adapted controls (Table 16) (Pařízková and Staňková 1964a).

Using the above described load the body composition was from the morphological aspect most markedly influenced by the increased energy turnover. The ratio of body fat in the organism can, however, also be influenced in addition to activity and muscular work by other factors associated with the daily load on the treadmill. We must consider for instance the *possible effect on the frequency of food intake* which alone has a marked effect on the lipid metabolism (Cohn 1957, Fábry

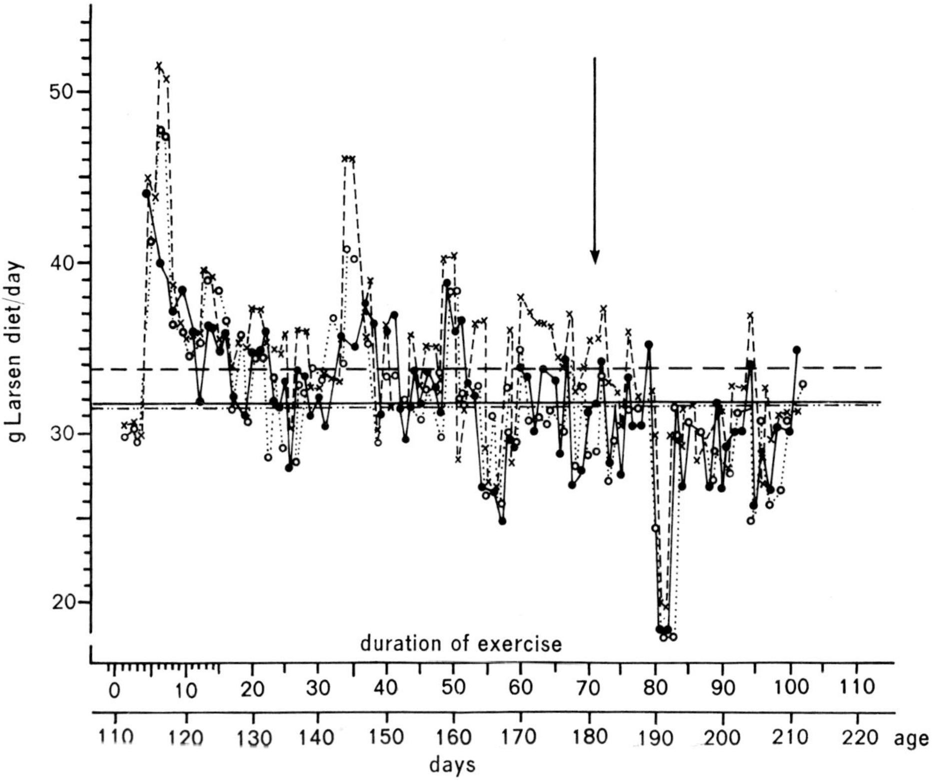

Fig. 28. Caloric input (g, Larsen diet day – ordinate) in male rats of different motor activity regime; interrupted line – daily run during 1.5 hour; full line – controls; dotted line – daily run as above interrupted at the age of 182 days (*see* arrow). Straight direct lines in the middle – mean values for the whole experiment. Abscissa – age in days and duration of exercise resp.

et al. 1962, Fábry 1969). The induced regime of exercise may interfere with the normal frequency of caloric intake and thus the effect of the regime of physical exercise would be in that case only mediated (or result from a combination of both stimuli—exercise and frequency of food intake). Systematic assessment of the food intake in a similarly arranged experiment during the 12th, 17th and 27th week of life, after two-hour intervals (food was always available in groups of exercised and control animals from 2 p.m. to 8 a.m. of the following day) however did not reveal any differences between exercised and control animals (Fig. 29). *The frequency of food intake was not affected by the daily exercise on the treadmill* (Pařízková et al. 1966b).

In the group of 360-day-old animals (*see* Fig. 24, 25) once during the period between the 250th and 270th day of life the possible preference of certain nutrients

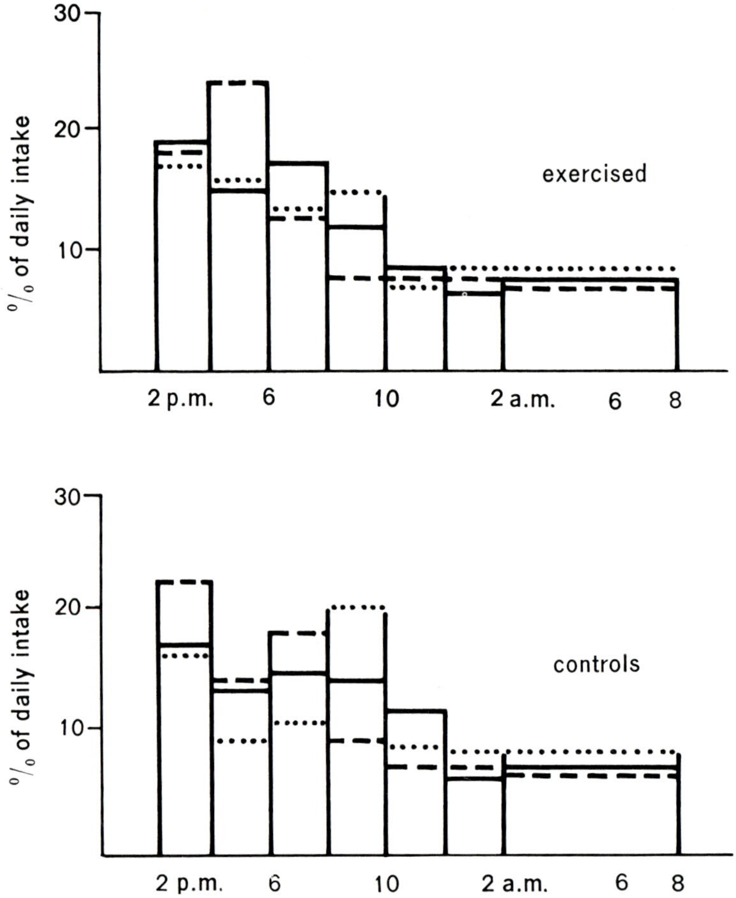

Fig. 29. Frequency of caloric intake (expressed in % of total daily caloric input – ordinate) during a day (hours – abscissa) in male rats adapted to different motor activity regime (daily run – columns in the upper part) and controls (lower part) at the age of 12 (full lines at the top of the columns), 17 (interrupted line) and 27 weeks (dotted lines) (Pařízková et al. 1966a).

was tested in relation to the intensity of exercise based on self-selection of a diet enriched with different nutrients (Larsen mixture mixed at a ratio 1 : 2 with starch or casein or margarine). The controls ingested double the amount of food with added starch or fat. Both groups ingested the same amount of the high casein diet (Table 17). The differences were relatively small. The conclusions of this investigation are again difficult to compare with data from other authors in view of the nature of the load used. *It does not appear that the medium load described above leads to a preference for a dietary constituent* (Pařízková and Staňková 1964a).

TABLE 16
Mean values ($\bar{x} \pm SD$) of oxygen consumption (in ml/100 g body weight/2 min) at rest and immediately after 20 min exercise (run on a treadmill) in exercised and control rats (Pařízková and Staňková 1964a).

	Rest		After 20 min work load	
	$\bar{x}$	SD	$\bar{x}$	SD
Exercised (n = 8)	4.4	0.7	4.5	0.7
Controls (n = 7)	4.3	0.9	5.3	0.9

TABLE 17
Average amounts of different diets ($\bar{x} \pm SD$) self-selected by exercised and control male rats per day during a period between the 250th and 270th day of life, and ratio of different diets in total caloric intake (Pařízková and Staňková 1964a).

	Starch diet		Casein diet		Fat diet	
	$\bar{x}$	SD	$\bar{x}$	SD	$\bar{x}$	SD
Exercised (n = 11)						
Diet eaten (g/100 g body weight)	2.16	0.97	1.09	0.80	2.24	0.91
Caloric intake (Kcal)	5.8	—	2.9	—	14.1	—
As % of total	25.5	—	12.7	—	61.8	—
Control (n = 11)						
Diet eaten (g/100 g body weight)	1.44	0.64	0.81	0.47	2.90	1.15
Caloric intake (Kcal)	3.8	—	2.1	—	18.3	—
As % of total	15.7	—	8.7	—	75.6	—

As apparent from the data presented, the caloric intake during a medium load is adequately regulated. In subsequent experiments we used an even more intense load (three-hour run supplemented by 3 hours hanging on a vertical ladder) from the 18th to the 285th day. At the age of 7–8 months we found significant differences between the caloric intake of running, control and hypokinetic animals (*see* Fig. 26). The animals adapted to the load had the highest caloric intake, the hypokinetic ones the lowest intake (this finding of the lowest caloric intake in this group explains the lower body weight and body fat ratio as compared with controls (*see* p. 65-7,

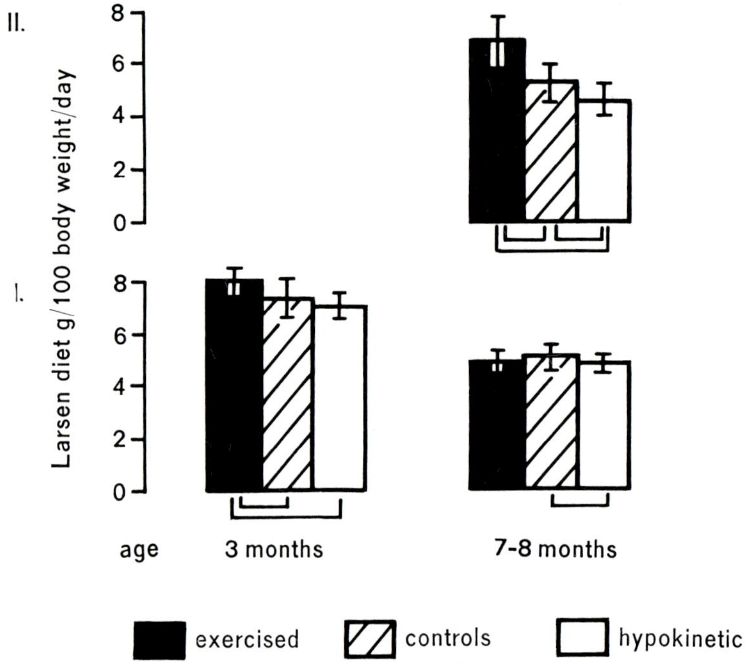

Fig. 30. Caloric intake (Larsen diet, g/100 g weight/ day – ordinate) in male rats adapted to different motor activity regime (black – active, exercised male rats = 2–3 hours running + 3 hours of static work load; hatched – controls; white – hypokinetic) either during their whole life (II.-upper part) or only temporarily up to the 65th day of life when the induced physical activity regime was interrupted, and the animals were then kept as controls (I.-lower part). Measured at the age of 3 months (I.) and 7–8 months (II., I.) (Pařízková et al. 1972c).

Fig. 26). As is apparent, *restriction of movement cannot be fully compensated by caloric restriction—the percentage of body fat in hypokinetic animals is still higher when compared with values in active animals with a substantially higher caloric intake.*

At the same time similar groups were investigated (exercised, controls, hypokinetic from the 18th day) where, however, the regime of exercise induced at the age of 65 days was discontinued and during their subsequent life all animals were kept as controls. During the period when the different regime of activity still persisted the gradation of the caloric intake was similar to that in previous groups (lower half of Fig. 30). After discontinuation of this regime at the age of 7–8 months the caloric intake was practically the same in all groups. The persistence of the slightly but significantly reduced caloric intake in the originally hypokinetic animals compared with controls is of interest (Fig. 30) (Pařízková et al. 1972c).

After a certain period on the same regime, i.e. that used in controls (which, however, also differs from the natural activity of these animals) the caloric intake did not differ (Pařízková 1972b, Pařízková et al. 1972c). At the end of the experiment we did not find therefore significant differences in mean values of body weight nor in the percentage of body fat between different groups which at the onset of ontogenesis had a different regime of physical activity. Individual values were very scattered. A more detailed analysis of results revealed that *discontinuation of the originally induced regime of physical activity produces in different animals a different response: in some after discontinuation of daily runs the body fat ratio increased, while in others it did not.* In our opinion the different responses are due to a different individual characteristic of spontaneous physical activity level and excitability of the central nervous system (CNS). With regard to above mentioned changes of body weight, caloric intake, weights of organs including adrenals we tried to investigate what changes at the level of excitability of CNS and of catecholamine metabolism can be caused by adaptation to various physical activity regimes, and what is their relationship to modifications in body composition.

3. Catecholamine synthesis and degradation in relation to physical activity and body composition

Increased catecholamine secretion in *trained athletes* was ascertained e.g. by Kagi (1956) who found that noradrenalin secretion increased six-fold after 45 – 70 min effort during gymnastic competition. Similar increase was observed by Elmajian and Hope (1958) in hockey players and boxers. Also Mikulaj et al. (1975) reported the augmentation of catecholamine secretion in trained subjects (who were moreover characterized by increased aerobic capacity etc.) during a work load. Wolf et al. (1970) found an increased amount of vanil mandelic acid in the urine of mount-climbers.—*In normal untrained subjects* plasma level of noradrenalin increased correspondingly with increasing work load, and was greater in humans with low level of fitness and performance capacity (Kozlowski et al. 1972).

Ostman and Sjöstrand (1971) showed significant increase in total adrenalin content expressed as microgram per pair of adrenals of *animals trained during 15 weeks.* Brown and VanHuss (1973) found increased concentration of noradrenaline in the brain of trained rats. The adaptation to increased work-load changes obviously the level of activity of the adrenergic system (Métivier 1975); long-term adaptation to exercise tends to decrease in the immediate catecholamine excretion after work load (Bernet and Denimal 1974).—We were therefore interested whether in our experimental model of exercised and hypokinetic rats (characterized so far by above-mentioned changes in growth, body composition, caloric balance etc.) the synthesis and degradation of catecholamines will be influenced, and how this will be related to body composition.

The adrenals of male rats were rapidly removed from the decapitated animals, weighed and homogenized in ice cold isotonic sucrose. An aliquot portion (100 μl) of the homogenate was added to 2.4 ml 0.4 N perchloric acid for assay of catecholamines (Anton and Sayre 1962). Another aliquot (30 μl) was diluted by

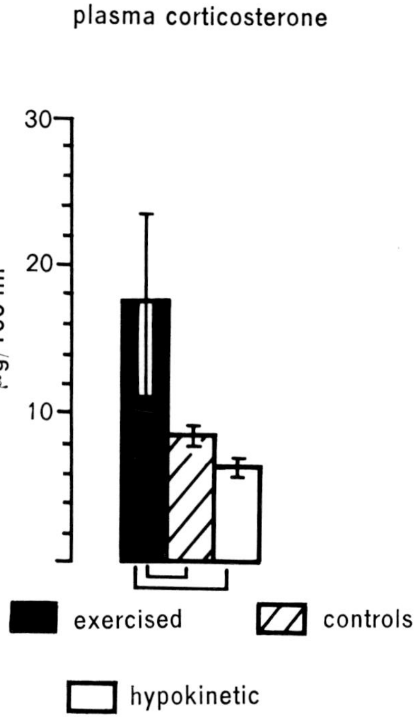

Fig. 31. Mean plasma corticosterone levels ($\bar{x} \pm SD$) in male rats (90 days) with different physical activity regime (Kvetňanský, Pařízková et al. 1975).

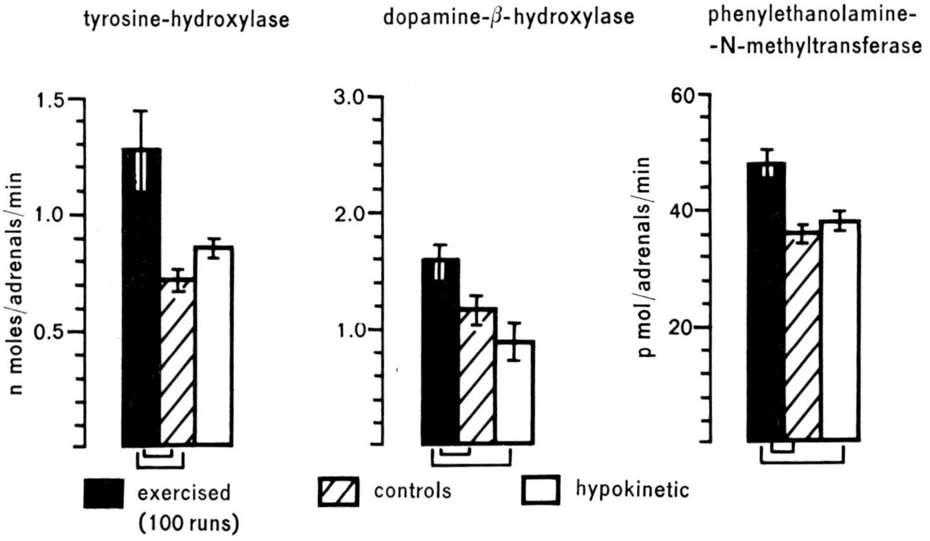

Fig. 32. Mean values ($\bar{x} \pm SD$) of activities of catecholamine synthetizing hormones in male rats with different physical activity regimes (Kvetňanský, Pařízková et al. 1975).

tris-triton buffer (0.3 mg/100 µl) for dopamin-ß-hydroxylase assay (Molinoff et al. 1971) and the remaining homogenate was centrifuged at 10,000 g for 20 min. The supernatant fraction was removed and the aliquot portions of the supernatant fluid were assayed for tyrosine hydroxylase using the method of Nagatsu et al. (1964) and phenylethanolamine-N-methyl transferase using the technique described by Axelrod (1962). The plasma corticosterone level was also estimated (Guillemin et al. 1959).

In this experiment 90- and 150-day-old animals were used 24 hours after the last work load in the exercised group. As apparent from Fig. 31, the *plasma corticosterone level in the exercised animals was significantly raised* indicating that even after long-term adaptation the daily work load on a treadmill implied a stress situation for the full grown animals. The amount of catecholamine in the adrenals and in the heart of the *exercised animals,* however, remained unaltered, while the *activity of catecholamine synthetizing enzymes—tyrosine hydroxylase, dopamine-β-hydroxylase and phenylethanolamine-N-methyl transferase in the adrenals was significantly elevated* (Fig. 32). In adult life there were no differences in that respect between control and hypokinetic animals. Prolonged hypokinesia to which the animals were adapted gradually since weaning no longer represented a stress in adult life (Kvetňanský et al. 1975). But a sudden complete restriction of activity in adult age repeated daily increased the level and secretion of catecholamines (Kvetňanský and Mikulaj 1970) and their biosynthesis (Kvetňanský et al. 1970).

In our animals the assessed activities of *catecholamine-degrading enzymes* also displayed changes as a result of the regime of physical activity. The *activity of monoamine oxidase* was measured in the liver and heart using the method of Wurtman and Axelrod (1963). *In exercised animals the activity* of this enzyme *was reduced.* It appears that the *exercised animal possesses a larger amount of catecholamines* than the control and in particular the hypokinetic animals. This again recalls the state found as a rule in younger organism: the activity of monoamine oxidase e.g. in the heart rises (Robinson 1975) and the amount of available catecholamines declines with age. Adrenocortical responsiveness to stress diminishes with age (Hess and Riegle 1970). This may be one of the reasons for the reduced adaptability of the organism in old age. *Larger amounts of catecholamines in the organism help to cope with the stress of the daily work load* on the treadmill and are also *partly responsible for other changes in the organism* incl. the *increased oxygen uptake,* the *increased level of metabolic turnover,* etc.

The analysis of the relationships between the level of activity of catecholamine-synthetizing and degrading hormones on the one hand, and percent of body fat on the other showed e.g. significant negative correlation between the activity of dopamin-β-hydroxylase in the adrenals and per cent fat ($r = -0.543$, $p < 0.05$) and a positive correlation between the activity of liver monoamine oxidase and per cent fat ($r = 0.547$, $p < 0{,}01$). As follows, an *organism with a high activity of catecholamine synthetizing hormones contains low proportion of fat* (as e.g. exercised animals) and *vice versa for an organism with high activity of catecholamine degrading hormones.*

4. Excitability of the central nervous system in relation to physical activity and body composition

Spontaneous physical activity declines during ontogenesis, concurrent with the excitability of the central nervous system (CNS) (Lát 1963) within a very wide range of interindividual variability; we may therefore assume a certain mutual relationship. From this ensues that a certain regime of physical activity induced in different stages of ontogenesis may also influence in a significant way the level of excitability of the CNS immediately and also remotely. Changes in the level of excitability of the CNS may be related in a significant way with other investigated parameters (caloric intake, body weight, body fat ratio, metabolic activity of tissues, etc.). The *excitability of the CNS was investigated by means of the habituation test* in groups of animals whose caloric intake (*see* Fig. 30), growth curves (*see* Fig. 26) and body composition (*see* p. 65-7) were already described. The response was assessed to a regime of physical activity altered permanently for prolonged periods (6-hour dynamic and static work-load, i.e. run and hanging on a ladder; restricted movement; control—II) from the 18th to the 285th day as well as to the later consequences of the same regime lasting, however, only from the 18th to the 65th day (group I) at the age of 285 days.

As part of the habituation test which is based on the evaluation of exploratory reactions in a special cage 70 × 50 × 30 cm the number of standing upright responses and passing squares into which the floor of the cage was divided, was assessed. The observation lasts 25 min. During this period the rats are stimulated six times by putting out the light for one minute followed by three minutes of light. The following are evaluated: (1) the sum of all exploratory reactions, (2) the maximum frequency per minute, (3) the time when this maximum takes place, (4) the rate of habituation, i.e. adaptation to the conditions of the test. These parameters make it possible to evaluate the level of excitability of the CNS and the intensity of inhibitory processes (Lát and Gollová 1969).

The sum of exploratory reactions was highest in animals whose activity was permanently restricted and lowest in animals permanently exposed to work loads, i.e. running and hanging on a ladder. The controls were intermediary. In the group with a temporarily altered regime of physical activity the conclusions of the investigation were similar, the differences between groups were, however, less marked. All other parameters of the *level of excitability of the CNS* investigated also suggested that the *level was lowest in animals permanently subjected to a load:* the *lowest sum of all exploratory reactions, later attainment of this peak, more rapid process of habituation. The highest level of excitability of the CNS was found in hypokinetic animals.* The values of both control groups could be combined in view of their homogeneity (Fig. 33).

Next we analyzed changes which take place after discontinuation of a certain regime of activity induced during early ontogenesis with regard to excitability of the CNS and body composition. *Analysis of the variability of groups* which as a whole did not differ in mean values at the end of the experiment (*see* p. 76-7) revealed that *the values of excitability indicators and the percentage of body fat are distributed in the control group regularly according to a Gaussian curve. In groups originally adapted*

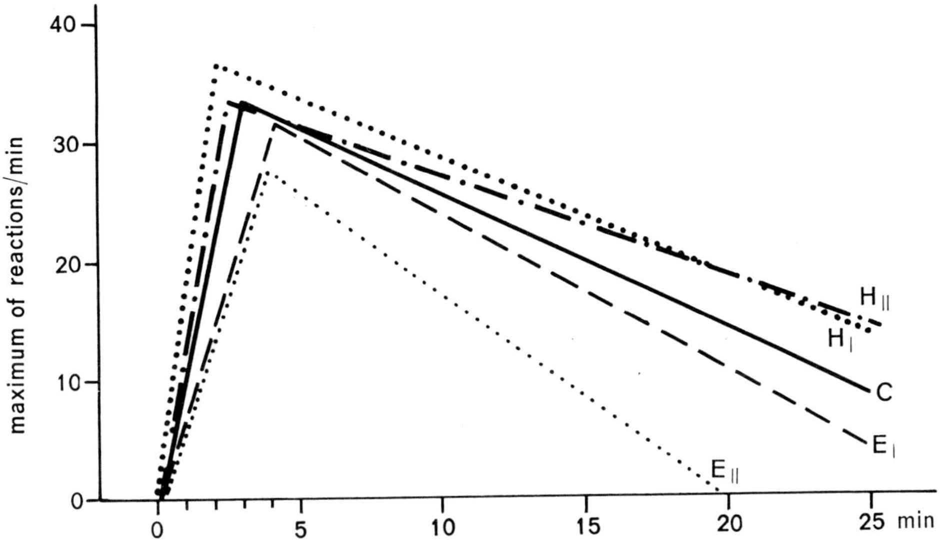

Fig. 33. Comparison of parameters characterizing the level of central nervous system excitability in male rats (age 285 days), adapted to different motor activity regime (E – active, exercised; C – control, H – hypokinetic animals; I – temporarily changed motor regime up to the 65th day of life and then as controls; II – permanently changed motor activity regime). Number of reactions per min (ordinate) during habituation test, time when peak (i. e. maximal number of reactions per min) was achieved, the speed of habituation, i. e. the adaptation to the habituation test. Abscissa – time in min (Pařízková and Lát 1973a).

to exercise and in those with restricted exercise the distribution was bimodal (Fig. 34). This means that some animals reacted to the discontinuation of the daily load by an increased excitability of the CNS while others did not. The same applies to the ratio of body fat—in some but not in others the discontinuation of the daily run leads to enhanced deposition of body fat. *Analysis of the above parameters in animals where a certain regime of physical activity was induced permanently throughout the experimental period* up to the 285th day *displayed a unimodal distribution of values* which means that *the group was more homogeneous as regards excitability of the CNS and body composition* due to adaptation to a certain regime.

The general confrontation of all results mentioned above revealed that some characteristics—e.g. *body weight, caloric intake, percentage of body fat responded to the increased intensity of the physical activity regime by maintaining the level usually found in earlier developmental stages.* As regards indicators of *excitability of CNS* the *tendency during an intensive load was reverse: animals adapted to a daily dynamic and static load diplayed a lower excitability of the CNS, resembling thus rather older animals* (Pařízková and Lát 1973a). The reduced intensity of response in test situations can also be interpreted as an increased economy of functions in an unknown stress

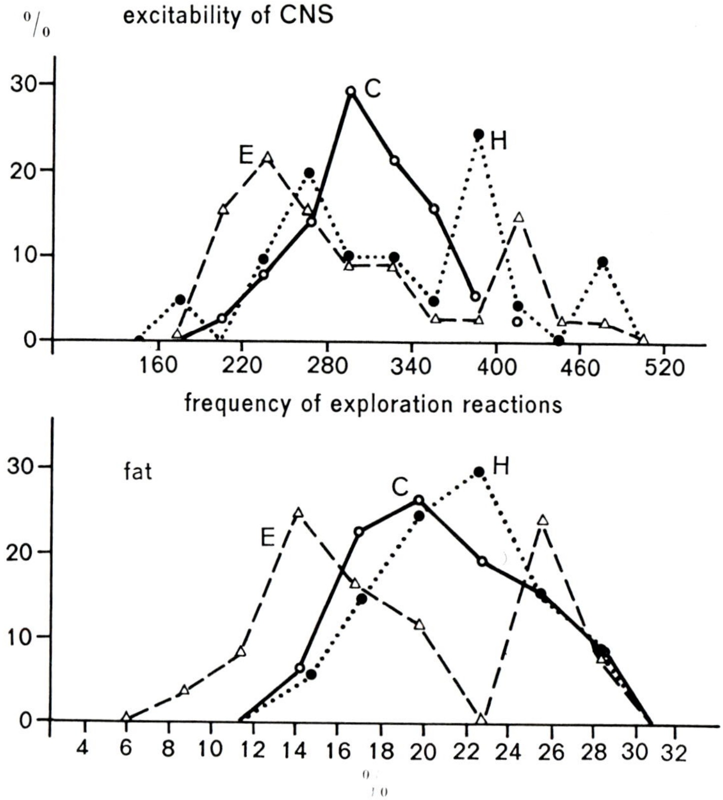

Fig. 34. The disposition of the values of parameters characterising the level of CNS excitability (upper part – frequency of the exploratory reactions) and percentage of body fat (lower part) in male rats adapted only temporarily (I) i. e. up to the 65th day of life to a different motor activity regime (E – active, exercised; C – control; H – hypokinetic animals) (Pařízková and Lát 1973a).

situation due to previous adaptation to physical load. The conclusions of investigations of the CNS are for our further investigations of considerable importance because it may be assumed that—in view of the manifestations of a reduced excitability of the CNS—there is a direct effect of adaptation to an increased load on the lipid metabolism which was investigated in subsequent experiments.

The different types of reaction to the discontinuation of a certain regime of activity induced in early ontogenesis again provides evidence of marked individual differences in the constitution pertaining to the level of spontaneous physical activity. For some animals obviously the stimulus of activity is very intensive, for others not; discontinuation therefore causes different metabolic changes and different changes in the CNS. On the other hand, a permanently altered regime of activity in the positive or negative sense induces marked changes in the energy turnover, body composition and level of excitability of the CNS which are fairly homogeneous in the groups investigated.

V. Influence of adaptation to increased muscle work on body composition in relation to caloric intake in man

1. Changes in body composition after adaptation to increased muscle work

Increased muscle work, e.g. sports training, exerts a similar effect on LBM and fat as physical activity in experimental animals. The *effect of physical strain and work is manifested in every period of human ontogenesis: comparison of groups of children and adolescents, adults and elderly subjects with normal and increased physical activity reveals an increased ratio of LBM at the expense of fat in subjects with increased physical activity* (Fig. 35), although subjects with the same relative body weight were compared (Pařízková 1963a). The *differences are greatest in adult life* (3rd decade) where the difference in intensity of the muscular load is also greatest. The athletes compared (wrestling, gymnastics) were members of the representative national teams of Czechoslovakia with a regimen of physical activity which differed as much as possible from that of the compared control groups. Similar differences in body composition of trained and untrained subjects were found by other authors (Behnke et al. 1942, Behnke and Royce 1966, Behnke and Wilmore 1974, Wilmore and Haskell 1972 etc.).

In view of the high energy requirements of sports training for champion athletes the caloric intake is also correspondingly increased. It may reach a range of 5000 to 7000 kcal/day e.g. in cyclists during the Peace Race etc. These cyclists belong, however, among athletes with the highest ratio of LBM. Athletes as a rule have a lower body fat ratio than people from the normal population with a caloric intake of less than half; the high energy turnover, i.e. the high energy intake as well as output leads to a high ratio of LBM at the expense of body fat.

This high caloric intake is essential in particular during periods of intensive preparation before decisive sports contests etc. It often happens that after discontinuation or substantial restriction of training the body weight increases and body fat is deposited even when the athletes try to maintain their weight and eat less (Paříz-

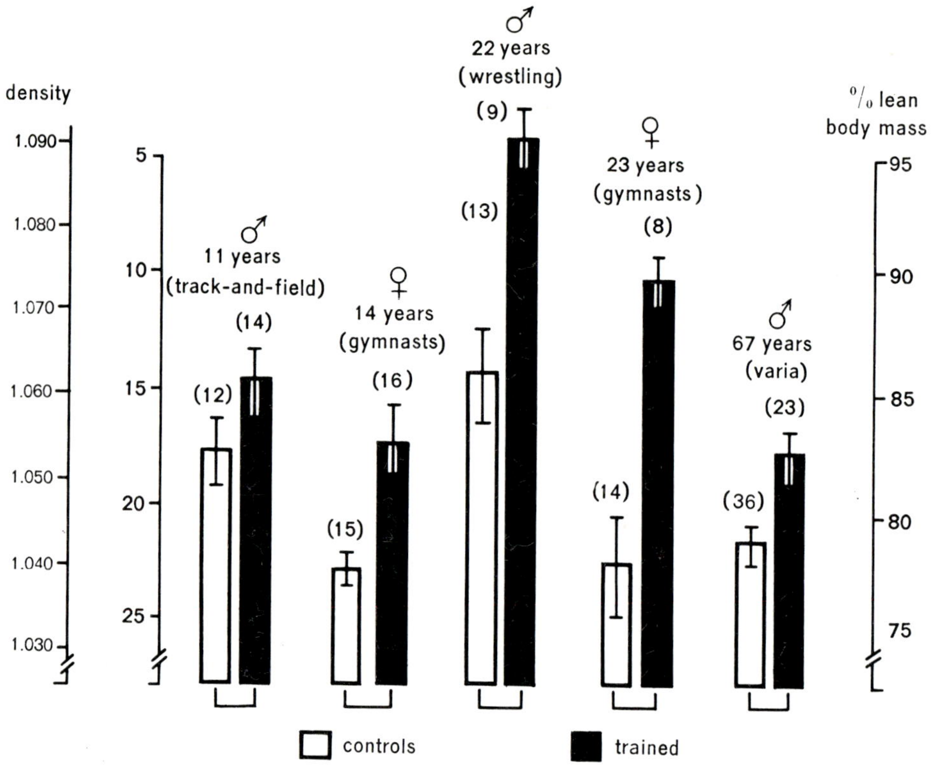

Fig. 35. Comparison of body density, or % depot fat (x̄ ± SD – ordinate left) and lean body mass (right) in groups of different age adapted to increased work load, i. e. sports training, and inactive controls of the same age, height and weight (Pařízková 1963a).

ková 1965, 1966). The question arises to what extent man is able to regulate his food intake adequately with regard to changes in the regime of physical activity which take place in periods with a different intensity of training. In man the position is more complicated because with the regulation of energy intake further factors interfere such as taste preferences and tendencies which are not present in animal experiments where standard Larsen mixture is fed.

We had the opportunity to investigate this problem in a group of adolescent girls, members of a special gymnastics school (Pařízková 1966, Pařízková and Poupa 1963). Along with changes in body weight, body composition and skinfolds we also investigated the caloric intake during periods of different activity (mean training intensity—end of school year-A; increased intensity—summer training camp-B; period of reduced physical activity—discontinuation of training during remainder of vacations and at the beginning of school year-C).

During the period of mean and increased physical activity the body weight remained the same, after discontinuation of training it increased (Pařízková 1960b, 1962b). The *body fat ratio declined during the period of increased intensity together with the skinfold thickness and increased during the period of reduced intensity* (Table 18); all changes were statistically significant.

TABLE 18
Changes of body weight, percentage of fat and skinfold thickness in girl gymnasts during periods with different intensity of physical exercise (n = 10) (Pařízková 1963c, 1966)

	Mean intensity of training A		High intensity of training (summer camp) B		Interruption of training C	
	$\bar{x}$	SD	$\bar{x}$	SD	$\bar{x}$	SD
Weight (kg)	52.9	1.1	53.1	1.0	53.6	1.2
Fat (%)	16.8	0.9	11.3	0.8	15.3	1.1
Sum of ten skinfolds (mm)	78.8	8.0	68.8	6.0	88.8	8.0

2. Caloric intake during periods with different physical activity

The increase of body fat ratio could be easily explained if during the period of reduced training the same or even a higher caloric intake persisted as during the period of high training intensity. Investigations of the caloric intake, however, did not confirm this.

The girls recorded their caloric intake during the experimental period and entered all foods consumed in the course of the day. These data were evaluated according to food tables. At the onset of the investigation and particularly during intensive training the entries were checked against the food issued by the camp kitchen and the food actually consumed. This check revealed the reliability of entries. The girls were interested in the results of the survey in order to avoid weight increments when discontinuing training.

The intake of calories and different nutrients—protein, carbohydrate and fats varied depending on the intensity of the regime of physical activity (Fig. 36); e.g. *during the period when training was discontinued, the caloric intake declined roughly by 25%*. Both changes in the caloric level were significant. At the same time *minor changes in the ratio of different food constituents occurred*—during the most intense training the gymnasts ingested relatively more carbohydrate (significant increase as compared with previous period by 2.7%) and somewhat less protein (decrease by

2.1 %). The fat intake did not change (Fig. 36). This change in the composition of the diet which was ingested during the period of very high or markedly reduced physical activity was, however, relatively small and therefore not very important from the biological aspect and could not lead in view of the reduced caloric intake to an increase in body weight as a result of excessive deposition of body fat (Table 18). Investigations of the caloric intake thus revealed that the *food intake in the girls was regulated so that it corresponded to the reduced energy output* and that *body fat deposition was not primarily due to impaired regulation of food intake* (Pařízková 1963a, Pařízková and Poupa 1963). It is *again apparent that reduction of the caloric intake cannot fully compensate reduced physical activity (as in experimental animals—see* p. 76)—and the amount of body fat increases.

It was therefore necessary to seek another explanation for the enhanced accumulation of body fat. It has been known that during intensive work the utilization of lipids (Christensen and Hansen 1931—*see* Åstrand 1972b) and especially of fatty acids in muscle is enhanced (Fredricson and Gordon 1958, Fritz 1961, Issekutz et al. 1965, Paul 1975 etc.), in the same way as in different animal species (George and Jyoti 1955, George and Naik 1958, Drummond and Black 1960 etc.). Long-term adaptation to increased muscular work can lead to adaptive changes pertaining to mobilization as well as utilization of fatty acids (Paul 1975, Leusing 1972 etc.). It may be assumed that fatty acid utilization and also utilization of other lipid metabolites is restricted during reduced energy output whereby the deposition of fat for a given metabolic stereotype in an organism adapted to a high energy turnover predominates over its mobilization even when the caloric intake is reduced. By discontinuing training the usual balance established during a high turnover even at cellular level is impaired and this concerns adipose tissue as well as muscles. We were, however, unable to study these problems under our conditions in human subjects. We again used experimental models of laboratory animals adapted to different amounts of physical activity.

Fig. 36. Changes in intake of total calories (Kcal, left) and of calories derived from proteins, fats and carbohydrates (right) by girls from sports school of gymnastics in the periods of routine training (A), intensive training (B) and after cessation of intensive training (C). Hatched areas = SE. Relative intensity of training is shown below the abscissa; after B, training was interrupted and then resumed with moderate intensity at the beginning of the school year (Pařízková and Poupa 1963). ▶

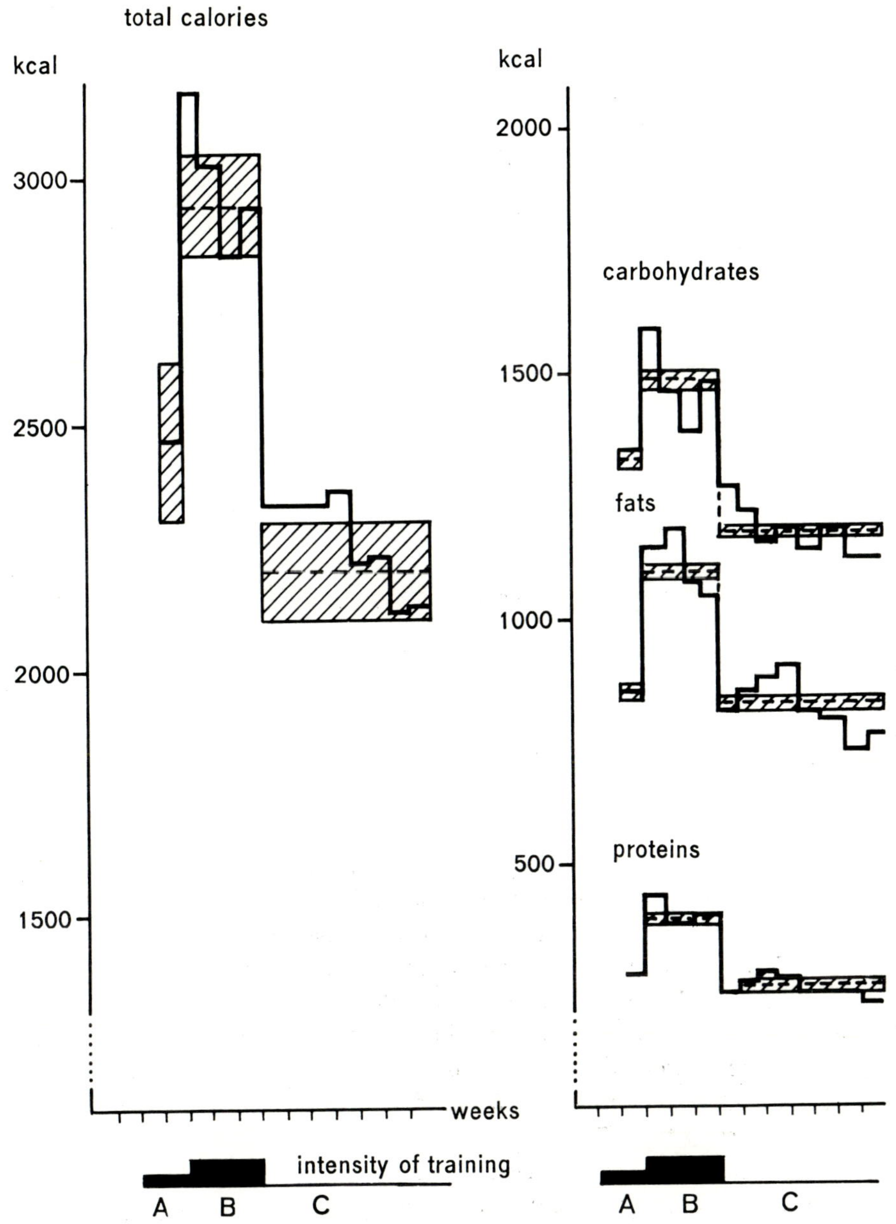
total calories
kcal
3000
2500
2000
1500
weeks
intensity of training
A
B
C
kcal
2000
1500
1000
500
carbohydrates
fats
proteins
A
B
C

VI. Adaptation to increased muscular work: consequences in adipose tissue

Lipid metabolism during muscular work was studied by a number of authors (Friedberg et al. 1960, Fritz 1961, Havel et al. 1963, Havel 1971, Carlsson 1967, Yakovlev et al. 1962, Leshkevitch 1960, Issekutz and Spitzer 1960, Issekutz et al. 1962, 1965, 1966, Carlsson and Mossfeld 1964, 1971, Nikkilä et al. 1963, Hagenfeldt and Wahren 1971, Paul 1975 etc. etc.) and was focused mainly on its changes during a single work load. Consequences of prolonged adaptation to increased regular muscular work have been studied more rarely from this aspect (e.g. Issekutz et al. 1965, Gollnick and Simmons 1967, Gollnick et al. 1970, Molé and Hollossy 1970, Paul 1975, Tipton 1974, Palmer and Tipton 1974 etc.).

Metabolic studies during a work load revealed that during brief intense work performed in oxygen debt carbohydrates are utilized. During prolonged work performed in a steady state with an adequate oxygen supply the participation of lipid metabolites increases and carbohydrates are spared. They are present in the organism in limited amounts and are needed for perfect function of the CNS. Wahren et al. (1971) believe that e.g. insuline decrease during exercise serves to limit blood glucose uptake by muscles thereby increasing its availability to the brain. Adaptation to a certain type of work (aerobic or anaerobic) can obviously influence also the participation of different energy sources used for muscular work (Young and Price 1961, Paul and Issekutz 1967).

Fatty acid levels vary in an inverse ratio to the intensity of their utilization (Dole 1956, Paul 1975 etc.). A negative correlation has been described between fatty acid and lactic acid levels which implies a *low mobilization, and obviously also utilization, of fatty acids during anaerobic work* or *when the organism is not adequately supplied with oxygen* (Issekutz and Miller 1962, Paul 1975).

Comparative physiology also provides some examples of increased lipid utilization during prolonged muscular work (Drummond and Black 1960, George and Vallyathan 1964a,b). The flight muscles of *migratory birds* adapted in the course of phylogenesis to long seasonal flights are equipped as regards enzymes and their microstructure for the predominant utilization of fats (George and Naik 1958) from body depots as during that period they are practically unable to ingest any food (Drummond and Black 1960). The lipolytic enzyme activity depends on the premigration and postmigration stage (George and Vallyathan 1964a,b). At the same time not only the fat content of muscles changes but also the body composition—before the seasonal migration the organism of these birds contains as much as 45% fat, after the flight only 8% (George and Jyoti 1955, Drummond and Black 1960).

All carbohydrate sources must not be used up during prolonged muscular work as without them the CNS cannot perform its normal functions; *efficiency may depend in that case on the ability to mobilize and utilize rapidly and sufficiently intensely other energy sources,* in particular *depot fat. These adaptive changes are related above all to the aerobic capacity of the organism; its high level is the decisive factor for the high efficiency and ability to use lipids more readily as an energy substrate and this is associated with variations of lipid reserves in the organism.* Although in man such liminal situations as in migratory birds are not encountered, these changes in the proportionality of energy sources for muscular work are also obviously important and typical for various stages of adaptation to an increased muscular load, in particular when this is of aerobic character.

Data on changes of the caloric intake during the period of discontinued training revealed that the increase of the body fat ratio in that case is not due to impaired regulation of food intake (*see* Fig. 36 and Table 18). Experiments in animals also reveal the ability to adapt the caloric intake correspondingly to the energy output (*see* Fig. 28 and 30). We must also take into account further *more profound adaptive changes in the metabolism at a cellular level—in adipose as well as muscular tissue—which in that case are induced by a prolonged load during ontogenesis.* A particularly *important part* may be played in this respect by an *increased load in the earliest stages of ontogenesis,* as has been demonstrated e.g. by Oscai et al. (1974). They investigated the development of male rats swimming from the age of five days. Training was terminated at the age of 28 weeks. The animals then remained sedentary without exercise for 34 weeks. Swimming in early life caused the body weight to remain even at the age of 62 weeks lower than that of sedentary freely eating controls. Body fat, epididymal fat pads and the number of its fat cells were significantly lower in animals exercised in early life. Mild food restriction during the same period had little effect on fatness and adipose tissue cellularity. The above results demonstrate that exercise in early life is effective in significantly reducing the rate of fat cell accumulation in epididymal fat pads of rats and results in a significant reduction of body fat in later life. By exercise during this period of life which is a critical one the organism can be influenced more substantially than at other times resulting not only in immediate but also in long-term changes. In connection with the above data we investigated selected metabolic indicators in adipose tissue together with others in the described experimental model.

1. Metabolic activity of adipose tissue and fatty acid utilization during adaptation to different loads

We investigated adipose tissue during periods of varying adaptation to increased or reduced muscular work associated with changes in the body fat of rats of different age (*see* Fig. 24 and 25). Previous work indicates that age and the size of the organism (Altschuler et al. 1962), different diets (Robinson 1960), obesity (Marshall and Engel 1960), adaptation to cold (Hannon and Larson 1962, Himms-Hagen 1972) will be manifested in metabolic properties of adipose tissue, e.g. in the ability to release fatty acids *in vitro*. When the ratio of adipose tissue is markedly influenced by adaptation to exercise further changes in its metabolic activity may also be assumed. In conjunction with a higher energy turnover during work we focused our attention again on the ability of adipose tissue to release FFA *in vitro*, spontaneously as well as after addition of adrenaline to the medium (Wenke et al. 1963) as the latter plays an important role in lipid mobilization during muscular work (Shafrir and Steinberg 1960, Carlsson 1967 etc.).

Adipose tissue of animals adapted to an increased load (running on a treadmill) always spontaneously released more FFA (Mosinger and Wenkeová 1963) *compared with hypokinetic and control animals after varying periods of incubation in Krebs-Ringer phosphate buffer with 3% albumin* (Fig. 37) (Pařízková and Staňková 1964a,b, 1967). Also *after addition of adrenalin the amount of released FFA was always greater in exercised animals* (Fig. 38) *with a lower body fat ratio* (*see* Fig. 24 and 25) (Pařízková 1963 – 1965). During the growth period (85 days) the difference between exercised animals and controls was not significant. From both these groups the hypokinetic animals differed significantly in their lower amount of released FFA. At the age of 125 days the controls and hypokinetic animals no longer differed, the adipose tissue of exercised animals again, however, released the largest amount of FFA. The same applied to 360-day-old animals. At that age we did not investigate the effect of hypokinesia as it did not manifest itself at the age of 125 days (Pařízková 1966, 1968e,f,g).

If we confront these changes with differences in body composition (*see* Fig. 25), we also find that in percentage of fat there is no difference between controls and hypokinetic 125-day-old animals. From this it follows that *during the growth period restriction of movement is a much more important stimulus (which is opposed to the natural spontaneous tendency of the organism at that age*—see Fig. 1) and *causes an increase in the body fat ratio and a reduction of its metabolic activity. In adult life, on the other hand, the reverse is an important factor, i.e. an increased intensity of physical activity which leads to restriction of the body fat ratio and to an increase in its metabolic activity* (Pařízková 1968f,g, 1969).

Comparison of exercised 125-day-old animals and 85-day-old controls does not reveal any difference in the percentage of fat nor in the ability to release FFA *in vitro* after adrenalin. The same applies to a comparison of the percentage of fat and FFA release in exercised 360-day-old animals and 125-day-old controls (*see* Fig. 25 and 38).

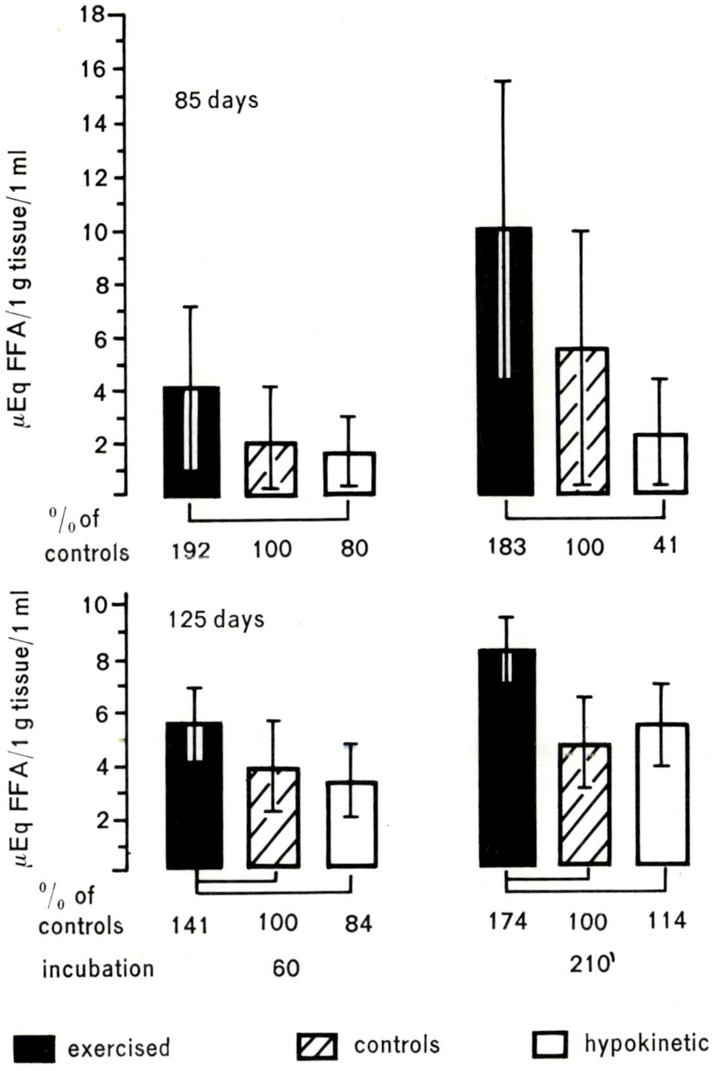

Fig. 37. Comparison of the metabolic activity of adipose tissue, i. e. spontaneously released free fatty acids ($\bar{x} \pm$ SD of FFA) *in vitro* from the epididymal adipose tissue of male rats of different age adapted to different motor activity regime (Pařízková and Staňková 1967).

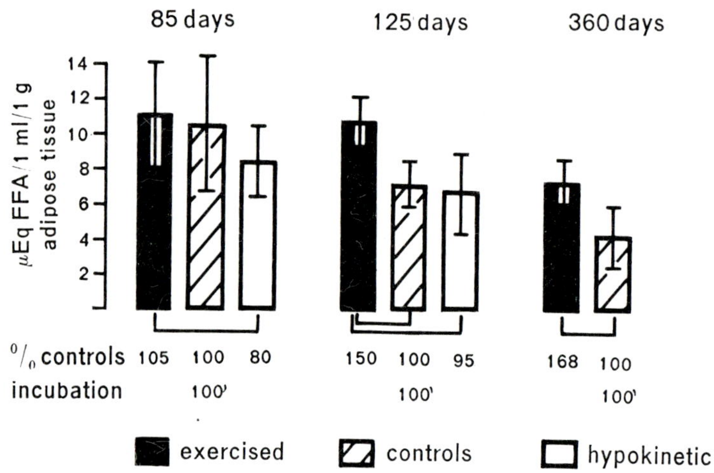

Fig. 38. Comparison of released free fatty acids after adrenalin (2 μg/100mg) from the epididymal adipose tissue of male rats adapted to different motor activity regime (Pařízková and Staňková 1967). (FFA; $\bar{x} \pm$ SD.).

It appears thus that *the properties of adipose tissue in the organism adapted to regular prolonged work loads are maintained as a result of this adaptation at a level which is usually encountered in a younger developmental stage.*

Next we investigated the effect of heparin which also plays an important part in lipid metabolism. A tendency to enhanced FFA release *in vitro* from adipose tissue of exercised 185-day-old animals was found (where also the body fat ratio was lower compared with controls. FFA release after adrenalin was enhanced). The differences were, however, not statistically significant (Pařízková et al. 1966b).

In older and hypokinetic animals resp. a higher body fat ratio was found as well as a lower ability to release FFA *in vitro* after adrenalin. The same was reported by Marshall and Engel (1960) and Trémolières (1971a) in hyperglycaemic obese mice. The reverse was found in young animals or those adapted to increased activity. We analyzed therefore the relationship of the percentage of body fat and the amount of released FFA in a specimen of adipose tissue *in vitro*. The correlation was significantly negative: *the higher the body fat ratio, the lower the ability to release FFA from adipose tissue, which implies a lower metabolic activity of a certain volume of adipose tissue* and thus a relatively lower capacity to provide lipid metabolites as energy substrate. This relationship was, however, significant only in full grown i.e. 125-day-old and 360-day-old animals (Table 19). During growth the ability to release FFA is generally very high (obviously as a result of the action of growth hormone which also enhances FFA mobilization—Winkler et al. 1964 etc.) and in animals with a higher body fat ratio.

We made furthermore a theoretical calculation: FFA released from 1 mg of an incubated specimen was calculated for the total amount of fat extracted from the organism. This total amount of theoretically released FFA was related to the fat-free body mass. The calculation revealed that the amount of FFA in the organism would not differ substantially in animals with a different body composition, age, degree of adaptation to a load, etc.; this would thus suggest that in the adult organism which has food *ad libitum* during the action of adrenalin the FFA release is regulated in such a way that total supply to tissues which need it is ensured as part of the energy requirements during the load. The above conclusion is also supported by findings at the same FFA level in blood which was collected in the experiments in both exercised and control groups; release and utilization were in equilibrium. But from these reflections we may also conclude that *in adipose tissue of animals which have a low body fat ratio (e.g. after adaptation to exercise) there is a more rapid turnover and higher metabolic activity.*

It was also shown that athletes have a somewhat higher blood flow in the splanchnic region (where important body fat depots are situated) during exercise as compared to untrained individuals (Rowell 1969, 1974). During prolonged exercise, redistribution of the blood volume to the body surface occurs to increase heat loss. Greater vascularization of the splanchnic region and the body surface where major fat depots are located may well be of crucial importance in enhancing mobilization and transport of FFA to the working muscles.

The above position in adipose tissue is further closely associated with the raised aerobic capacity, i.e. increased ability of the organism to supply tissues with oxygen which is a consequence of adaptation to exercise (Åstrand and Rodahl 1970 etc.); it is also *relatively high in the young organism* (*see* Fig. 20). The above data from the literature pertaining to the relationship between plasma lactate and FFA (Issekutz and Miller 1962) indicate that increase in lactate and reduction of FFA have a common cause, i.e. an inadequate oxygen supply (Peterson et al. 1964). Ischaemia of the untrained muscle leads to competition between pyruvic acid and dihydroxyacetone phosphate for reduced nicotineadenine dinucleotide (NADH), and to an increase in lactate and alpha-glycerophosphate. It may be assumed that a similar competition also exists in adipose tissue. Accumulation of alpha-glycerophosphate can lead to a reduction of the amount of released FFA (Paul and Issekutz 1967, Paul 1975).

In tissues of an organism adapted to prolonged increased loads due to the raised aerobic capacity of the organism (Åstrand and Rodahl 1970, Buskirk and Taylor 1957, Fischer et al. 1965, Šprynarová 1966, 1974, Shephard 1969 etc.) *a sufficiently high* P_{O_2} *is maintained which prevents a major shift in NADH/NAD.* This means that *reduction of dihydroxyacetone phosphate cannot increase sufficiently to match the accumulation of released FFA during the work load.* This results in an *increased FFA turnover in adipose tissue.* On the other hand, in the case of oxygen shortage, i.e. when the *aerobic capacity of the organism is low,* as it is when *not adapted to increased activity, NADH accumulates,* anaerobic glycolysis provides *more glyceraldehyde phosphate* and thus also more dihydroxyacetone phosphate produces *sufficient*

TABLE 19.
Correlation coefficients (r) of the relationship between percentage of body fat and the amount of released FFA *in vitro* after adrenalin from epididymal adipose tissue of rats of different age (Pařízková and Staňková 1967)

Incubation (min)	60		210		60		100		210	
Adrenalin (μg/ 100 mg	0		0		2		2		2	
adipose tissue)	r	sign.	r	sign.	R	sign.	r	sign.	r	sign.
A — 85 days (n = 36)	—0.452	0.05 > p > 0.02	—0.220	n.s.	—0.158	n.s.	—0.347	n.s.	—0.351	n.s.
B — 125 days (n = 24)	—0.792	p > 0.001	—0.305	n.s.	—0.702	p < 0.001	—0.719	p < 0.001	—0.783	p < 0.001
C — 360 days (n = 14)					—0.395	n.s.	—0.541	0.05 p < 0.02	—0.494	p < 0.001

TABLE 20
Oxidation of free fatty acids (FFA) during palmitate-^{14}C infusion into the femoral vein of anaesthetized 110-day-old male rats with a different physical activity regime (Poledne and Pařízková 1975a,b)

	Expired $^{14}CO_2$ (as % of applied activity/hour)	
	$\bar{x}$	SD
Exercised	10.87	1.41
Controls	6.40	0.31
Hypokinetic	5.50	0.45

amounts of alpha-glycerophospate to meet the catecholamine-induced hydrolysis of triglycerides and FFA release. Then *reesterification predominates* and *fatty acid turnover declines.* The organism adapted to an aerobic load, when performing the same work, can use (as energy source) to a greater extent adipose tissue due to the increased ability of the transport system to supply required amounts of O_2. This also spares carbohydrates and *expands the functional* and *metabolic abilities of the organism.* But this manifests itself only as *an adaptational consequence of* a *long lasting dynamic work load of aerobic character.*

The more rapid turnover in adipose tissue prevents more ample deposition of fat depots (Pařízková 1963–5, 1968g). These properties of adipose tissue are in the organism adapted to a load and with a high aerobic capacity related to a greater ability to utilize fatty acids in muscles: e.g. Issekutz et al. (1965) found a higher turnover of injected palmitate-^{14}C and larger amounts of ^{14}C in expired CO_2 during physical exercise in dogs adapted for prolonged periods to running on a treadmill compared with untrained animals.

But there is evidence that this increased ability to utilize fatty acids is not manifested only under conditions of increased energy output, as was demonstrated by some further measurements.

A continuous infusion of free fatty acids bound to albumin and labelled with palmitate-^{14}C was administered into the femoral vein of anaesthetized trained, control and hypokinetic rats. Oxidation of the free fatty acids was assessed by collecting the expired CO_2 in which the activity was measured (Poledne and Pařízková 1975a,b).

Oxidation of palmitate-^{14}C *was greater in the exercised animals* (Table 20) and *lowest in the hypokinetic animals.* This confirms further the *increased capacity of the organism adapted to an increased load to utilize fatty acids as a source of energy;* as suggested by these results this increased ability is not manifested only during a load but *also under conditions of rest and even under anaesthesia.*

2. Deoxyribonucleic acid content in adipose tissue during adaptation to different loads

For reasons given above we analyzed the adipose tissue of animals with a different intensity of physical activity from the aspect of fat cell size which can be roughly evaluated from DNA concentration in adipose tissue. *In exercised animals we found a higher ratio of DNA/100 mg adipose tissue* (investigated by the method of Slabochová and Placer 1962) *than in controls or hypokinetic animals.* When we *referred the released FFA to DNA the difference between groups with different physical activity disappeared* (Fig. 39). The level of metabolic activity and *ability to release FFA* is obviously closely *related to the number of cells in adipose tissue and their enzymatic apparatus.* When the *energy turnover is greater* as a result of adaptation to daily

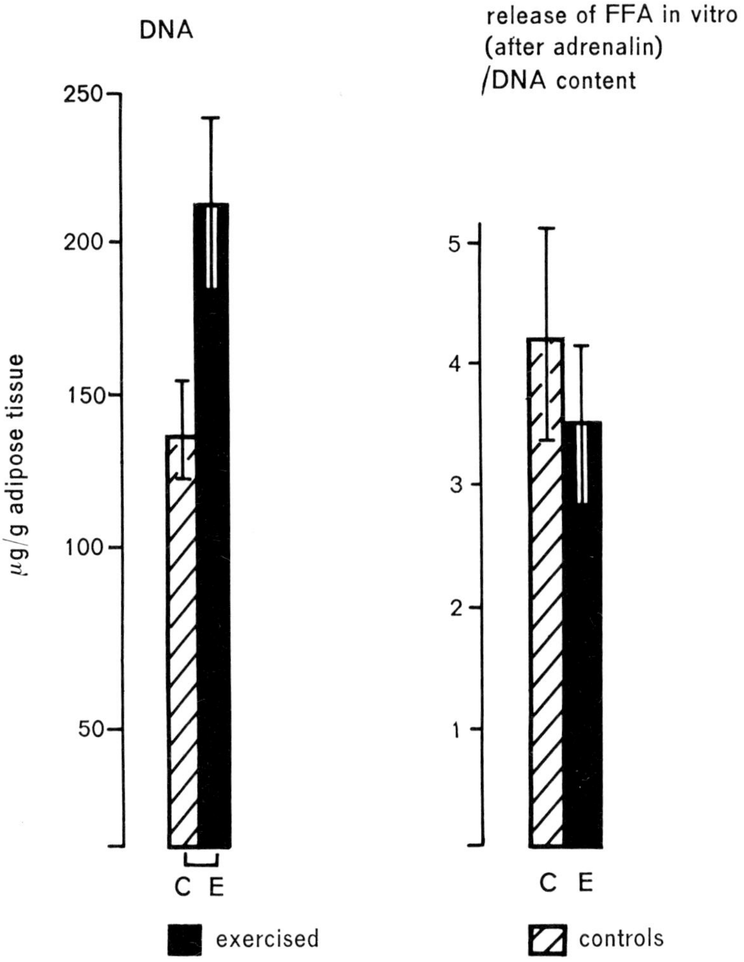

Fig. 39. Mean values ($\bar{x}$ ± SD) of deoxyribonucleic acid (DNA) content in adipose tissue (left side) in active, exercised male rats (black columns) as well as controls (hatched columns), and released free fatty acids related to the content of DNA (right) (Pařízková et al. 1966b).

exercise, the *fat cells do not hypertrophy and are maintained in a state corresponding to a younger ontogenetic stage* (Pařízková 1966, 1968e,f,g etc.).

In this connection it is important to draw attention to the *significant negative correlation between the body fat ratio and the percentage of DNA in adipose tissue:* the larger the adipose tissue, the lower the percentage of DNA. This applies in particular to old and hypokinetic animals (Pařízková et al. 1966b). Growing animals and those adapted to physical activity are at the opposite pole (Fig. 40).

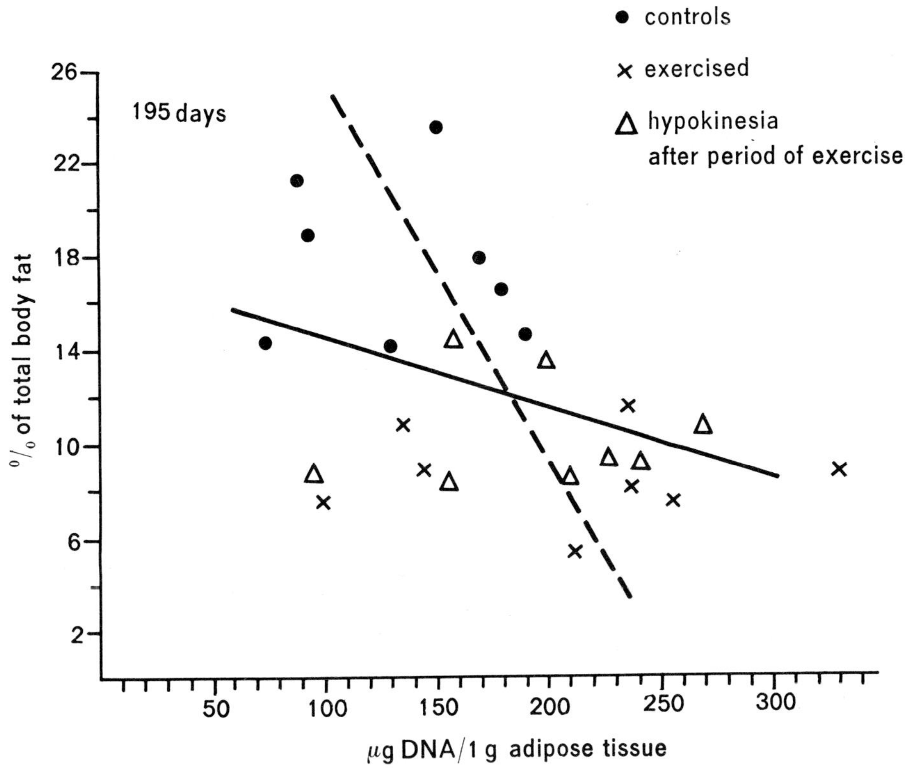

Fig. 40. Relation between percent body fat (ordinate) and DNA content (μg/1 g epididymal adipose tissue – abscissa) in subgroups of male rats adapted to different motor activity regime (x = active, exercised; ● = control; △ = animals with interrupted training; age 195 days) (Pařízková et al. 1966b).

In another experiment we compared the amount of released FFA in relation to the protein content; the difference between exercised, control and hypokinetic animals (125 days) declined but was still significant in favour of exercised animals. In 85-day-old animals the protein content of adipose tissue was in all groups higher than in the two older groups which is also in keeping with findings of a higher cellularity of adipose tissue in the growing organism. In this age group FFA released calculated per protein content was equal in all groups regardless of physical activity (Pařízková and Staňková 1967).

The higher DNA concentrations in adipose tissue of exercised animals indicate that their adipose tissue as in growing animals is not only more cellular but also metabolically more active and *capable,* if necessary, *of providing more rapidly lipid metabolites as an energy substrate for muscular work* (Pařízková 1968g).

3. Fatty acid uptake and their inflow rate into adipose tissue in animals with different levels of activity

Changes in the amount of adipose tissue in relation to different levels of physical activity may ensue from a different degree of fatty acid release or from a different ability to incorporate fatty acids into triglycerides. We investigated therefore the FFA uptake by adipose tissue from the medium.

The FFA uptake was investigated in the same medium, i.e. Krebs-Ringer phosphate buffer with 3 % albumin after addition of excess oleic acid (10 mEq/ml) and insulin (substance SPOFA — 500 i.u./ml medium) or glucose (0.9 mg/ml medium) after 180 min incubation (Raben and Hollenberg 1960). FFA were titrated according to Dole et al. (1956), the decrease of FFA was related to 100 mg adipose tissue. This comparison was also made in the subsequent experiment in groups of exercised and control animals aged 195 days.

Fig. 41 compares the results of FFA uptake from the medium after addition of insulin alone, glucose or both. *Only after addition of glucose alone was the FFA uptake lower in the animals adapted to physical activity* which differed from the two other groups. The same conclusion was reached when calculating the FFA uptake from the medium in relation to DNA in adipose tissue. Adaptation to a different regime of physical activity thus did not alter the ability of adipose tissue to take up FFA from the medium and obviously also to build triglycerides under the influence of insulin (although it cannot be ruled out that the dose used was excessive and this may have masked possible differences which would be found after smaller doses). The smaller FFA uptake in the presence of *glucose* alone indicates that *its excess in the medium is a much weaker stimulus for the FFA uptake by adipose tissue and obviously for lipogenesis also in animals adapted to regular activity* than in the remaining groups. This may, however, also be the consequence of the fact that glucose is utilized in the organism adapted to exercise more adequately than in the organism which is relatively inactive, and it is also deposited to a greater extent in the form of glycogen as was shown e.g. in the skeletal muscles or liver of trained animals. Although we cannot completely rule out the effect of different degrees of FFA adsorption on the surface of the specimens investigated *in vitro,* these results seem to suggest, along with a greater capacity of adipose tissue to release FFA, its higher metabolic activity focused in particular on the provision of necessary energy substrates (Pařízková et al. 1966b).

These conclusions were later supplemented by investigations of the *fatty acid outflow rate from the plasma and their inflow rate into adipose tissue* of animals adapted to daily exercise on a treadmill starting on the 18th day, compared with controls and also with animals adapted to hypokinesia from the 30th day, as described above. First group was followed up to 90th, second until 150th day of life. Again in these animals in addition to body composition the caloric intake, organ size etc., were also assessed.

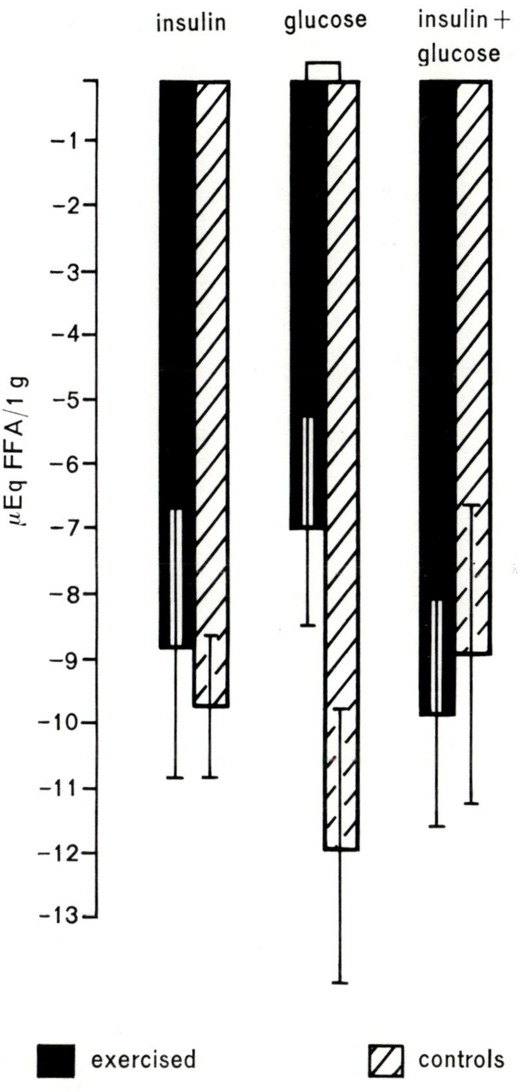

Fig. 41. Uptake of free fatty acids by epididymal adipose tissue *in vitro* – ordinate; in μEq, FFA/1 ml/1 g from the medium after the addition of insulin, glucose, and both. Black columns – active, exercised; hatched columns – control male rats: $\bar{x} \pm$ SD; age 195 days (Pařízková et al. 1966a).

Outflow rate of the plasma free fatty acids and their distribution resp. inflow rate into individual tissues was measured by means of albumin-bound palmitate-^{14}C (3 μCi Amersham England) injected in 0.2 ml of rat serum into the tail vein together with albumin^{131}I (Baker and Rostam 1969). As activity of the albumin in the plasma decreases the specific activity was calculated from the value extrapolated to zero

TABLE 21.
Mean values ($\bar{x} \pm$ SD) of body composition, caloric intake, outflow rate of plasma free fatty acids and their inflow rate into the adipose tissue in groups of male rats of different age and different physical activity (Poledne and Pařízková 1975a,b).

Age (days)		90			150		
Group		Exercised	Control	Hypokin.	Exercised	Control	Hypokin.
n		11	13	12	12	12	12
Weight (g)	$\bar{x}$	342.2	380.7	345.1	430.3	445.3	487.5
	SD	11.8	25.1	26.9	27.3	44.3	43.8
Fat (%)	$\bar{x}$	5.9	12.7	12.1	9.3	16.2	18.4
	SD	1.3	3.0	2.9	2.5	2.8	3.0
Calor. intake (g Larsen		55—65			85—105		
diet/100 g body	$\bar{x}$	9.9	9.9	9.2	7.9	7.3	6.6
weight/1 day)	SD	0.8	0.7	1.0	1.2	0.5	0.8
(days of measurement)		66—76			130—150		
	$\bar{x}$	9.7	9.0	7.5	6.1	4.7	4.8
	SD	0.8	0.9	0.8	0.7	0.5	0.4
		77—87					
	$\bar{x}$	8.0	8.0	7.3	—	—	—
	SD	1.0	1.3	1.2			
Plasmat volume (ml)	$\bar{x}$	13.15	12.00	12.00	15.80	13.62	14.90
	SD	1.09	1.12	0.81	1.25	1.20	1.05
Plasma FFA (μmol/ml)	$\bar{x}$	0.49	0.51	0.29	0.87	0.92	0.60
	SD	0.23	0.13	0.07	0.15	0.20	0.17
FFA pool (μmol)	$\bar{x}$	6.62	6.12	3.36	13.75	12.53	8.94
	SD	1.43	1.22	0.85	1.14	2.82	1.43
Outflow rate (μmol/min) R	$\bar{x}$	8.27	7.65	4.40	14.47	13.19	9.41
	SD	—	—	—	—	—	—
Inflow rate adip. tissue (mμmol/min/g tiss.)	$\bar{x}$	1.96	4.15	1.86	3.11	6.46	3.86
	SD	0.55	0.82	0.33	0.62	0.85	0.41

time: plasmatic volume $= \frac{\text{total activity injected}}{\text{activity zero time / ml}}$. From plasmatic volume and concentration of FFA the FFA pool in the organism was evaluated. Outflow rate (Schotz and Baker 1969) of FFA from the plasma was subsequently calculated: $R = \frac{PV \times [FFA]}{y_i(t)}$ (PV = plasmatic volume, [FFA] = concentration of free fatty acids; $y_i(t)$ was determined from the exponential decrease of radioactivity $y_i(t)$ of plasma FFA.

This function expresses the area under the curve of decreasing FFA activity in plasma
$y_i(t) = c_1e^{-a_1t} + c_2e^{-a_2t} + c_3e^{-a_3t}$).
Finally the inflow rate of FFA to individual tissues was evaluated as I = R . % of distribution (R = outflow rate of plasma FFA, distribution of activity is expressed in per cents of activity in the particular organ from the total dose applied, which equals 100 %) (Poledne and Pařízková 1975a,b).

Weight, relative fat and caloric intake differed according to the regime of physical activity as usually (Table 21). *Plasmatic volume was greatest in exercised animals in both age groups, FFA concentration was significantly lowest in the hypokinetic group* as compared with both exercised and control animals. *The same applied to FFA pool and FFA outflow rate* which were also *smallest in the hypokinetic group* (Table 21). The evaluation of *inflow rate of FFA to the adipose tissue* displayed *the lowest values in the active, exercised animals, the highest one not in the hypokinetic, but in controls* in both age groups (Table 21). Lower values of inflow rate to the adipose tissue in the exercised animals were caused first of all by smaller distribution of FFA, but in the hypokinetic animals by lower outflow rate (R). As apparent from the comparison, the *greatest fat accumulation in the organism, in particular* striking *in older hypokinetic animals, was found not only with the lowest caloric intake but also at a lowest inflow rate of FFA into adipose tissue,* compared with controls (Table 21) (Poledne and Pařízková 1975a,b). From this ensues the *important role of enhanced lipolytic processes in the adipose tissue metabolism resulting from optimal physical activity* which cannot be replaced by any natural factor; as is apparent from the results, a *reduction of the caloric intake does not compensate for the lack of activity.* On the other hand, increased activity reduces fat deposition even at a higher level of caloric intake, and this is not only due to higher fatty acid utilization etc. (Table 20) but also primarily to the fact that in the organism adapted to activity fatty acids are distributed to a lesser extent into adipose tissue (Table 21). The different inflow rate of palmitate-^{14}C seems to indicate inter alia a mechanism rendering a more or less efficient uptake of FFA possible as a consequence of a different regime of physical activity.

4. Ratio of individual fatty acids in adipose tissue

Another question associated with the effect of adaptation to different loads of activity on adipose tissue was its composition from the aspect of individual fatty acids. Diet and hormones influence in a significant way the fatty acid composition of triglycerides in adipose tissue. Less was known about the fatty acid composition of adipose tissue under conditions where their release and peripheral utilization are increased (Kohout et al. 1965).

Adipose tissue from the two above mentioned groups of 125-day and 360-day-old rats was analyzed in exercised and control animals (*see* Fig. 24, 25 and 38) using gas chromatography. The acids were methylated according to Stoffel et al. (1959), methyl esters of fatty acids were separated on a Pye chromatograph with an ionizing detector (RaD) at 192 °C. The stationary phase was Reoplex 400 on Celit 545, mesh 60—80 (Kohout et al. 1965).

The results were evaluated as the ratio of individual fatty acids in adipose tissue (Table 22). *Only palmitoleic acid differed significantly* in individual groups. *Its ratio in adipose tissue of animals adapted to exercise was significantly reduced. The same applies to its content in the heart muscle* (Fig. 42). These differences are obviously associated with the preferential release and utilization of this acid caused by the action of adrenalin during muscular work.

This is suggested also by the *significant negative relationship between the amount of released FFA from adipose tissue in vitro into the medium and the percentage of palmitoleic acid in adipose tissue* (Table 22). The greater the capacity to release FFA, the lower the ratio of palmitoleic acid in adipose tissue and vice versa. There existed moreover also a *significant positive relationship between the total fat content of the organism* (and its total weight resp.) *and the percentage of palmitoleic acid in adipose tissue* (Table 23) (Kohout et al. 1965).

The reduction of the palmitoleic acid content in adipose tissue of the organism adapted to prolonged muscular work may be due not only to preferential mobilization but also to slower synthesis. A low ratio of this acid is found in an organism with low lipogenesis (e.g. on a high-fat-diet) or in alloxan-diabetic rats. The palmitoleic

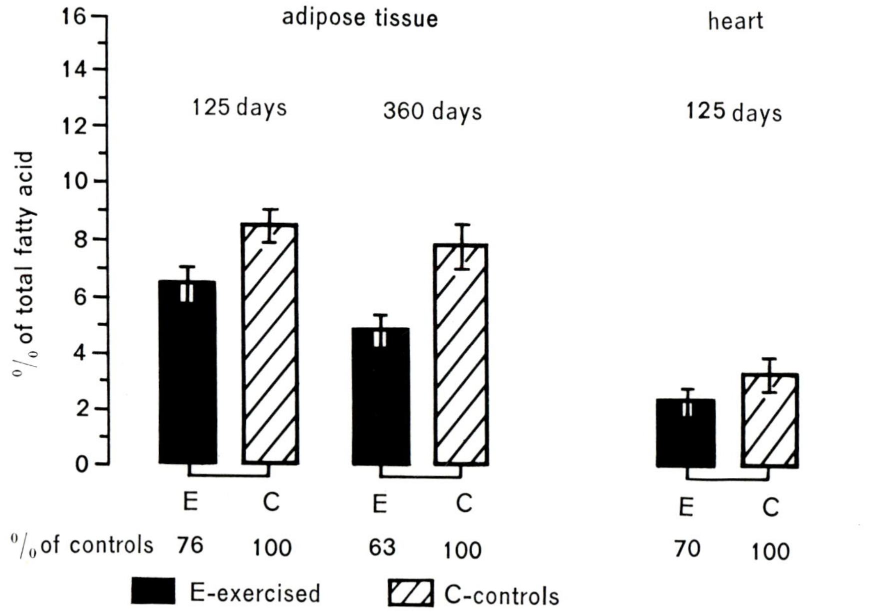

Fig. 42. Comparison of the content of palmitoleic acid $C_{16:1}$ (expressed in % of total fatty acids; $\bar{x} \pm SE$) in the epididymal adipose tissue of male rats adapted to different motor activity regime (black columns – active, exercised animals; hatched columns – controls; age 125 and 360 days) and in the cardiac muscle (only 125 days old male rats; Kohout, Braun and Pařízková 1965).

acid content also reflects the degree of lipogenesis in the organism, as demonstrated by a positive correlation between the ratio of this acid in adipose tissue and the total lipid content of the organism, as well as by findings of a lower inflow rate to adipose tissue (Table 21) and lower FFA uptake from a medium with an excess of glucose by adipose tissue of animals adapted to increased physical activity (Fig. 41).

TABLE 22.
Fatty acid composition in epididymal adipose tissue of male rats aged 125 days (Kohout, Braun and Pařízková 1965)

Chain length	Controls			Exercised	
n	10			10	
	$\bar{x}$	SE		$\bar{x}$	SE
C 12	0.46	0.08*		0.56	0.15
C 14	2.76	0.12		3.28	0.24
C 15	0.69	0.03		0.76	0.05
C 16	24.26	1.19		22.39	0.80
C 16 : 1	8.59	0.41	$p < 0.01$	6.49	0.55
C 17 : 1	1.10	0.09		0.92	0.09
C 18	3.31	0.22		3.51	0.24
C 18 : 1	39.50	0.87		40.86	0.96
C 18 : 2	16.39	0.68		18.46	0.42
C 18 : 3	2.93	0.26		2.75	0.24
Body weight (g)	341.0	16.2		353.0	14.6
Body fat (%)	14.7	1.01	$p < 0.001$	9.0	0.7

*The values are expressed as the mean percentage of the total fatty acids present.

TABLE 23
Relationships between body fat ratio and the percentage of palmitoleic acid (as % of total fatty acids in the epididymal adipose tissue of male rats aged 125 and 360 days – Kohout, Braun and Pařízková 1965)

	Correlation coefficients r	significance
Male rats 125 days old:		
Body fat (%): $C_{16:1}$	+ 0.623	$0.01 > p > 0.02$
Body weight (g): $C_{16:1}$	+ 0.545	$0.05 > p > 0.01$
Male rats 360 days old:		
Body fat (%): $C_{16:1}$	+ 0.353	$0.02 > p > 0.01$
Body weight (g): $C_{16:1}$	+ 0.432	$0.02 > p > 0.01$

VII. Adaptation to different loads: consequences in the lipid metabolism of skeletal and heart muscle and other organs

One of the most striking manifestations of adaptation to an increased load is muscular hypertrophy (Roux 1905, Yakovlev et al. 1962, Goldberger 1967 etc.). Its degree may, however, differ considerably in different types of work load as exemplified by representatives of different sports disciplines of a predominantly dynamic or static character. Great hypertrophy of the muscles need not always be associated with adaptation to intensive muscle work (e.g. in long distance runners, etc.). Various observations in animals and humans indicated that fat reduction participates relatively more than muscular hypertrophy in differences of body composition during a more intense regime of physical activity, in particular if it is not focused specifically along a certain line. It seems also that the response to a load differs not only according to the type of work but depends also on age and the type of muscle. In the experimental model mentioned we were able to study in greater detail the problem of hypertrophy of some skeletal muscles along with some aspects of the lipid metabolism.

1. Weight, fibre size and percentage of fat in muscles during different activities and in different age groups

In groups of 85-day, 125-day and 360-day-old male rats with a different regime of physical activity (exercised, controls, restricted activity) together with growth curves (*see* Fig. 24) and body fat ratio (*see* Fig. 25), metabolic activity of adipose tissue (*see* Fig. 38) the fresh weight and fat content in the tibialis anterior muscle and m. soleus (i.e. a mixed muscle with a predominance of the dynamic component, and a postural, red muscle) were investigated. In the youngest animals the weight of the tibialis muscle did not differ in relation to physical activity (Table 24). The soleus muscle was heaviest in the 85-day and 125-day exercised animals. In the oldest

TABLE 24
Mean values ($\bar{x} \pm SD$) of weights and fat content in skeletal muscles of male rats with different age and different physical activity regimes (Pařízková et al. 1966a)

		Tibialis muscle			Soleus muscle		
				WEIGHT (mg)			
Age:		Exercise	Control	Hypokin.	Exercise	Control	Hypokin.
85 days (n = 36)	$\bar{x}$	427.0	405.3	437.3	115.0	102.5	93.4
	SD	41.0	38.0	44.0	12.0	18.0	15.0
125 days (n = 30)	$\bar{x}$	681.0	553.0	572.0	153.0	115.0	109.0
	SD	61.0	63.0	80.0	22.0	15.0	9.0
360 days (n = 14)	$\bar{x}$	752.2	677.0	—	148.8	147.2	—
	SD	71.2	33.2	—	17.1	26.7	—
				FAT (%)			
85 days	$\bar{x}$	1.6	2.0	2.0	2.3	3.4	4.46
	SD	0.4	0.9	0.5	0.6	0.9	2.5
125 days	$\bar{x}$	1.72	1.88	1.95	2.04	2.71	4.12
	SD	0.28	0.38	0.33	0.69	0.64	1.03
360 days	$\bar{x}$	2.49	2.65	—	3.66	3.70	—
	SD	0.39	0.55	—	0.60	0.80	—

animals the weight of the soleus muscle did not differ. The tibialis muscle was heaviest in the exercised animals only at the age of 125 and 360 days. *The increased intensity of exercise seems to affect the weight of the dynamic muscle only at more advanced age, while it affected the weight of the postural muscle during growth and early adult life* (Pařízková and Koutecký 1968).

In another group of animals the *fibre size* in the soleus muscle measured in groups of 90- and 150-day-old male rats was compared.

The diameter of the muscle fibres from the primary fascicle was ascertained microscopically always in two rectangular projections. At least 600 measurements were made for one animal. Relative changes were expressed as values of controls taken as 100% (Puzanová and Pařízková 1976).

As apparent from Fig. 43, *the effect of exercise was manifested relatively more markedly in younger animals where the fibre size of exercised animals was almost 20% greater;* in adult life, i.e. in the 150-day-old animals, the relative increase of fibre size was smaller, i.e. only 5–10%. The effect of hypokinesia was less marked, i.e. present only in some animals (Puzanová and Pařízková 1976). Restricted activity thus did not produce a marked reduction of fibre size even though the weight of the whole soleus muscle in absolute and relative values was lowest.

The soleus muscle contained significantly more fat than the tibialis muscle at the age of 85 and 125 days (Table 24). *The fat content was significantly influenced only in the soleus muscle* at the age of 85 and 125 days (Pařízková and Koutecký 1968), which contains mostly red fibres in contrast to the tibialis muscle which contains predominantly white fibres. *In the tibialis muscle the fat content did not change under the influence of adaptation to exercise; in both muscles the percentage of fat increased significantly with age.*—Also Fröberg (1971a,b) found in trained rats lower plasma and intramuscular triglycerides while liver triglycerides were raised. Reitman et al. (1973) found after exhaustive exercise the greatest decrease of triglycerides in red muscle (70%), smaller (25%) in an intermediate muscle and no change in white portion of the quadriceps muscle.

Muscles with a different function were thus affected by the same load (running) in a different way, the consequences in earlier life being more marked. This may be associated with a greater adaptability as well as with the possibility of applying a more intensive load.—A higher fat ratio was found also in muscles of domesticated species, compared with wild-living animals (Crawford 1968) in which higher motor activity is supposed. Mentioned changes demonstrate the participation of muscle triglycerides as a source of energy during work load. Carlson et al. (1971) using the method of needle biopsy clearly showed the participation of intramuscular substrates including triglycerides also in energy expenditure of man.

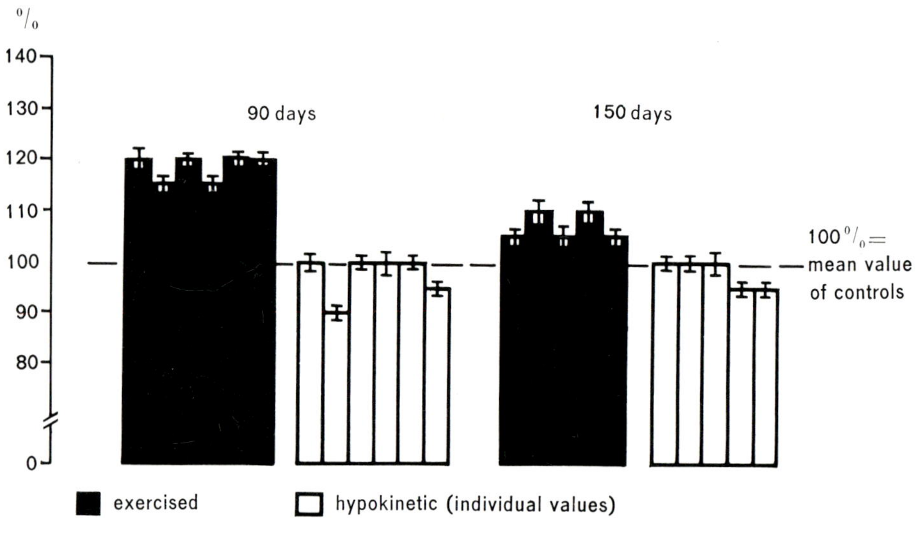

Fig. 43. Mean fibre size in soleus muscle of individual exercised (black) and hypokinetic male rats with restricted activity (white columns) expressed in values of controls (which equal thus 100%) (Puzanová and Pařízková 1976).

2. Lipoprotein lipase activity in heart and skeletal muscle after adaptation to different loads

Along with findings of changes in the body fat ratio of birds before and after the period of migratory flights comparative physiology provides some data on the lipid metabolism in muscles (Drummond and Black 1960). During the premigratory period the fat content in the pectoralis muscle of migratory birds increases (George and Jyoti 1955) along with a decline of the lipase activity (George and Vallyathan 1964b); these changes are associated with an increase of the body fat ratio and of total body weight. The capacity for fatty acid oxidation in the breast muscle homogenate is reduced during this period (George and Vallyathan 1964a). On the other hand, during the post-migration stage when this capacity increases along with an increase of lipase activity the fat content in this muscle and the organism as a whole declines. George and Jyoti (1955) had previously demonstrated that the pectoralis muscle e.g. in pigeons utilizes fat as the main energy source during electric stimulation. The flight muscles of migratory birds have, contrary to domesticated birds, a high lipase and succinic dehydrogenase activity (George and Vallyathan 1964b). These changes are conditioned by prolonged adaptation to very intensive muscular work during phylogenesis.

Adrenalin increases lipoprotein lipase (LPL) activity in the heart *in vitro* (Mallow and Alousi 1969). Nikkilä et al. (1963) proved an increased LPL activity after a single work-load in the heart and skeletal muscle of the rat. In this connection we were interested in the problem whether and to what extent adaptation to prolonged exercise and hypokinesia resp. is manifested during ontogenesis. LPL activity which may provide an indirect information on the intensity of the lipid metabolism in muscles was used as an indicator of lipid metabolism (Crass and Meng 1966, Pette 1966).

The LPL activity was investigated again by the method of Cherkes and Gordon (1957) in the heart muscle, tibialis and soleus muscle and in adipose tissue. In the first series of experiments the LPL activity was compared in the above mentioned organs of exercised and control rats and finally in those where the original adaptation to daily running on a treadmill from the 32nd day was replaced at the age of 105 days by a regime of restricted movement by keeping the animals in small cages to the end of the experiment, i.e. up to the age of 195 days. We found a *significant reduction of LPL activity only in the heart muscle of animals where secondary restriction of movement i.e. hypokinesia was enforced* (Pařízková et al. 1966a,b). In the other tissues different levels of physical activity did not cause any differences. Comparison of mean values in the other tissues suggests a possible relationship between the fat content and LPL activity—the soleus muscle has a higher fat content and also a higher LPL activity than the tibialis muscle.

The results indicate that it is possible to influence the LPL activity by the intensity of exercise, in particular by hypokinesia. The question arose whether by prolonged restriction of activity starting at the earliest stage of ontogenesis (where restriction

TABLE 25
Mean values ($\bar{x} \pm SD$) of body weight, percentage of fat and lipoprotein lipase activity (LPL) in the heart and skeletal muscles (expressed in µEq FFA/1 g tissue) in male rats of different age and different physical activity regime (Pařízková and Koutecký 1968)

		Weight (mg)	Fat (%)	LPL
		HEART		
Young	$\bar{x}$	358.60	2.62	11.54
(n = 10)	SD	41.02	0.30	2.72
Exercise	$\bar{x}$	808.25	2.58	13.37
(n = 12)	SD	98.34	0.57	2.07
Control	$\bar{x}$	815.50	2.85	10.10
(n = 9)	SD	94.38	0.50	3.06
		TIBIALIS MUSCLE		
Young	$\bar{x}$	184.0	1.87	3.05
	SD	27.0	0.37	0.61
Exercise	$\bar{x}$	517.0	1.67	2.39
	SD	82.36	0.47	0.50
Control	$\bar{x}$	540.4	1.49	2.08
	SD	57.0	0.26	1.16
		SOLEUS MUSCLE		
Young	$\bar{x}$	41.8	2.81	12.30
	SD	7.6	0.58	3.18
Exercise	$\bar{x}$	149.0	2.22	8.11
	SD	31.0	0.79	1.93
Control	$\bar{x}$	114.2	1.87	4.38
	SD	18.7	0.47	1.01

of activity has the most marked effect—*see* Fig. 25 and 38), it would be possible to achieve more marked results. In the next series the rat pups were therefore placed in small cages immediately after weaning. *At the age of 160 days an increased fat content was found in the heart muscle;* the absolute and relative weight of the heart, however, did not differ. *The LPL activity in the heart of the hypokinetic animal was by 31% lower than in controls.* In the *tibialis muscle* as a *result of prolonged hypokinesia* the *percentage of fat was also somewhat higher and the LPL activity significantly lower* (i.e. less than half). But in this experiment, however, no changes in the soleus muscle were found (Pařízková and Koutecký 1968).

In the subsequent series of experiments we again compared absolute and relative weights of the heart and skeletal muscles along with the percentage of fat and LPL activity in animals adapted to a different regime of activity. Adaptation to daily exercise was started immediately after weaning and the load was increased according

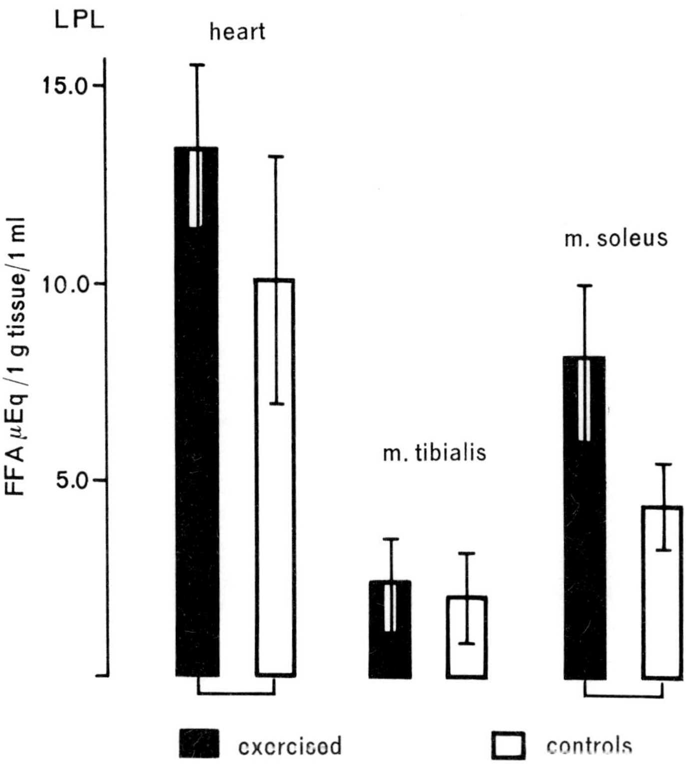

Fig. 44. Comparison of the activity of lipoprotein lipase ($\bar{x} \pm SD$) in the heart, tibialis and soleus muscles of male rats adapted to daily running (black columns) and of controls (white columns; age 160 days). Expressed in μEq FFA/1 ml/1 g – ordinate (Pařízková and Koutecký 1968).

to the pattern described previously (see p. 61-3). For comparison the results obtained in growing animals are also presented (Table 25), where the values were highest. These were followed by values of exercised and finally by values of 160-day-old control animals. The differences were in all instances significant. *During adaptation to increased muscle work and a higher level of energy turnover the LPL activity was thus also increased in the heart and soleus muscle* (Fig. 44); in this respect it differed from mean values of LPL activity in growing animals much less than in controls.—Askew et al. (1962) did not find after shorter period of adaptation to daily run (using a slightly greater speed combined with 30 s sprint at 1.8 mph every 15 min) any change in LPL activity in the heart and quadriceps muscle. Obviously the type of work-load, lenght of its duration and also the type of engaged muscles (white or red) differ as regards the results of adaptation to exercise (Reitman et al. 1973).

Pette (1966) demonstrated that e.g. the soleus muscle which displays a relatively high LPL activity has also a high activity of enzymes involved in beta-oxidation of fatty acids. *Along with our findings of a greater capacity to release fatty acids from adipose tissue in young as well as exercised animals, the higher LPL activity may be considered as indicating the ability to use a greater proportion of lipid metabolites—in particular fatty acids—as energy source for muscular work*. (This ability is generally associated with the high aerobic capacity in relation to LBM) (*see* Fig. 20). Therefore animals exercised for prolonged periods to dynamic exercise have a *lower body fat ratio even at a more advanced age*. Opposite results are produced by adaptation to reduced physical activity, manifested in body composition. Hellander (1959) demonstrated atrophy of the muscles of the hind limb and lipomorphosis after immobilization by means of a plaster bandage. A marked reduction of LPL activity in the pectoralis muscle was also found by Vallyathan et al. (1966) during drastic restriction of physical activity by means of a plaster bandage. But even the effect of restriction to a small space in our experiments produced a significant effect (Pařízková 1969).

There exists a certain relationship between values of the percentage of total body fat and LPL activity: we found a significant negative correlation between LPL activity (only in the heart muscle) and the total body fat ratio ($r = 0.336$): the higher the body fat ratio the lower the LPL activity in the heart and vice versa. This finding may imply a reduced ability to assimilate fat by the heart muscle in connection with enhanced fat deposition in the body which predominates in hypokinetic or elderly organism.

The greater ability of skeletal muscle to utilize fatty acids as an energy source was also provided by investigation of the *fatty acid inflow rate*. In the previous chapter (*see* p. 100) the method used was described and evidence was provided of a lower inflow rate of palmitate-^{14}C to adipose tissue of male rats adapted to increased activity (*see* Table 21). In these animals on the other hand *an enhanced inflow rate of palmitate-^{14}C to skeletal muscle, i.e. the soleus muscle, was demonstrated* which was manifested in particular in 150-day-old animals after a prolonged period of training. In hypokinetic animals at that age the inflow rate of palmitate-^{14}C to the soleus muscle was lowest (Table 26).

Table 26 also shows that under the influence of adaptation to exercise the *inflow rate of palmitate-^{14}C to the heart muscle is also increased* and *is lowest in hypokinetic animals*. These results indicate that *under the influence of prolonged adaptation to different loads marked changes in the lipid metabolism* of different tissues occur which are also *manifested under conditions of rest*.

We further investigated the *distribution of administered activity from palmitate-^{14}C in different fractions of myocardial lipids*. As apparent from Table 27, the distribution of activity between esterified fatty acids (triglycerides and phospholipids) and non-esterified (intracellular) free fatty acids was identical in all compared groups. This could imply that even when the distribution of FFA in the exercised animals is increased the esterifying system in the heart cells is activated sufficiently to maintain the proportion of intracellular FFA unchanged. FFA must be first transferred from plasma albumin to the proteins of the cellular membrane before they enter the intracellular space through the lecithin-lysolecithin pump which is fast enough and cannot be the rate-limiting step. Finally FFA must be esterified before they can be used as an energy source. Therefore in the next experiment (male rats with different activity, 110 days old) the first transfer step was measured *in vitro* on skeletal muscle preparations under anaerobic conditions, as we found previously that the FFA transfer from plasma albumin to the protein of the cellular membrane is energy independent. The activities of labelled palmitate transferred from albumin in the incubation medium to the protein membrane of the muscle cell within 10 min in an atmosphere of nitrogen were identical, i.e. 1.35% in the exercised animals, 1.23% in controls and lower in hypokinetic animals (1.17%). From these results we may conclude that the *increased inflow rate of plasma FFA to the cell of the contractile system can be due inter alia to an increased esterification rate inside the cell* (Poledne

TABLE 26
Mean values ($\bar{x} \pm SD$) of inflow rate of free fatty acids (FFA) into the soleus muscle and the heart (Pařízková and Poledne 1974a,b, Poledne and Pařízková 1975b).

Age (days)		90			150		
Groups		Exercised	Control	Hypokinetic	Exercised	Control	Hypokinetic
Inflow rate: (mμmol/min/ /organ)							
Soleus muscle	$\bar{x}$	2.39	1.19	0.96	6.96	4.35	2.08
	SD	0.33	0.42	0.25	1.21	0.25	0.35
Heart	$\bar{x}$	—	—	—	191.10	145.10	73.30
	SD				22.93	16.80	9.91

TABLE 27
Mean percentage values ($\bar{x} \pm SD$) of activity from palmitate-^{14}C in myocardial lipids in groups of male rats with different physical activity regime (age 110 days) (Poledne and Pařízková 1975b).

	Phospholipids %		Free fatty acids %		Triglycerides %	
	$\bar{x}$	SD	$\bar{x}$	SD	$\bar{x}$	SD
Exercised	14.98	3.38	2.37	0.32	82.64	3.1
Control	13.09	3.34	2.51	0.48	84.39	4.2
Hypokinetic	15.79	3.89	3.5	0.46	80.73	4.73

and Pařízková 1975b; in press). A higher esterification rate takes up FFA from the bound places of the proteins of cellular membranes and further FFA can be moved from the plasma albumin to the free places in the cellular membrane. The uptake of fatty acids is more rapid thus promoting their greater utilization (as indicated already by increased activity of LPL—*see* Fig. 44), which is further demonstrated by the above-mentioned lower content of triglycerides in the soleus muscle of exercised animals (*see* Table 24) in spite of the higher inflow rate of FFA (*see* Table 26). Higher activity of LPL indicates higher activity of beta oxidative enzymes as shown by Pette (1966). Bass et al. (1976) found indeed higher activity of hydroxyacyl-CoA dehydrogenase in biopsies from the quadriceps femoris muscle of athletes compared to sedentary subjects. After endurance training (cross-country skiers) the activity of this enzyme increased and after speed training it decreased.

3. Cholesterol formation during different levels of physical activity

Findings of the effect of increased physical activity on the cholesterol level in serum and liver are so far controversial. Some authors show reduced cholesterol levels after hyperkinesia (Keys et al. 1956. Campbell 1965, Hebbelinck and Casier 1966, Hoffman et al. 1967, Gollnick and Simmons 1967, Šimko and Charvátová 1968, Gollnick and Taylor 1969, Ahrens and Broxton 1970 etc.), others, however, found no changes (e.g. Nikkilä and Kontinen 1962, Carlsson and Mosfeld 1964 etc.). The position as regards the cholesterol level in liver is similar. One of the causes of this controversy may be, however, the great differences in the size of the load used. Not only the duration of the load per day differs (15 min to 8 hours/per day) but also the total period of training (4 – 200 days) and its type (swimming, running on a motor driven treadmill, etc.). The main attention was paid to cholesterol degradation and not to its synthesis. Information on the action of marked restriction of movement was also lacking. This was the subject of subsequent experiments.

We again used Wistar strain male rats adapted to daily exercise on a treadmill (from the 18th to the 120th day) or hypokinesia from the 30th—120th day. Cholesterogenesis was investigated using Na-acetate-1-^{14}C in liver slices, as described by Avoy (1965). The cholesterol level was assessed by Abell's chemical method (1951).

As usual the animals of different groups differed in their body weight (lowest in exercised animals, highest in hypokinetic ones) and the percentage of body fat which had the same trend as the body weight. The food intake (g/100 g body weight) was again highest in the exercised and lowest in the hypokinetic animals. This suggested the highest metabolic level in animals adapted to running which was confirmed also by the higher oxygen consumption per day (*see* Table 15). In a similar way as the daily oxygen consumption also the *level of lipogenesis and cholesterogenesis was altered* (Fig. 45). *The acetate incorporation was significantly raised in exercised animals, the lowest values being found in hypokinetic animals.*

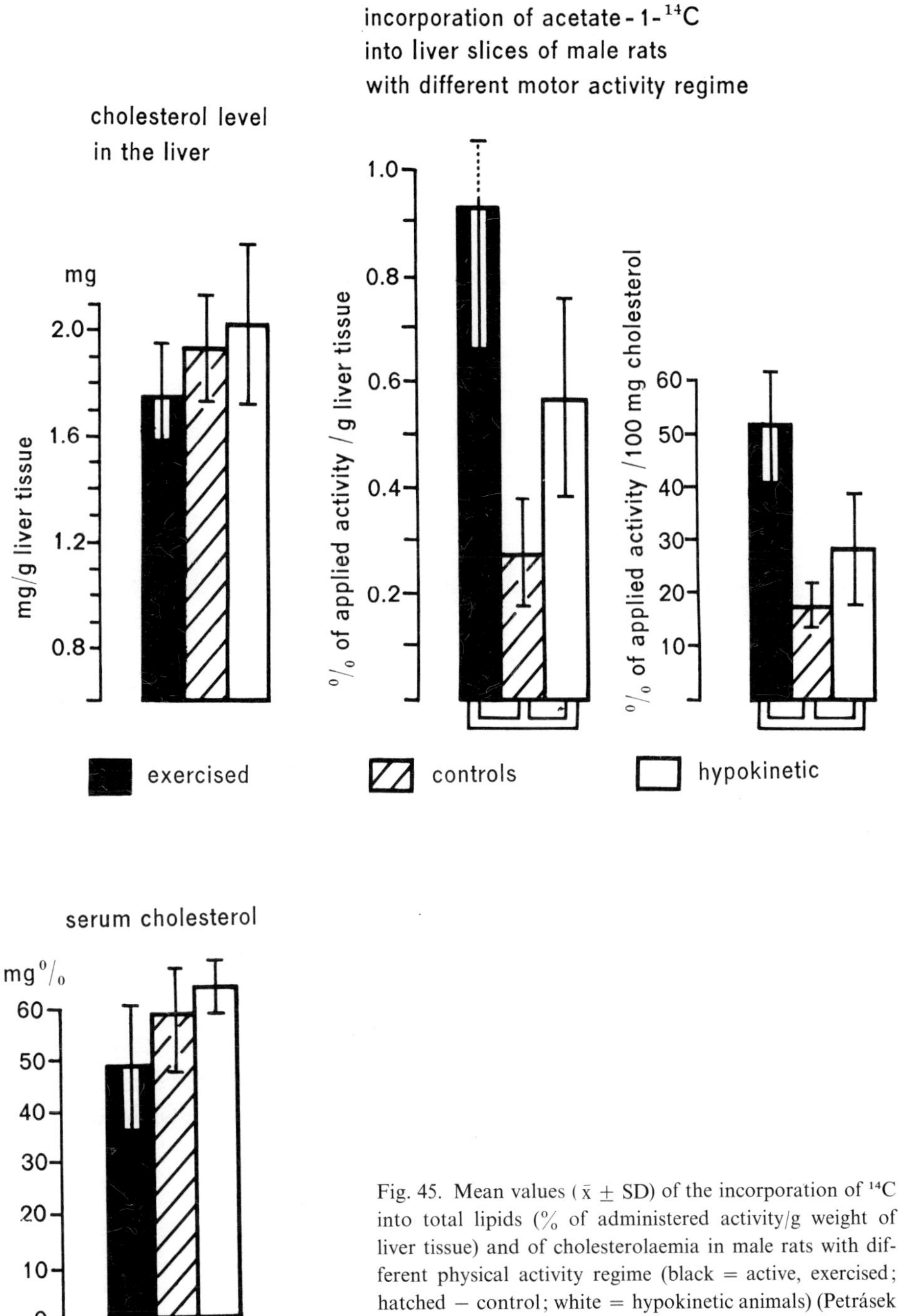

Fig. 45. Mean values ($\bar{x} \pm$ SD) of the incorporation of ^{14}C into total lipids (% of administered activity/g weight of liver tissue) and of cholesterolaemia in male rats with different physical activity regime (black = active, exercised; hatched – control; white = hypokinetic animals) (Petrásek and Pařízková 1975, 1976).

Although the above results indicate the *highest level of cholesterogenesis after long-term adaptation to an increased load*, the *cholesterol level in the liver and serum was lowest*. On the other hand, after *adaptation to hypokinesia leading to the lowest cholesterogenesis the cholesterol levels in the liver and serum were highest* (Fig. 45) (Petrásek and Pařízková 1975). As apparent, the differences in the cholesterol level of serum and in liver do not reflect changes of its formation. In hyperkinetic animals the general metabolic level is higher whereby, however, catabolic processes clearly predominate. Increased exercise thus leads, even when the cholesterol synthesis is increased, to enhanced cholesterol degradation to bile acids and its metabolites are excreted in the faeces, as was demonstrated e.g. by Hebbelinck and Casier (1966), Simko and Charvátová (1968).—Decreased excretion of cholesterol was also found in ageing animals characterized inter alia by a reduced level of metabolic activity, low spontaneous physical activity and reduced oxygen consumption/day, etc.

The above results—in particular the concomitantly raised fatty acid and cholesterol formation in exercised animals and the reduced synthesis in hypokinetic animals—are to a certain extent in disagreement with the hypothesis of Foster and Bloom (1963) on the indirect relationship between fatty acid and cholesterol formation found by these authors during starvation, but in other instances, e.g. in young animals or infrequently fed animals (where the metabolic level is also raised), this indirect relationship does not apply. This indicates that *adaptation to an increased load also brings the organism with respect to the level of selected parameters closer to a condition usually encountered at an earlier age*. It was also shown that long-term restriction of activity may lead to changes in the lipid metabolism which are typical for the development of serious disorders of the cardiovascular system. Link and Pedersoll (1972) showed in a study with swine that long exercise and an atheromatic diet increased blood lipids in both exercised and non-exercised groups, but atheromas and fatty streaks (which in various human populations correlate, when occurring in the young, with raised lesions in the elder—Restrepo and Tracy, 1975) appeared predominantly in the non-exercised group. Finally the finding of raised level of cholesterogenesis in the hyperactive organism which by increased degradation maintains reduced cholesterol and lipid levels leads to the conclusion that e.g. *sudden discontinuation of intensive activity might lead in the adapted organism to more adverse consequences than a steady minimal regime of activity* (as e.g. in our controls). From the aspect of medical prevention it is thus necessary to maintain a balanced and steady regime of physical activity without major variations throughout life.

4. Influence of increased physical activity during prenatal ontogenesis on the lipid metabolism in the offspring

The important effect of nutrition in the initial stage of ontogenesis on the development of the number of fat cells in the organism of the rat and thus also the possible different development of adiposity and of lipid metabolism in subsequent periods of life

(Knittle and Hirsch 1968, Lemonnier et al. 1973, Johnson et al. 1973, Berglund et al. 1974, Moser and Berdanier 1974 etc.) has already been mentioned, similarly as the effect of swimming from the 5th day of postnatal life (Oscai et al. 1974). Also the diet of the lactating mother can influence the cellularity of the adipose tissue of the offspring (Knittle 1972). Metabolic reactions to various stimuli in the pregnant organism show certain characteristic differences which are reflected not only in the mother, but may be manifested also in the organism of the offspring. Foetal adipose tissue development has an important relationship to maternal levels of free fatty acids (Szabo et al. 1975), which can be transmitted to the foetus during pregnancy (Dancis 1975). The glucose rise in the 180 minutes following oral carbohydrate loads is greater and more prolonged antepartum than postpartum, and associated with a greater increase in immunoreactive insulin (Freinkel and Metzger 1975).

Regular work loads change significantly the level of various metabolites in the blood (glycaemia, free fatty acids, lactate etc.), increase the release of catecholamines and so forth. In conjunction with all abovementioned findings arose the question how selected parameters of lipid metabolism of the offspring could be influenced by the daily work load of the pregnant mother.

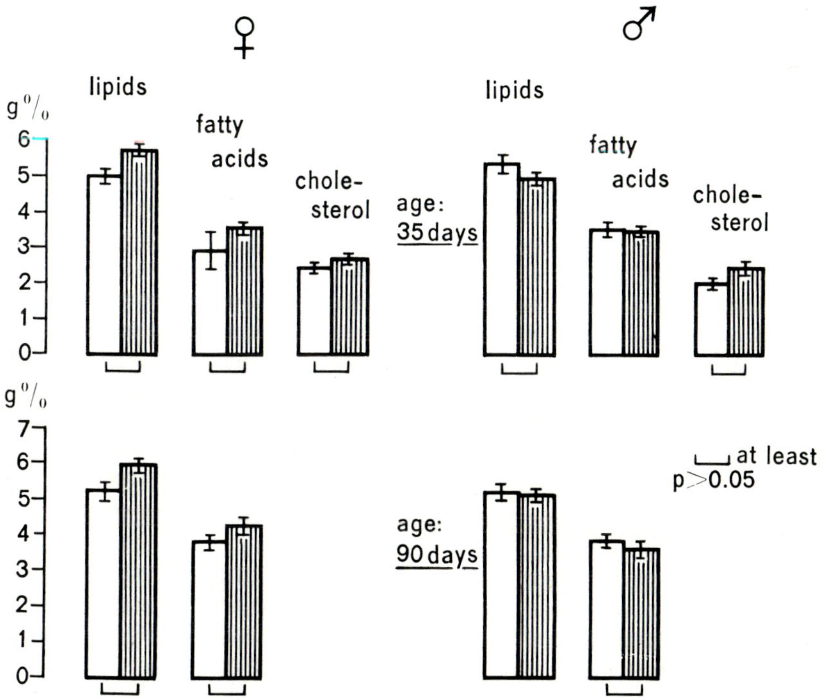

Fig. 46. Mean values (x̄ ± SD) of total lipid, fatty acid and cholesterol concentration in the liver of female and male offspring of exercised (hatched) and control, inactive rat mothers (white columns; Pařízková and Petrásek, 1976.) at the age of 35 and 90 days.

Young female rats were selected and mated with males (always 4 females with 2 males in one cage) at the age of approximately 120 days. The mean weight of the females at the beginning of the experiment was 230 g, that of males cca 400 g. Half of the females were exercised on the treadmill during the whole period of pregnancy starting 2—3 days after mating, for 1 hour per day, at a speed of 14—16 m/min (i.e. mild exercise of an aerobic character). 9 to 12 littermates were born to one mother, but only 8 were left in one nest during weaning period which lasted until 30th day of life. Four groups of the offspring were followed up in this series of experiments, and always 6 males and 6 females were selected at random from 4—6 exercised and 5—6 control mothers for our analyses at different ages (35, 90, 100, 108 days). No further change in the physical activity regime during postnatal ontogeny of the offspring was induced.

The concentration of total lipids and fatty acids in the liver and small intestines was assessed gravimetrically. The cholesterol level was ascertained in the liver by a chemical method (Abell et al. 1951). The total lipid, fatty acid and cholesterol synthesis in the liver was investigated *in vivo* based on ^{14}C incorporation from injected Na-acetate-$1^{14}C$ and *in vitro* by incubation of the liver slices using again Na-acetate-$1^{14}C$ as mentioned above (Avoy et al. 1965).

The weight of the pregnant rat mothers at the end of pregnancy increased to 290–310 g and did not differ in exercised and control mothers. The birth weight did not differ either; weights of all 35-day-old offspring of exercised mothers were significantly higher, and those of 90- and 108-day-old offspring were significantly lower in male offspring of exercised mothers. Differences in the weights of the liver varied.

Total lipid and fatty acid concentrations in the liver of female offspring of the exercised mothers at the age of 35 and 90 days were significantly higher than in the liver of the offspring from control mothers as measured *in vivo* (Fig. 46). In 35-day-old female and male offspring also the *level of cholesterol was significantly higher in the liver of the offspring of exercised mothers* compared to those from control mothers. Lipid and fatty acid concentrations in the liver of male offspring either did not differ, or the differences were reverse compared to female offspring of exercised mothers.

The free fatty acid serum level was significantly higher in both male and female offspring of exercised mothers.—The synthesis of total lipids and fatty acids was significantly lower in female offspring of exercised mothers at the age of 35 days; in the following series when measuring female offspring of the same age no significant differences were found, but *at the age of 90 days the total lipid and fatty acid synthesis was also significantly lower.* The synthesis of fatty acids in the male offspring at the age of 35 days was higher, that of total lipids lower. In 90-day-old male offspring there were no differences, with the exception of cholesterol synthesis which was higher in male offspring of exercised mothers, similarly as in female offspring of exercised mothers (Pařízková and Petrásek, 1976).

Another experiment in 108-day-old males (in vitro study) showed also a *reduced concentration of lipids in the liver of the offspring of exercised mothers,* and in this case also *lowered fatty acid concentrations;* cholesterol concentration in the liver did not differ. Lipid synthesis in the liver did not differ according to physical activity regime of the pregnant mother.

The analysis of lipid concentration in the small intestine (in vivo study) *of male offspring of exercised and control mothers* at the age of 100 days showed *no differences* between groups as regards total lipid and fatty acid concentrations. Again *higher values of cholesterol in male offspring of exercised mothers were found.* Synthesis of fatty acids was significantly higher and that of cholesterol lower in the offspring of exercised mothers (Pařízková and Petrásek, 1976).

The presented results suggest that *regular exercise of the mother during pregnancy has a marked impact on selected parameters of the lipid metabolism.* The most regular change was the increase in lipid concentration in the liver which was proved in females. In males such changes were either not apparent, or were of reverse character. Only in cholesterol the changes were similar, i.e. in 35-day-old animals there was an increase in its concentration in the liver of the offspring of exercised mothers. This change differed from those induced by exercise during postnatal ontogeny which resulted in reduced cholesterol concentration in the liver with simultaneously increased cholesterol synthesis (Petrásek and Pařízková, in press). As apparent, synthetic processes and concentrations of certain substances do not always change in a corresponding manner, due to many other interfering processes.

Increased lipid concentrations in the liver in female offspring may be related to a possible sexual dimorphism in lipid metabolism (about which very little is known until now) due to the action of female sex hormones, and a different role of fat depots in the female organism (increased as compared to males—see Fig. 2) considering especially pregnancy and lactation.

Also lipid synthesis was influenced by a different physical activity regime of the mother, but in this case changes induced by this factor were not as homogeneous as those concerning the lipid concentrations in the liver. Also the trend of changes seemed to be again of an opposite character compared to that of lipid concentrations. The differences were relatively small and thus of lesser biological importance. The synthetic processes which are of a more dynamic character manifest obviously the modifications in a less apparent way in one individual measurement than the resulting lipid concentrations in the liver.—The mechanisms of mentioned changes in lipid metabolism in the liver of the offspring could be caused by a number of factors, e.g. by fluctuations in blood glucose level (which influence the insuline release), changed release of catecholamines etc. during exercise. As mentioned above during long-lasting aerobic exercise mobilization of lipid metabolites—especially of free fatty acids occurs (Paul 1975) together with further changes in lipid metabolism (Pařízková and Poledne 1974). Increased free fatty acid levels were also found in the offspring of both sexes of exercised mothers.—The increase in the blood levels could concern, however, also further lipid metabolites in the mother and this could persist also in the offspring due to induction of necessary mechanisms during prenatal ontogeny (mainly during its last part) even without any subsequent change in the physical activity regime after birth. This might be the cause of a changed concentration of lipids in the liver.—The importance of these findings for *possible differences in the development of lipid metabolism later in life* is therefore further investigated, together with additional exercise during postnatal ontogeny. The mentioned data seem to indicate a *significant impact of a regular work load of the mother on the foetus which can be relevant in both physiological and pathological sphere.*

VIII. Effect of increased physical activity on body composition during growth in different groups of children (longitudinal studies)

Increased spontaneous motor activity is one of the most marked characteristics of the developing organism during the growth period. Maintenance of an increased motor activity during later periods of life when there is already a natural tendency towards its reduction leads to the maintenance of some selected properties in the organism which correspond to earlier developmental stages—e.g. those pertaining to lipid metabolism. The question arises how changes in the regime of activity, i.e. an increase (in keeping with the natural trend) or conversely its reduction during the growth period can influence body composition in relation to other characteristics of the human organism in which we can investigate these changes from some aspects in more detail.

The effect of physical exercise on the development of young people has been investigated so far mainly in cross-sectional studies comparing various indicators in children engaged or not engaged in physical training during adolescence and early school life. The results of such comparisons are, however, difficult to interpret as we cannot elimitate constitutional and genetic factors: it is very probable that children participate in these physical training groups who are more interested in physical activity, who are keener on physical training and who may already differ from the somatic, functional etc. aspects before they engage in physical exercise.

A more suitable approach to investigation of this problem is longitudinal study of groups of children where it is possible to compare the course of changes of somatic, functional and motor development during the action of physical training and compare it with children not engaged in organized physical training. It is, however, essential to ensure that at the onset of the investigation the groups are homogeneous and comparable. It is very difficult to meet this condition because at the end of the trial we can evaluate only those children who were followed up from the onset. It would also be necessary to analyze factors which cause some children to participate in physical exercise successfully for some years while others soon discontinue (also from the psychological, metabolic aspects, etc.). In any case it is possible to investigate in detail in a longitudinal survey how children engaged in regular physical exercise develop as compared with those with a relatively low activity (Pařízková 1965-6, 1968a,d, 1970a,b).

Very few data are available on preschool children where optimal stimulation by physical activity is a very important factor for the desirable somatic, functional and motor development. It is also important to take into account that in some sports nowadays at this age a certain type of training has already started (e.g. figure-skating, gymnastics, swimming). So far we do not know, however, the effect of intensive training at an early age as regards immediate and late sequelae which may be positive as well as negative.

1. Somatic and functional development of preschool children

The body composition and its changes in preschool children were investigated primarily by assessment of the skinfold thickness which is the most readily available method. Data also exist obtained by means of ^{40}K using a whole body counter (e.g. Burmeister and Fromberg 1970, Novak et al. 1970 etc.). Comprehensive studies which comprise both somatic and functional development are very rare. We therefore focused our attention not only on anthropometric indicators but also on characteristics of the circulation and motorics in children with different regimes of physical activity.

We investigated groups of children aged 3—6 years in the Prague population, from children attending nursery schools in different parts of the capital (boys n = 127, girls n = 112). The children had a relatively constant daily regime as regards occupation and diet and came from a homogeneous family and hygienic environment. In these children we examined selected morphological indicators, skinfold thickness by means of a modified Best caliper (1954) and Harpenden caliper. We used also the modified step test (height of step 25 cm, rate of mounting 30/min) (Čermák et al. 1973). As children at that age are not yet able to keep the necessary rhythm, the experimental worker always mounted the step with two children holding their hand lightly and thus regulated the rate and duration of the load. From the pulse rate during the step test Brouha's step test index was calculated. — We also investigated the performance in selected disciplines such as running, jumping and throwing a ball and finally the strength of the hand grip using a special dynamometer based on tensometric principles (Sukop 1966).

The basic anthropometric characteristics are presented in Table 28. The birth weights and actual body weights of the boys were higher as usually found in different child populations in other age categories (Tanner 1962, Pařízková 1962a, Suchý 1971 etc.). The mean values corresponded in all instances to the national standard according to Kapalín (1967).

The biacromial and biiliocristal diameters and bicondylar humerus and femur were mostly somewhat greater in boys. The same applied to the circumference of the chest and abdomen. The arm circumferences were practically identical while the circumference of the thigh was greater in girls. The most marked increase in values with age was apparent between the age of 4–5 (Pařízková et al. 1974a).

The only somatic indicator which did not increase at that age was subcutaneous fat.

TABLE 28

Mean values ($\bar{x} \pm SD$) of anthropometric parameters in boys and girls aged 3—6 years (Pařízková et al. 1974a)

		x̄	SD	x̄	SD	x̄	SD	x̄	SD
Age	♂	3.519	0.279	4.548	0.339	5.552	0.269	6.363	0.247
(years)	n	(34)		(28)		(39)		(25)	
	♀	3.481	0.322	4.471	0.331	5.460	0.302	6.333	0.226
	n	(25)		(28)		(34)		(25)	
Birth weight	♂	3350	567	3382	425	3337	463	3425	333
(g)	♀	3273	435	3370	442	3205	497	2931	574
Actual	♂	16.46	1.75	19.18	2.86	20.85	2,76	22.21	2.86
weight (kg)	♀	15.88	2.21	18.27	3.42	19.53	2.50	21.59	2.81
Height	♂	101.93	4.62	109.0	3.96	113.52	5.87	119.50	4.18
(cm)	♀	100.18	5.03	107.59	5.87	112.56	4.58	118.68	4.94
Sitting	♂	57.82	2.95	62.0	2.39	63.84	2.73	65.66	2.62
height	♀	56.73	3.34	59.92	2.49	62.41	2.68	64.77	2.82

TABLE 29

Mean values ($\bar{x} \pm SD$) of skinfold thicknesses measured both by modified Best and Harpenden calipers in boys and girls aged 3—6 years (Pařízková et al. 1974a)

Age (years)		3—4		4—5		5—6		6—7	
		x̄	SD	x̄	SD	x̄	SD	x̄	SD
Triceps	♂	9.2	2.1	9.3	1.9	8.9	1.9	7.2	1.7
(mm) (Harp.)	♀	10.0	2.6	10.2	2.4	8.6	2.1	9.4	2.0
Subscap.	♂	5.5	1.9	4.6	0.6	4.8	1.6	4.1	0.5
	♀	6.2	2.0	5.2	1.2	4.8	0.8	5.6	2.3
Suprail.	♂	4.0	1.4	3.6	1.2	4.0	1.7	3.1	0.7
	♀	5.4	2.6	4.7	1.7	3.5	0.9	4.9	3.2
Calf	♂	4.8	1.1	4.6	1.0	5.3	2.1	4.0	1.0
	♀	5.8	1.9	5.5	1.5	4.3	0.9	5.0	1.8
Biceps	♂	4.5	1.2	4.4	1.1	3.9	0.7	3.0	0.6
	♀	4.6	1.3	4.5	1.0	4.0	1.0	4.2	1.3
Sum of ten skinfolds (Best's calip.)	♂	44.7	11.6	41.6	9.6	43.1	17.0	38.4	9.9
	♀	53.8	20.2	50.4	11.8	45.7	14.9	49.4	18.1

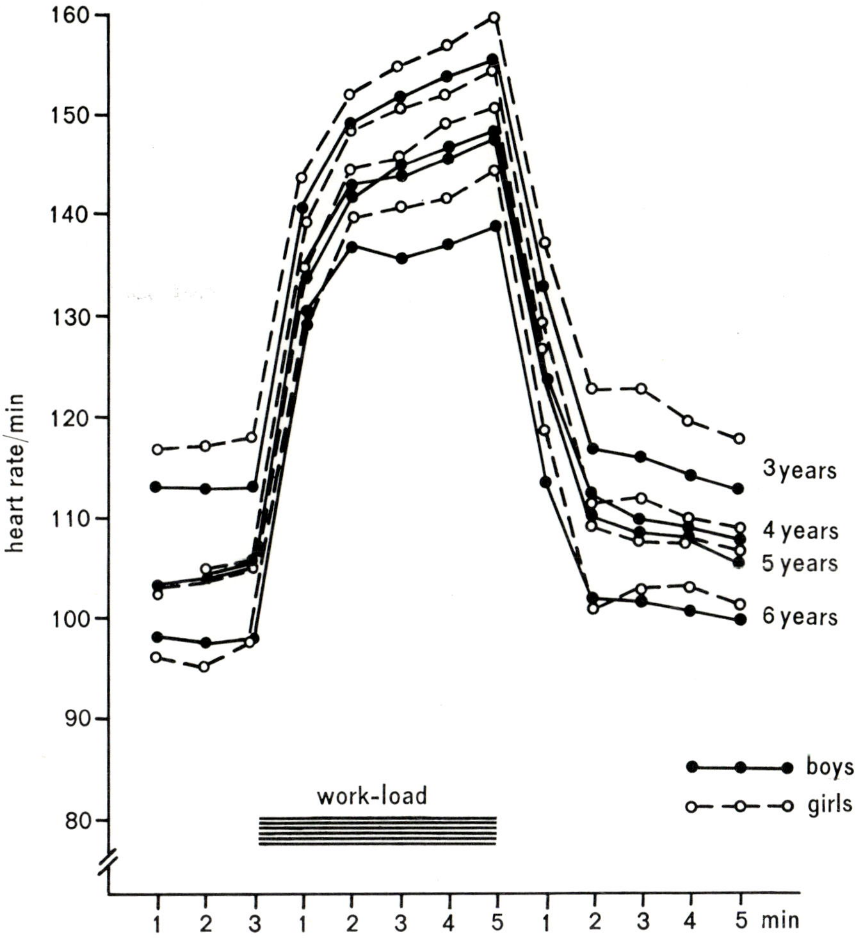

Fig. 47. Mean values of pulse rate during 3 min rest, 5 min work-load during a step-test, and during 5 min recovery period in groups of preschool children from 3 to 6 years of age (Pařízková, Čermák and Horná 1974a).

As apparent from Table 29, the thickness of selected skinfolds measured by means of a Harpenden caliper were smaller in older children which corresponds with values obtained by a modified Best caliper (1954) (sum of ten skinfolds) obtained in the same children and previous measurements of other Prague children (*see* Fig. 6a, 7), (Pařízková 1959a, 1962a). *In the great majority the skinfold thickness was greater in girls.*

The pulse rate at rest, during the step test and recovery declined with advancing age (Fig. 47). In this respect we did not reveal any sexual differences. *The work economy of the cardiovascular system improved at that age*, as was also shown by a special quotient described by Čermák (1969). The same conclusion was reached by an analysis of Brouha's step test index: e.g. at the age of 3.519 the index in boys equalled 87.0 (SD ± 8.00) and at the age of 6.363 to 99.39 (SD ± 9.94). The same was found in girls. It is known that in younger children the regulation during a load is due, in particular, to an increase of the pulse rate and later the regulation also effected by an increase of cardiac output.

Performance in special disciplines also differed by sex—*the performance of boys in running* (i.e. a shorter time for 20 m), *jumping and throwing were better than in girls. The muscular strength of boys was also greater* (Table 30 and 31).

TABLE 30
Physical performance in selected disciplines (run, broad jump and cricket ball throwing) in boys and girls aged 3—6 years (Pařízková et al. 1974a)

Age (years)		3—4		4—5		5—6		6—7	
		$\bar{x}$	SD	$\bar{x}$	SD	$\bar{x}$	SD	$\bar{x}$	SD
Run 20m	♂	6.8	0.8	5.6	0.8	5.1	0.5	4.9	0.2
(cm)	♀	7.4	0.8	6.2	0.7	5.1	0.2	5.1	0.2
Broad jump	♂	60.7	15.4	82.6	13.8	95.8	14.4	103.4	18.7
(cm)	♀	59.1	18.6	71.6	15.6	90.9	17.7	96.2	16.4
Cricket ball	♂	419.4	143.3	562.5	199.9	813.1	209.3	1028.0	404.7
throw (cm)	♀	326.5	101.4	438.3	131.9	601.2	126.9	695.6	135.2

TABLE 31
Hand grip strength (kp) in boys and girls aged 3—6 years (Pařízková et al. 1974a)

Age (years)		3—4		4—5		5—6		6—7	
		$\bar{x}$	SD	$\bar{x}$	SD	$\bar{x}$	SD	$\bar{x}$	SD
Right hand	♂	7.6	1.5	10.5	2.2	12.0	2.5	13.7	2.2
	♀	5.6	1.4	7.5	2.4	9.6	2.4	11.3	2.2
Left hand	♂	7.4	1.6	10.0	2.0	11.6	2.7	13.0	2.6
	♀	5.4	1.4	7.2	2.5	9.6	2.4	10.7	1.9

The results indicate a *different morphological and functional development in preschool boys and girls in the majority of indicators.* Only the efficiency of the cardiovascular apparatus evaluated according to the modified step test displayed no differences. In motor tests and strength primary differences are apparently involved even when in the nursery school both sexes had the same regime of physical activity.

The above *differences were confirmed in a representative sample of boys and girls shortly before starting school* (6.4 years, boys n = 2866, girls n = 2765), measured

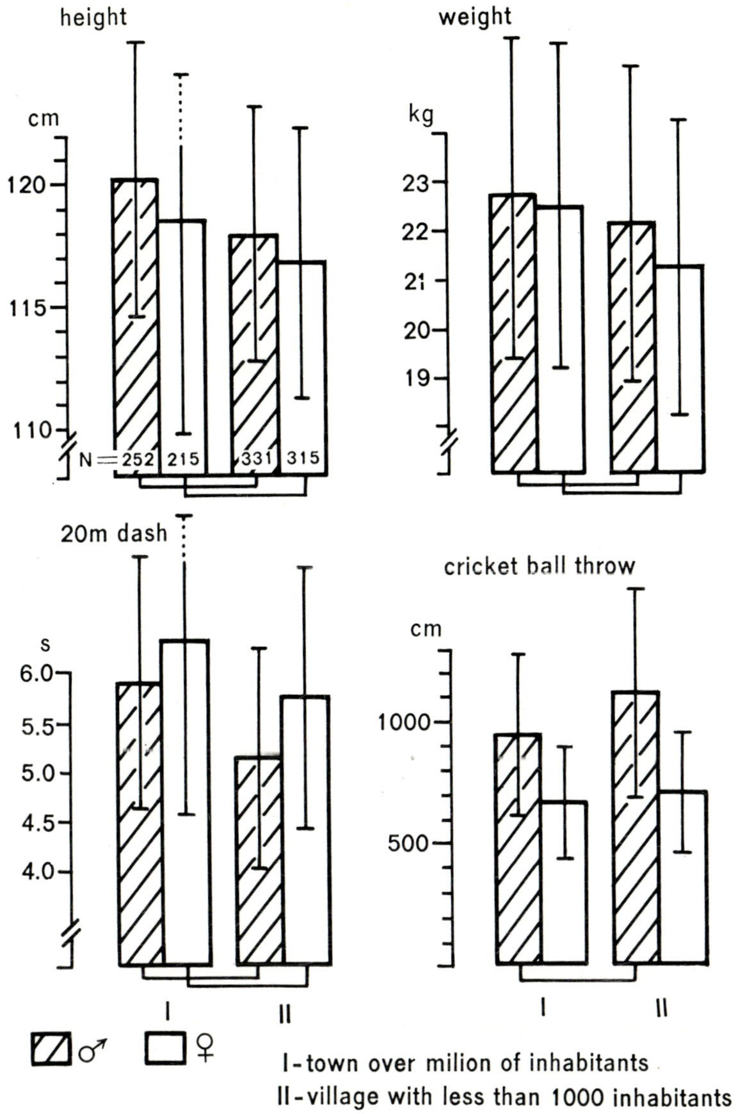

Fig. 48. Mean values ($\bar{x} \pm$ SD) of height, weight and performance in selected disciplines in preschool children living in communities with different number of inhabitants (Pařízková and Berdychová 1974, 1976). └──┘ p at least 0.05.

in Bohemia and Moravia (Pařízková and Berdychová 1974, 1976). This indicates that it is *necessary to use a differentiated approach in physical education of children of this age.*

TABLE 32.
Somatic development and physical performance in a representative sample of boys and girls (mean age 6.4 years) classified according to the period when engaged in systematic physical education (0 – 3 years) in preschool age (Pařízková and Berdychová 1976).

Physical education		0		1		2—3 years	
		$\bar{x}$	SD	$\bar{x}$	SD	$\bar{x}$	SD
Weight	♂	22.19	3.20	22.26	2.71	23.60	2.30
(kg)	♀	21.60	3.30	22.30	3.40	22.10	3.60
Height	♂	118.6	5.3	119.4	5.3	120.8	5.1
(cm)	♀	117.6	5.2	118.6	5.3	119.0	5.5
Chest	♂	59.2	3.3	59.6	2.9	61.0	3.4
circumf. (cm)	♀	57.9	3.7	58.5	3.6	58.2	4.1
20m dash	♂	5.4	1.1	5.6	1.3	5.5	1.2
(s)	♀	5.7	1.2	5.7	1.3	5.7	1.2
Broad jump	♂	108.0	20.9	109.9	17.9	119.9	22.3
(cm)	♀	100.7	20.4	105.0	20.1	110.6	18.4
Cricket ball throw	♂	1060	391	1075	421	1081	419
(right hand) (cm)	♀	676	220	722	235	717	240
Cricket ball throw	♂	672	240	683	287	752	302
(left hand) (cm)	♀	519	163	549	166	551	168

Investigation of this representative sample revealed some further *differences depending on oecological conditions*, e.g. *children from the capital* (i.e. a larger agglomeration with 1 million inhabitants where conditions for the physical activity of children are very restricted) *were taller and heavier but their motor development was on a lower level* (Fig. 48), i.e. the performance as regards running and throwing a ball was poorer. *More rapid somatic development thus did not create better prerequisites for functional development* (Pařízková and Berdychová 1976). The same applied to a comparison of groups of children classified by the *economic standard* of the family—boys and girls from families with a higher mean income per head were taller and heavier but their performance in the above discipline was poorer. *Bigger was not better in this case.* When we selected, however, from this sample *children who at this age were already engaged systematically for some time in physical education and exercise* and compared them with children not so engaged, the *taller children* (i.e. those who were *engaged in physical training* for the longest period) (Table 32) had a *better performance* except in running. Thus during systematic motor stimulation physical performance also reached the highest level. Although we cannot rule out

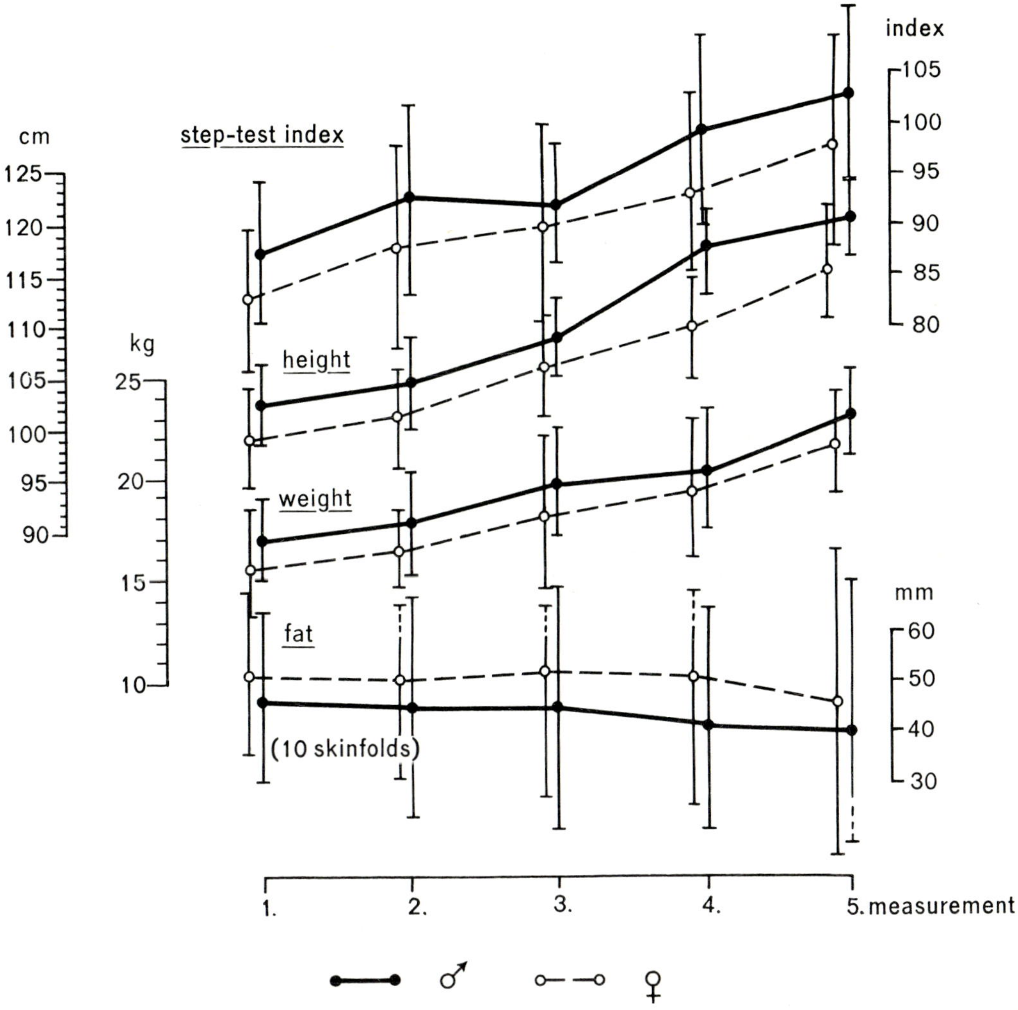

Fig. 49. Mean values ($\bar{x} \pm SD$) of step test index, height, weight and sum of ten skinfolds in groups of preschool children followed longitudinally. Mean ages ($\bar{x} \pm SD$) – boys: lst measurement = 3.48 ± ± 0.29, 2nd = 3.93 ± 0.34, 3rd = 4.54 ± 0.33, 4th = 5.10 ± 0.34, 5th = 6.02 ± 0.33 years. Girls: lst measurement = 3,53 ± 0.36, 2nd = 3.92 ± 0.35, 3rd = 4.48 ± 0.37, 4th = 5.02 ± 0.35, 5th = = 6.01 ± 0.36 years.

the influence of a certain selection (i.e. that somatically more advanced children and those more gifted for exercise became engaged in this activity) we may conclude in conjunction with the above comparisons that *regular physical training already exerts a favourable effect on the somatic and motor development at this early age* (Pařízková and Berdychová 1976). *The raised values of somatic indicators alone did not imply more favourable prerequisite conditions for physical performance but did so when associated with regular physical education.*

During a subsequent investigation we compared the skinfold thickness in children aged 2–5 years who attended special physical education groups together with their parents (Berdychová 1972), with children from the normal child population not engaged in physical training. At this age there was already a *tendency towards lower values of subcutaneous fat in children engaged in physical education* (Wolański and Pařízková 1976, Berdychová and Pařízková 1973).

The minority of children followed up in Prague (*see* p. 119) was measured repeatedly after 6-month intervals from 3–6 years of age (boys n = 34, girls n = 22). *The longitudinal study confirmed the developmental changes of morphological and functional indicators* (Fig. 49), i.e. a mild reduction of subcutaneous fat values (more marked in boys), while the other morphological indicators showed an increase. The work economy of the cardiovascular system evaluated by the step test index improved.— Comparison of the performance of children from nursery schools with different conditions for exercise revealed a tendency for more favourable development in children from nursery schools with better facilities.

2. Body build and body composition in boys engaged and not engaged in physical training

Body composition and the effect of systematic exercise on body composition during growth has only recently been studied systematically (Pařízková 1959b, 1960b,c, 1962a,b, 1963a,b, 1965, 1966, 1968a, etc.; Stupin 1964, Novak 1966 etc.). Changes in the LBM and body fat ratio are similar to those in other age groups (*see* Fig. 35) or in experimental laboratory model: the ratio of LBM increases at the expense of fat. In a longitudinal study of boys initially for five and subsequently eight years we investigated how these changes develop under the influence of a load in relation to chronological and bone age, other somatic changes (e.g. stature), physical fitness and aerobic capacity.

These boys who lived with their families (n = 96) under similar social, hygienic and nutritional conditions were divided during the period of 1961—1965 into four groups according to the amount of physical activity. Group I comprised boys who were engaged systematically in basketball or track-and-field athletics for more than six hours per week throughout the experimental period. Boys from group IV were engaged for less than two years in some unsystematic physical activity. The remaining groups were intermediary. It was not possible to find controls i.e. normal healthy boys who did not participate for at least two hours per week in physical education in schools. The latter activity was common to all children. With regard to known data about the activity of boys of this age the average population would correspond to group III. All measurements were made regularly in spring (April — June) after a detailed medical entrance examination. From the original 146 boys selected in 1961 (Pařízková 1964—1967) by 1965 with the same selected anthropometric indicators only 96 boys were left who were evaluated throughout the experiment (Pařízková 1968a,d, 1970b,c).

The development of height and weight by age was compared with standards for Czech boys according to Kapalín (1967), and also with standards for the English population (Tanner et al. 1966) and boys of similar age in the USA (Wetzel 1942).

TABLE 33.
Mean values ($\bar{x} \pm$ SD) of height, weight, chest circumference (rest), bone and chronological age in individual years of measurements (1961—5) in groups of boys with different physical activity regime followed longitudinally (Pařízková 1968a,b,c)

	1 1961		2 1962		3 1963		4 1964		5 1965	
	$\bar{x}$	SD	$\bar{x}$	SD	$\bar{x}$	SD	$\bar{x}$	SD	$\bar{x}$	SD
Height (cm)										
I	147.2	3.5	152.3	3.8	158.7	4.9	166.5	5.9	173.3	5.4
II	145.5	6.7	150.6	7.9	156.5	7.6	163.7	8.6	170.3	7.8
III	144.6	6.7	149.1	5.6	154.1	5.4	161.8	6.3	168.7	6.6
IV	144.4	5.2	149.3	5.7	154.5	6.4	161.4	7.3	169.6	7.0
Weight (kg)										
I	37.6	4.0	40.8	3.7	46.4	5.0	52.7	7.2	60.4	7.1
II	35.8	4.3	39.3	5.1	43.4	6.2	49.2	7.3	55.9	7.7
III	36.6	4.7	40.1	4.8	44.0	5.5	50.5	6.7	57.7	6.2
IV	38.4	6.0	42.3	7.2	46.0	7.7	51.6	8.6	59.5	9.6
Chest circumference (rest; cm)										
I	69.8	2.7	71.7	3.5	74.1	2.7	78.1	3.9	83.7	4.2
II	68.1	2.9	69.6	4.2	71.8	3.8	75.3	4.3	80.4	4.9
III	69.0	3.8	71.2	4.2	73.4	4.9	77.1	4.9	82.4	5.1
IV	70.7	4.9	72.1	6.0	74.5	6.0	77.6	6.1	83.1	5.9
Bone age (years)										
I	11.05	0.80	11.89	0.82	12.86	0.65	13.80	0.86	14.86	0.99
II	11.02	0.71	11.94	0.84	12.82	0.50	13.64	0.62	14.57	0.85
III	10.71	1.09	11.75	0.95	12.59	0.77	13.60	0.73	14.57	0.75
IV	11.00	0.68	11.85	0.71	12.69	0.73	13.51	0.71	14.44	0.98
Chronological age (years)										
I	10.76	0.39	11.73	0.37	12.74	0.38	13.74	0.38	14.64	0.37
II	10.90	0.33	11.89	0.36	12.81	0.32	13.89	0.31	14.77	0.32
III	10.83	0.29	11.90	0.29	12.87	0.31	13.89	0.28	14.81	0.30
IV	10.99	0.25	11.99	0.29	12.92	0.28	13.91	0.27	14.86	0.28

Table 33 shows the changes of height, weight and chest circumference. The results of the investigation, however, did not differ significantly from these control values nor from the other mentioned growth grids. Boys of group I tended to be slightly taller than the others.

The bone age was investigated by means of X-rays of the wrists and by evaluation according to standards of Greulich and Pyle (1959). Comparison with chronological age did not reveal any differences in any of the investigated groups in bone or chronological age in relation to physical activity (Table 33). The *investigated groups* were thus *homogeneous for basic somatic indicators* (Pařízková 1968a,d, 1970b,c).

Along with the characteristics mentioned we assessed some other anthropometric measurements—length, breadth, circumferences of trunk and extremities (a total of 28) from which relative dimensions were derived which characterize body build (Pařízková 1970b, 1972g,h). Comparison revealed no differences in the circumferences of the chest (rest, inspiration, expiration), biacromial, biiliocristal, bitrochanteric diameters, length and circumference of extremities. Also the robustness of the skeleton evaluated from the breadth of the wrist and bicondylar femur did not differ. During the period from 10.7 to 14.7 years this indicator changed relatively little—the bicondylar by cca 4.4% of the initial values, the wrists by 13.2% (Pařízková 1968a,d, 1970b, 1970c).

Gradually the *boys differed most markedly as regards body composition. LBM in per cent was highest in group I starting with the second year of the investigation,* while in group IV the LBM was lowest. Between the 1st and 5th year of investigation the percentage of LBM in group I increased significantly while in group IV it remained the same. *The absolute amount of LBM was also greatest in group I* (Table 34) (Pařízková 1968a,d). The reverse applies to the percentage of body fat. In the first year of the investigation there were no significant differences between groups with different physical activity but in the *last year the percentage of fat was lowest in group I* and highest in group IV (Table 34). *The absolute amount of body fat did not change in boys of group I,* despite the great change in total body weight, i.e. *body weight increased only as a result of the development of LBM*. In group IV the absolute weight of body fat increased significantly (Table 34) (Pařízková 1968a,d, 1970b,c).

The composition of weight increments in various years thus differed: in certain periods only LBM increased, in others fat also participated in the weight increments. There are, however, *also periods* where the *increment of LBM was greater than the weight increment because there was a simultaneous decline of body fat* (e.g. between 13–14 years).

Several tens of relative measurements characterizing body build were evaluated (Pařízková 1965-6, 1967, 1968a,d). It was revealed that the most typical relative dimension is the biiliocristal diameter (bicristal) expressed in per cent of the value of height or shoulder breadth (biacromial). *The most active and leanest boys of group I had the relatively narrowest pelvis*—in the last year the difference was statistically significant (Fig. 50).

The above changes in body composition confronted with total body weight also elucidate the absence of difference in circumferences of extremities (in those engaged in training usually greater circumference is assumed to be due to increased musculature). In inactive boys the smaller muscle mass was compensated by an increased body fat layer, the reverse being true in the active boys. This is also apparent from

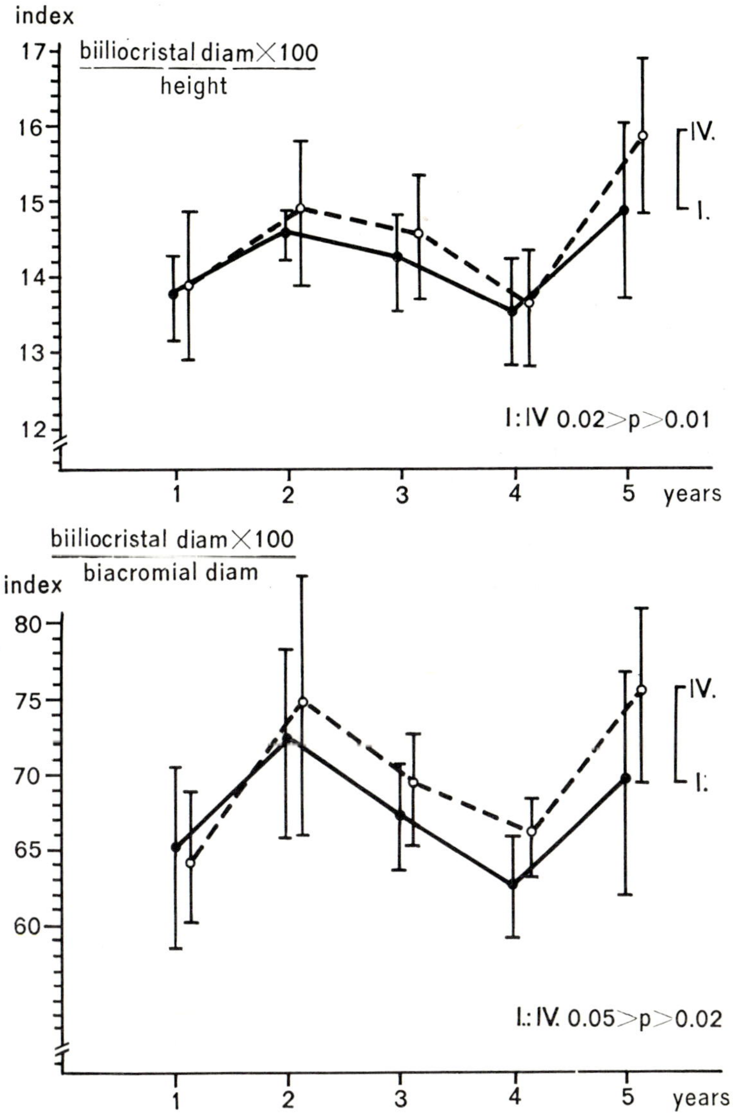

Fig. 50. Development of relative dimensions ($\bar{x} \pm SD$) characterizing the changes in relative pelvic breadth in groups of boys with different physical activity regime (—●——●——● I – highest physical activity; ○--○--○ IV = lowest physical activity followed from 10.7 (1) up to 14.7 (5) years (1961 – 5) (Pařízková 1968).

TABLE 34.
Mean values ($\bar{x} \pm$ SD) of relative fat (%) and absolute lean body mass (kg LBM) in groups of boys with different physical activity regime followed longitudinally during five years (from 10.7 up to 14.7 years of age — 1961—5; n = 96) (Pařízková 1968a,b)

Group		1 1961		2 1962		3 1963		4 1964		5 1965	
		$\bar{x}$	SD	$\bar{x}$	SD	$\bar{x}$	SD	$\bar{x}$	SD	x	SD
I	% fat	15.7	5.4	14.1	5.7	12.7	1.5	9.7	3.3	9.9	4.6
	kg LBM	31.6	3.3	35.0	3.8	40.4	5.4	45.5	6.8	54.4	7.1
II	% fat	15.5	5.6	13.5	5.9	12.4	4.7	11.4	4.1	12.5	4.1
	kg LBM	30.2	4.3	33.8	4.5	37.9	5.3	44.1	7.2	49.1	8.3
III	% fat	14.7	6.4	14.5	7.5	14.8	5.7	12.5	5.9	13.6	4.2
	kg LBM	31.0	3.1	34.1	3.4	37.3	3.6	43.9	5.1	49.7	5.4
IV	% fat	17.2	6.2	19.1	6.0	16.6	5.9	14.7	4.4	15.9	5.4
	kg LBM	31.4	3.3	33.8	3.9	37.8	4.6	43.8	6.3	49.6	6.6

skinfold thickness (Pařízková 1968a,b, 1970a,b,c). The described results seem to indicate that *increased physical activity during growth, during the prepubertal and pubertal period modified somatic development not only by promoting the development of LBM at the expense of fat but also promoted a typical "virile" stature* (i.e. a *relatively narrow pelvis*—Pařízková 1968a,d, 1970b,c).

3. Body composition in relation to aerobic capacity in boys

An intensive regime of physical activity and regular physical training along with changes in body composition leads to greater fitness of the organism: investigations of aerobic capacity by measuring the *maximum oxygen consumption* (max O_2) during a graded load on a treadmill (Šprynarová 1966) made together with other measurements revealed a *more marked development in the active boys of group I. The values of aerobic capacity in this group were highest when expressed in absolute figures and also in relation to body weight and LBM* (Fig. 51) (Šprynarová and Pařízková 1962, 1975). Differences between groups developed only after a certain duration of the regime of physical activity, i.e. during the 3rd investigation, i.e. at 12.7 years.

Differences in aerobic capacity were not caused merely by a greater LBM as was shown in group I but also by a higher value of the maximum oxygen consumption in relation to LBM (this difference was significant only in the third year of the investigation). In general the differences between groups were most marked in the

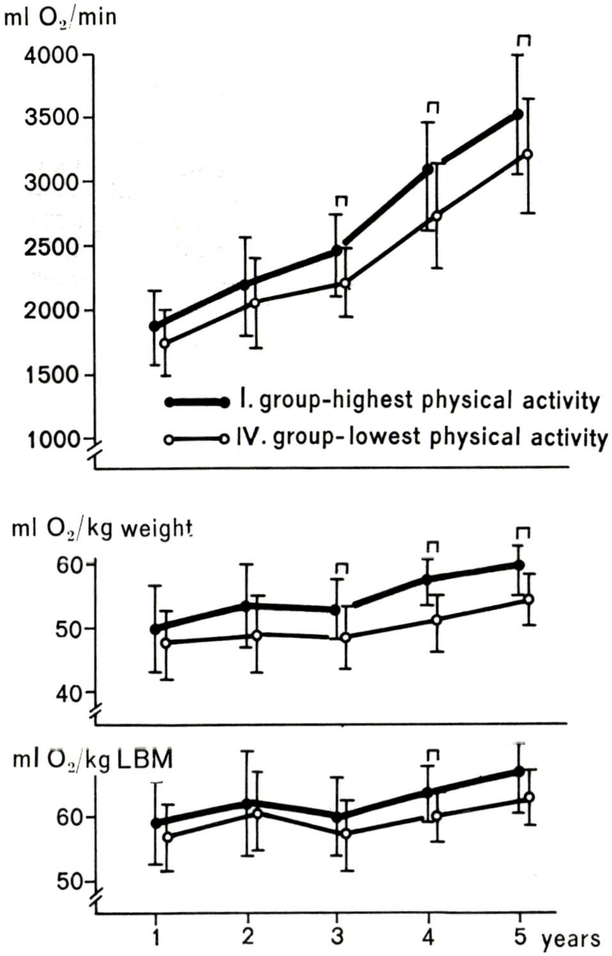

Fig. 51. Development of aerobic capacity, i.e. maximal oxygen uptake, expressed in absolute (above — ml O_2/min) and relative (middle — ml O_2/min/kg body weight; bottom — ml O_2/min/kg LBM) values in groups of boys with most intensive (I —●—●—●—) and least intensive physical activity regime (IV ○———○) followed from 10.7 (1) up to 14.7 (5) years (1961–5) (Šprynarová and Pařízková 1975, Pařízková and Šprynarová 1967, 1970). ⌐¬ p at least 0.05.

fourth year of the investigation when the differences in the regime of activity were also greates (Pařízková and Šprynarová 1968, 1975). Evaluation of increments of aerobic capacity revealed also the significantly greatest increase in group I (Šprynarová 1966).

The increased aerobic capacity in relation to LBM proves moreover a greater efficiency of the cardiovascular and respiratory apparatus (Buskirk and Taylor 1957),

TABLE 35.
Correlation coefficients (r) of the relationship between height, weight, lean body mass and oxygen consumption at rest, during standard and maximal work loads in boys from 10.7—14.7 years of age (n = 92) (Pařízková and Šprynarová 1968, 1970, 1975).

				1	2	3	4	5
			Year	1961	1962	1963	1964	1965
Oxygen consumption	Rest		Height	0.330	0.477	0.504	0.581	0.375
			Weight	0.376	0.453	0.629	0.615	0.505
			LBM	0.409	0.468	0.599	0.628	0.555
	Work load	Standard	Height	0.459	0.508	0.555	0.687	0.527
			Weight	0.722	0.765	0.862	0.861	0.790
			LBM	0.680	0.610	0.806	0.812	0.721
		Maximal	Height	0.571	0.531	0.663	0.755	0.718
			Weight	0.661	0.692	0.731	0.804	0.821
			LBM	0.599	0.680	0.779	0.868	0.850

which was manifested also by a *higher oxygen pulse in group I* (Šprynarová 1966). Ventilation, maximum pulse rate etc. did not differ in different groups, nor did various functional parameters (ventilation, oxygen consumption, pulse rate during a standard load of 60 W on a bicycle ergometer—Ulbrich 1971). *The maximum oxygen consumption, one of the most typical indicators of physical fitness along with LBM which both develop under the influence of physical activity, take a parallel course.* We analyzed therefore the relationship of these two indicators in more detail.

The relationship of maximum oxygen consumption was closer to LBM than to total body weight starting at the age of 12.7 (third year of investigation). During the first two years of the longitudinal study the relationship was closer with total body weight. In adults in the third decade Buskirk and Taylor (1957) demonstrated a much closer relationship between maximal oxygen consumption and LBM than with body weight. During growth this relationship obviously develops gradually in the course of puberty (Table 35) (Pařízková and Šprynarová 1968, 1970).

Next we analyzed the relationship of aerobic capacity per kg LBM and percentage body fat. In the above boys we found a negative relationship—the higher the maximum oxygen consumption per 1 kg LBM, the lower the percentage of fat in the organism. The high level of aerobic processes in LBM prevents more marked deposition of depot fat.

4. Functional characteristics and composition of weight increments in boys with different physical activity during adolescence

The longitudinal study of boys proceeded for another three years up to the average age of 17.7 years in a reduced number of boys (group I – III) who attended examinations (n = 41—Pařízková 1970a – c, 1972h). Analysis of indicators assessed during the 1st to 5th year in boys who remained in our experimental groups throughout the experiment from 10.7 – 17.7 years and in those who dropped out revealed that there were no significant differences in morphological or functional indicators, i.e. discontinued participation was not conditioned by lower fitness, retarded development, etc. (Šprynarová 1974). That means that the conclusions of the eight-year investigation in the smaller group correspond to the previous findings covering a shorter period of time and presented in Tables 33 – 35 and in Fig. 50.

The data were analyzed using the repeat measures analysis of variace (ANOVA) because of the dependence inherent in measuring the same subjects in eight test sessions. Post hoc comparisons of the differences between group means were made using the Student-Newman-Keul (SNK) procedure (Sokal and Rohlf 1968). Because of the unequal number of subjects in the groups each comparison between groups was done individually and involved a range of eight differences. The ANOVA results showed that for each parameter the groups were statistically different. As could be expected the years were significant due to growth. *The most active group (I) was clearly different from the least active group in that boys were significantly taller at each annual measurement* (Fig. 52); this group was significantly *heavier than the inactive group only during the last two years* (Fig. 53). *The greater body weight of the most active group was due to a greater lean body mass* (significantly greater since the third year of our study) *and less fat* (percentage of body fat significantly lower since the second year—Fig. 54 and 55). Skeletal age of the groups did not differ (Pařízková 1974b). Along with differences in body composition *differences in body build also persisted, characterized in particular by a narrow pelvis in the most active boys with the largest ratio of LBM and lowest body fat ratio* (Pařízková 1972h).

In this smaller group we analyzed separately the *composition of weight increments in individual years* (Fig. 56). In some periods LBM and fat increased in certain ratios, while in others the LBM increased. *Between the second and fourth, and sixth and eighth years the increments of LBM were greater than the total weight increments as the amount of body fat simultaneously declined.* The composition of increments differed also by groups—the most active boys of group I did not deposit any fat between the fourth and fifth year of the investigation, while we observed an increment between the sixth and seventh year, where in the remaining groups body fat declined. Group I displayed thus in this respect a more rapid development (Pařízková 1970a, 1972e,h).

Analysis of functional results also confirmed the significantly different development of aerobic capacity depending on the extent of physical activity in boys. Measu-

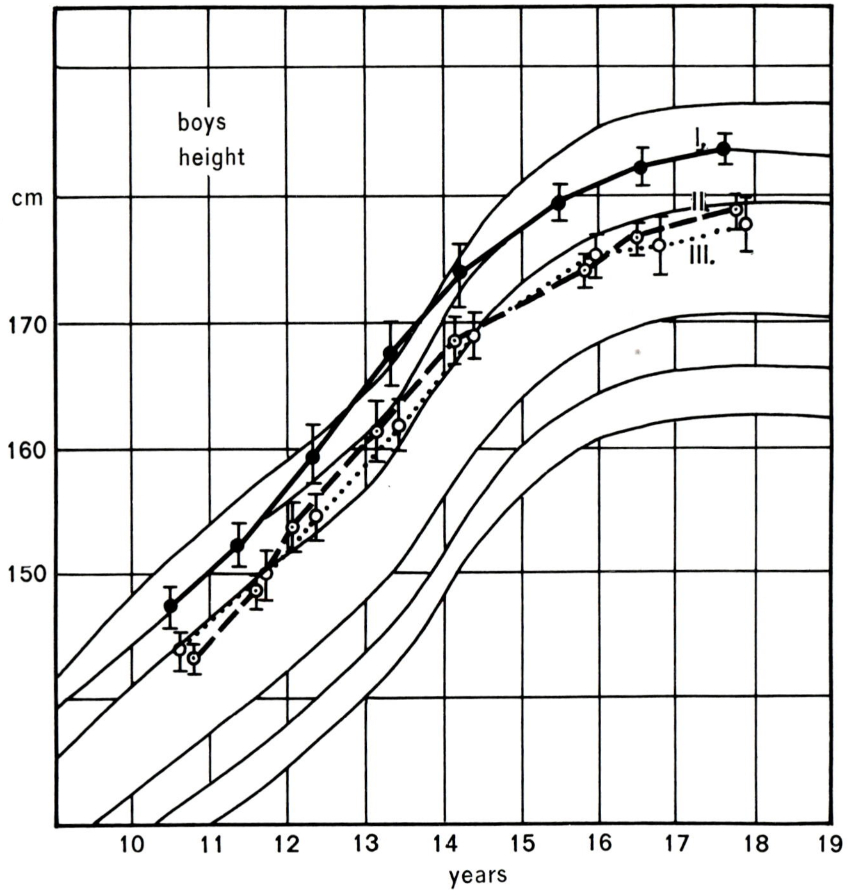

Fig. 52. Development of height ($\bar{x} \pm SE$) in groups of 41 boys with different physical activity regime (I. = highest intensity; III. = lowest intensity of exercise) followed longitudinally during eight years (1961–8). Presented on the background of growth grid of Tanner et al. (1966) (Pařízková 1972h).

rements during the first year revealed a wide range of initial values of max O_2/kg body weight in boys with the highest physical activity indicating that the group which was engaged regularly in training recruited boys with all levels of aerobic capacity and thus did not differ from the remaining groups. *In absolute values of maximum oxygen consumption significant differences were found in the last before one year and last year* (i.e. the *highest values in boys with the greater physical activity); in relation to body weight* (max O_2/kg *weight*) *the values recorded in the most active boys were significantly higher during the second, fifth and seventh year of the investigation. The highest values in all groups* were reached *in the 4th and 5th year. In active boys no marked drop was recorded;* it was, however, significant in boys with the lowest

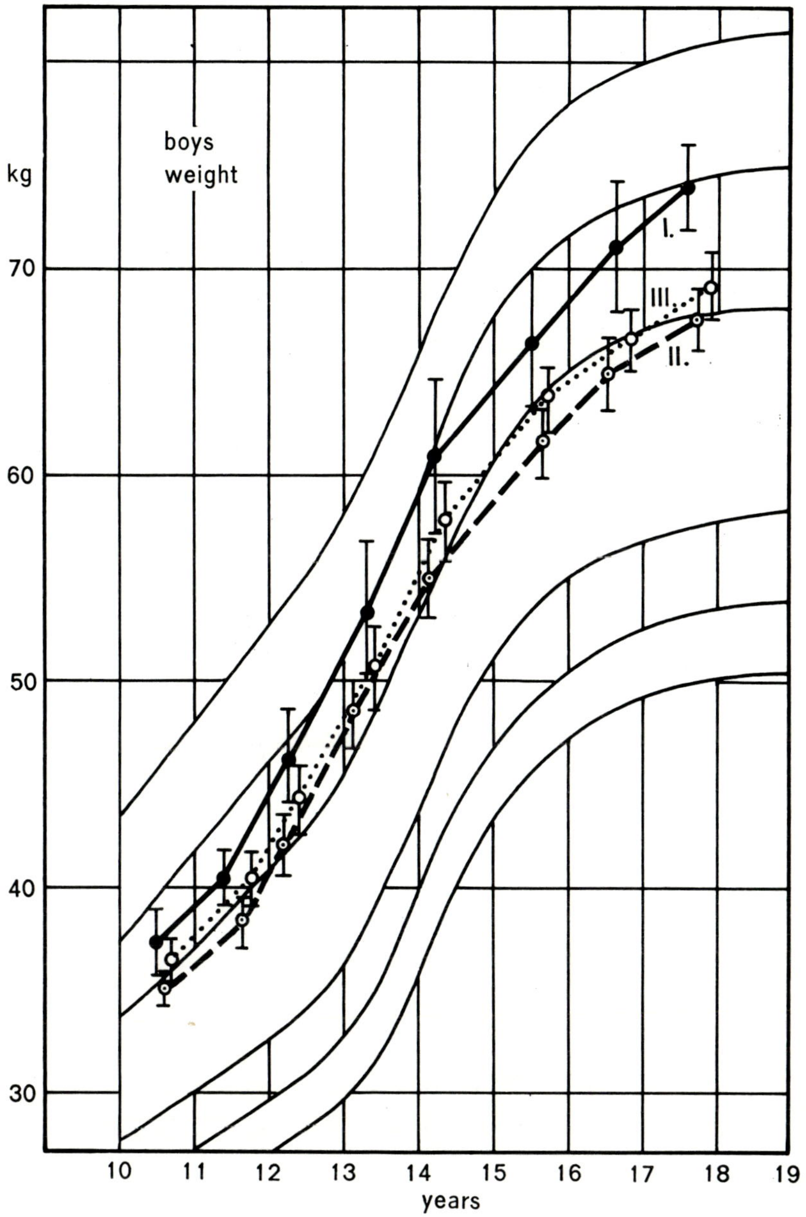

Fig. 53. Development of weight ($\bar{x} \pm SE$) in groups of 41 boys with different physical activity regime followed longitudinally (for explanation *see* Fig. 52), presented on the background of the growth grid of Tanner et al. (1966).

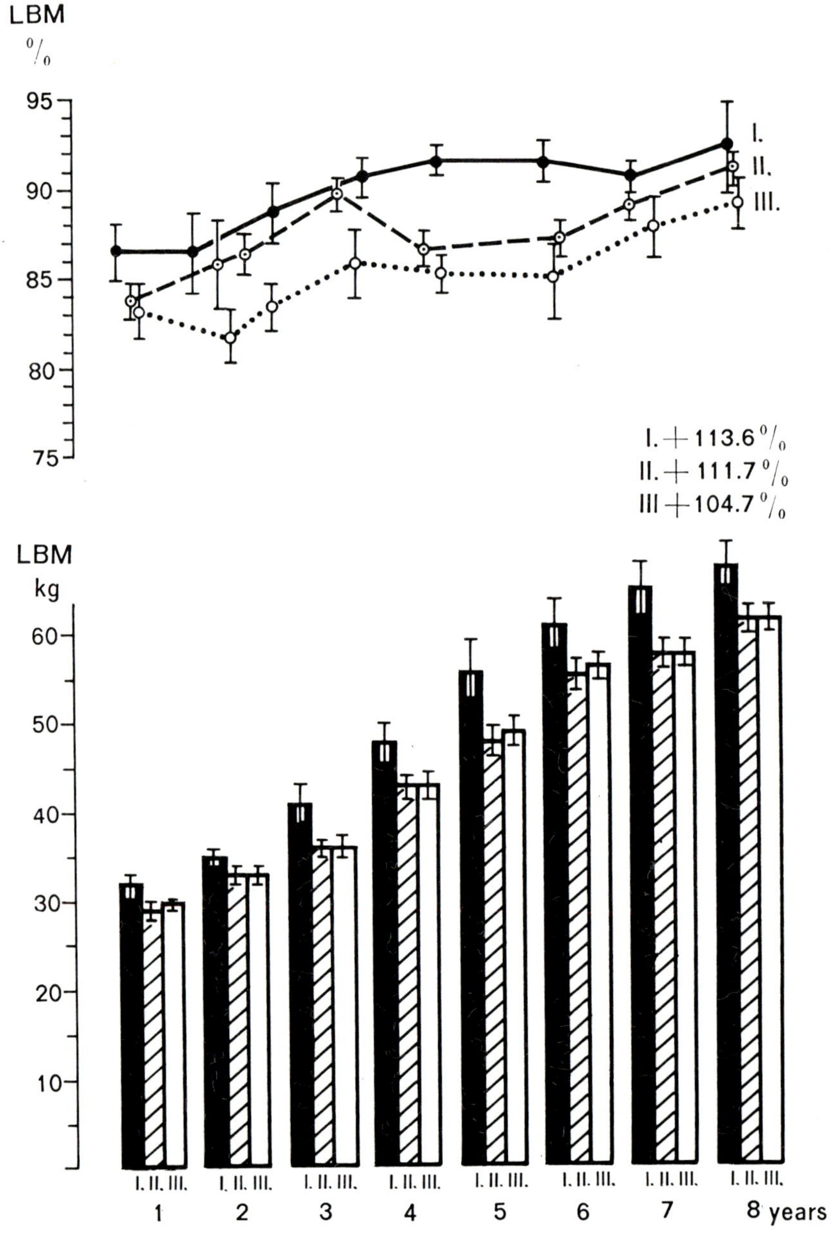

Fig. 54. Development of relative (% — upper part) and absolute (kg — lower part; $\bar{x} \pm$ SE) amount of lean body mass in groups of 41 boys with different physical activity regime (n = 41; I = highest intensity; III = lowest intensity) followed longitudinally during eight years (1st–8th, i.e. 1961–8) (Pařízková 1970a–c, 1972g).

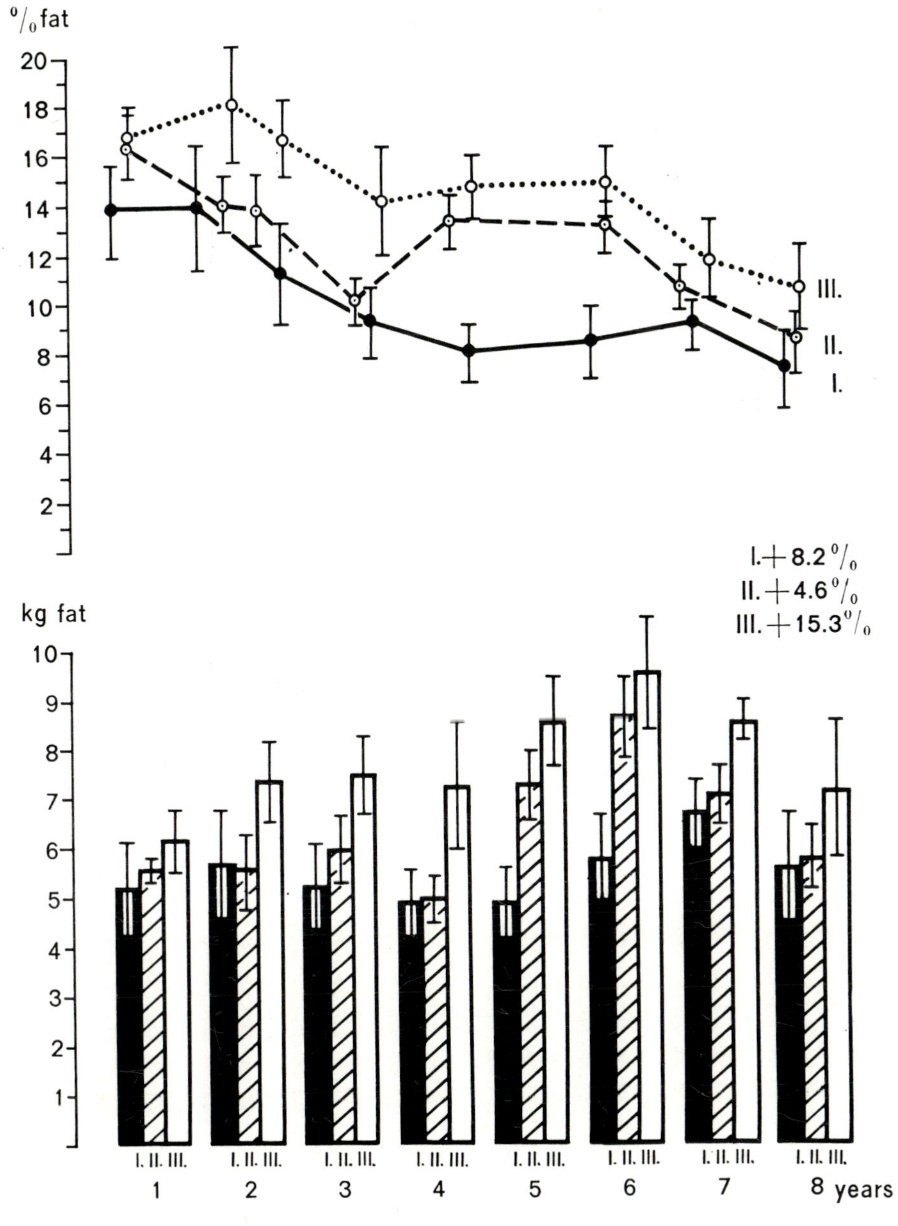

Fig. 55. Development of relative (% — upper part) and absolute (kg — lower part; $\bar{x} \pm$ SE) amount of depot fat in groups of 41 boys with different physical activity regime (for explanation *see* Fig. 54).

activity (Table 36). It was of interest that *before the peak values were reached 4–4.5 hours of sports training in the most active boys sufficed to increase the relative aerobic capacity; however, after that period six hours per week were needed to prevent a significant drop in the aerobic capacity* and to maintain significant differences between groups (Šprynarová 1974, Šprynarová and Pařízková 1975).

The *highest values of aerobic capacity* expressed as max O_2 in relation to total or lean body mass *were in agreement with the peak values of the relative heart volume* (assessed by teleroentgenography in a recumbent position at the end of expiration—Čermák 1969, and calculated according to Musshoff and Reindell—1956). Developmental changes of absolute and relative values of the heart volume are given in Fig. 57 which demonstrates the results in a group of boys mentioned previously but not differentiated by physical activity. *Comparison of boys with the highest and lowest physical activity indicates higher values of relative heart size in the most active boys* (values up to the age of 11.7 years are given) throughout the period of investigation. The differences remained almost the same (Table 37).

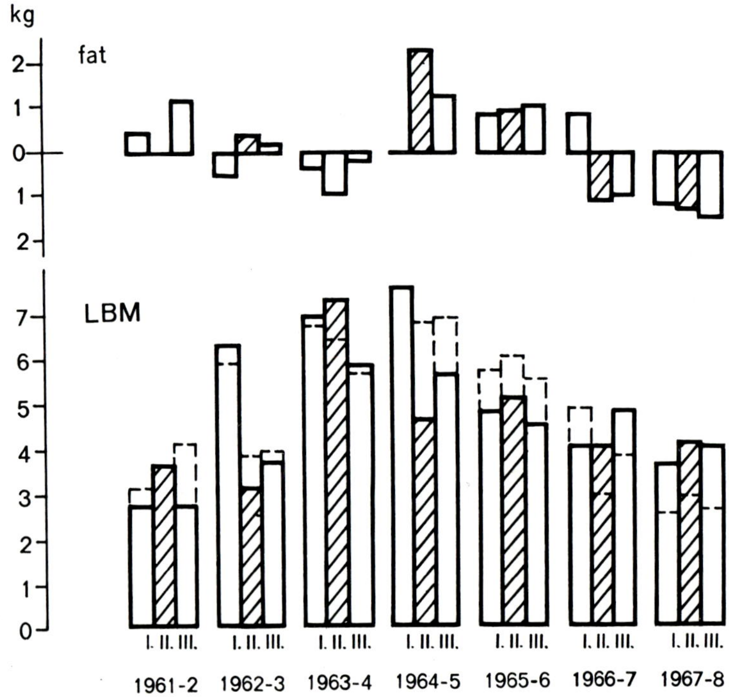

Fig. 56. Composition of weight increments in individual years (1961–8) in groups of 41 boys adapted to different motor activity regime (group I — highest activity; III — lowest activity). Fat increments — upper part; lean body mass increments — lower part; hatched lines in lower columns represent total body weight increments (Pařízková 1972a,g).

TABLE 36.
Mean values ($\bar{x} \pm SD$) of maximal oxygen consumption (ml/min/kg body weight or lean body mass) in groups of boys with different physical activity regime (I — highest intensity of training, III — lowest intensity of training followed up from 10.7 up to 17.7 years of age (1961—8)
(Šprynarová 1974; Šprynarová and Pařízková 1975)

Years		1 1961	2 1962	3 1963	4 1964	5 1965	6 1966	7 1967	8 1968
Max O_2/kg weight									
I	$\bar{x}$	48.9	52.8	51.6	58.3	58.4	57.3	54.7	55.4
(n = 8)	SD	7.75	4.71	5.27	2.54	3.35	4.78	3.34	4.65
III	$\bar{x}$	45.1	46.6	47.5	52.3	53.8	52.3	47.3	46.3
(n = 12)	SD	4.17	5.86	5.54	6.48	3.79	8.70	3.32	6.01
Max O_2/kg LBM									
I	$\bar{x}$	57.8	62.5	59.6	64.5	65.5	63.81	60.3	59.9
	SD	9.59	8.88	8.02	2.68	5.62	5.59	4.15	6.20
III	$\bar{x}$	53.8	57.0	57.4	60.6	63.7	61.79	53.6	52.1
	SD	4.82	7.50	5.08	4.01	4.28	8.08	3.23	6.81

TABLE 37
Changes in relative heart volume, i.e. ml/kg body weight ($\bar{x} \pm SD$) in groups of boys differing maximally in physical activity regime (I and III) followed from 11.7 to 17.7 years of age (Čermák 1976, in press).

		2 1962	3 1963	4 1964	5 1965	6 1966	7 1967	8 1968
group I	$\bar{x}$	11.93	12.62	13.46	13.15	12.58	12.76	11.76
	SD	1.34	0.68	1.05	1.63	1.47	1.20	0.75
group III	$\bar{x}$	10.64	10.84	11.56	11.60	10.56	11.18	10.34
	SD	0.96	1.20	1.09	1.42	1.17	1.24	1.13

It thus seems that *boys engaged in systematic training already displayed primarily certain, mainly morphological, differences (taller stature, greater relative heart volume) which may imply a certain disposition for greater activity and performance capacity.* The *body composition and aerobic capacity change more markedly only after a certain period of adaptation to a greater load* (Pařízková 1975c). Differences were moreover manifested in boys engaged and not engaged in sports (investigated only during the first four years of the longitudinal study in groups which were roughly equal to the groups mentioned in the five-year investigation (*see* Table 33–35 and Fig. 50) with regards to *muscular strength* and *performance in selected disciplines* (e.g. running, jumping etc.) (Sukop 1966, Juřinová 1968). *Interest in sports and the ability to persevere in long-term training is obviously conditioned among others by certain prerequisites and properties which develop* and *expand further in the course of regular*

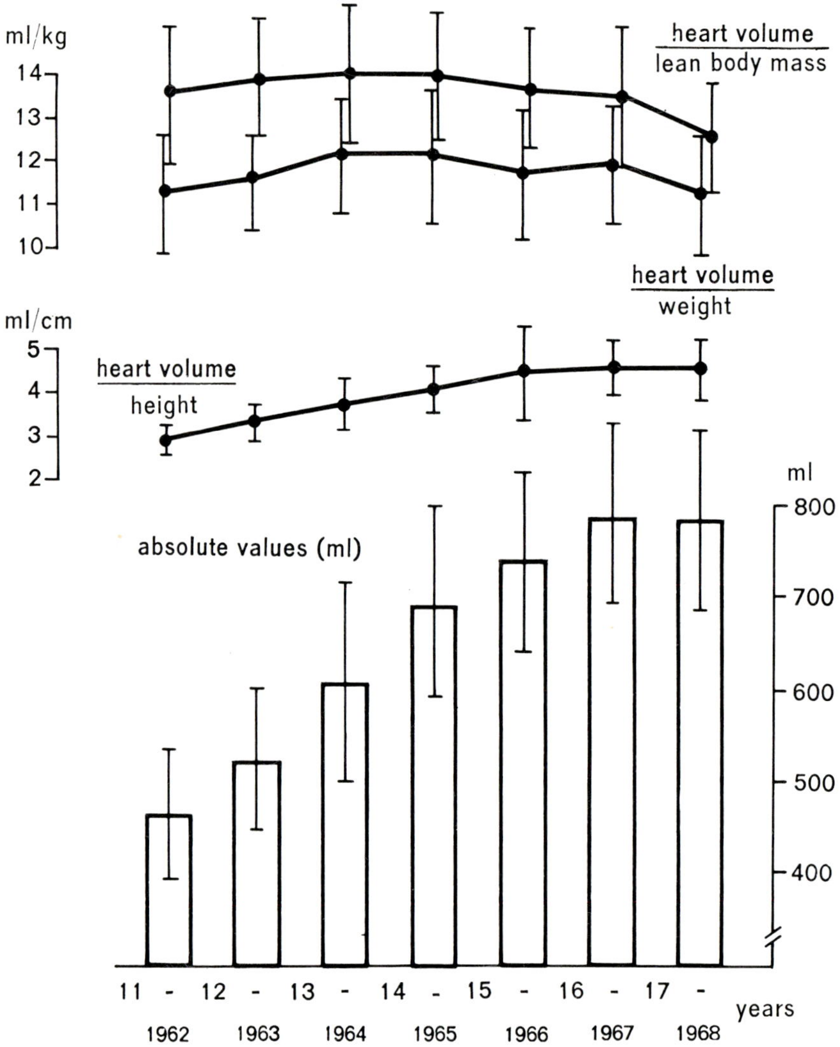

Fig. 57. Mean values ($\bar{x} \pm$ SD) of absolute (ml) and relative values of heart volume (ml/kg weight or LBM, and ml/cm height) in 39 boys followed up longitudinally from 11.7 up to 17.7 years of age (Čermák and Pařízková 1974; Pařízková and Čermák 1975).

training. This is essential in particular for *sports at a higher level*. Nevertheless *adaptation to an increased load is also manifested very clearly in individuals without this disposition* or even subjects handicapped in a certain sense, in body composition as well as aerobic capacity and performance which was demonstrated most clearly, e.g. in obese children (*see* chapter IX).

5. Stability of body composition characteristics in boys during adolescence

It is known that basic somatic characteristics such as height and weight display during development a considerable stability. On this various growth grids are based (Wetzel 1942, Tanner et al. 1966, Kapalín 1967 etc.). From the above growth data assembled in groups of boys (I – IV) during five years (n = 96) as well as eight years (n = 39 – 41) we analyzed the stability of height and weight as well as of selected characteristics of body composition. We used the method of correlation analysis of the relationship between values recorded during the first and fifth year and the first and eighth year. (Slightly differing numbers of boys are due to the fact that in some cases not all the boys had always all the measurements done).

After the shorter period the correlations were in all instances closer for height, body weight, percentage and absolute amount of LBM and fat (Table 38). The highest values of *r* were proved for height, body weight, absolute amount of LBM and fat. The relative values of LBM and fat correlated less closely. The conclusions from analyses of measurements made in 96 as well as 41 boys during the same period of time were in agreement (Pařízková 1972a,h).

After the longer time interval all relationships were less close. The *closest relationship between the first and eighth year was found between values of height and absolute amount of LBM in kg.* The lower *r* values in the first and eighth year were obviously due to the fact that the relationship between relative and absolute values of fat disappeared the latter being a very variable somatic component during this period.

TABLE 38
Correlation coefficients (r) of the relationships between anthropometric measurements assessed during the 1st and 5th, and 1st and 8th year of the longitudinal study (1961—8) in 96 and 41 boys resp. (Pařízková 1972e,h)

	11 : 15 (n = 96)	11 : 15 (n = 41)	11 : 18 (n = 41)
Height	0.83	0.86	0.68
Weight	0.80	0.80	0.50
LBM (%)	0.40	0.35	(0.20)
LBM (kg)	0.58	0.68	0.60
Fat (%)	0.33	0.35	(0.20)
Fat (kg)	0.66	0.51	0.25
Skinfolds:			
Triceps	0.65	0.65	0.37
Subscapular	0.59	0.75	0.30
Abdomen	0.66	0.76	0.54
Suprailiac	0.70	0.81	0.51
Calf	0.71	0.60	0.32

Values in parentheses are not significant

TABLE 39
Relationships between values of height, weight, lean body mass and fat measured repeatedly in 39 boys from 10.7 up to 17.7 years of age (1961–8) (Pařízková 1970b,c, 1972h) (cm, kg)

Years of measurement	1	2	3	4	5	6	7	8
	1961	1962	1963	1964	1965	1966	1967	1968
Correlation coefficients r:								
Height: weight	0.43	0.69	0.75	0.78	0.78	0.59	n.s.	0.41
Height: LBM	0.54	0.75	0.81	0.89	0.84	0.66	0.58	0.59
Weight: LBM	0.92	0.82	0.89	0.92	0.92	0.85	0.48	0.80
Weight: fat	0.71	n.s.	0.51	0.43	n.s.	0.46	n.s.	0.45

n.s. — not significant

The distribution and *absolute values of skinfold thicknesses proved also to be a very stable somatic characteristic* (Table 38). The correlation coefficients *r* were again higher for values assessed during the shorter period of time; *skinfolds on the trunk had a tendency to correlate somewhat more closely* than skinfolds on the extremities. In all instances the relationships were significant. *The pattern of subcutaneous fat distribution is thus a more constant sign than total body fat* (Pařízková 1972a,h).

The results indicate that *not only the most basic somatic characteristics* such *as height* but also *the absolute amount of LBM together with the distribution of subcutaneous fat are stable somatic signs during growth and development* and have *under normal stable living conditions a constant trend.* The relative amount of LBM and fat, on the other hand, are very variable, obviously because they depend on the actual energy turnover and equilibrium rather than constitutional factors.

As regards relations between height, body weight and individual components we found the *closest relationship between weight and LBM* (Table 39) which was constant throughout the period of investigation from 10.7 to 17.7 years. The other relationships were less close and more *age-dependent,* i.e. the *closest relationship was reached during the peak of puberty and growth* in the majority of boys (13.7 – 14.7 years). Least close was the relationship between weight and body fat (Pařízková 1972h, 1976). Similar relations were found e.g. by Forbes (1975), Falkner (1975) etc.

The increase in body weight and LBM is most closely related to height velocity: when we evaluated increments of body weight, LBM and fat with regard to the year when peak of the height velocity was reached (i.e. the greatest increment per year from the whole period of investigation) the *period of maximum weight and LBM increments was in agreement with the period of maximum height increments* (Fig. 58). Increments of body fat evaluated in the entire group regardless of physical activity varied insignificantly throughout the period of investigation without any obvious relationship to the peak height velocity (Pařízková 1976). Evaluation of these changes

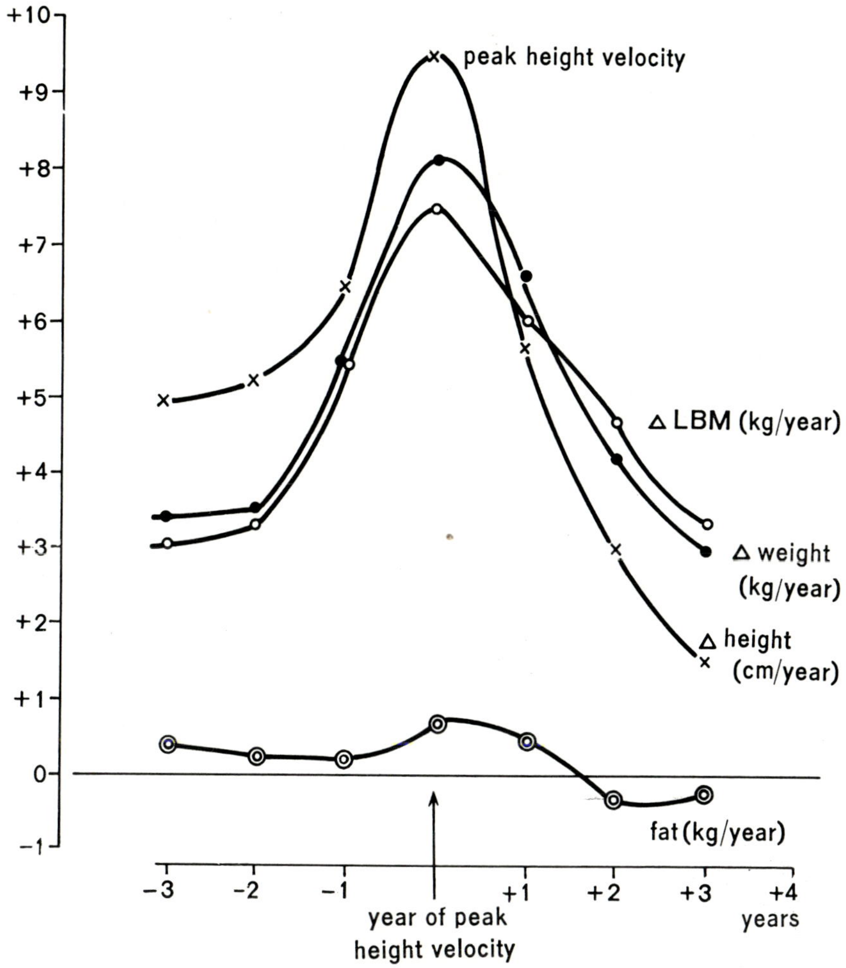

Fig. 58. Changes in increments of LBM, total body weight and fat (Δ in kg) by the year of peak height velocity in boys from 10.7 up to 17.7 years of age (n = 40; Pařízková 1976).

in different groups (divided according to physical activity) was made more difficult by the small number of subjects and their considerable variability.

Stability in the development of LBM ensues also from the evaluation of selected individuals in relation to mean values of LBM ($\bar{x} \pm SD$) calculated for the whole group of boys. Fig. 59 presents examples of longitudinal data of a boy with accelerated growth, i.e. higher values of height and bone age (from the group with the greatest physical activity—I), a boy with an average development and finally a boy who displayed as regards height and bone age slight retardation. As apparent from Fig. 59,

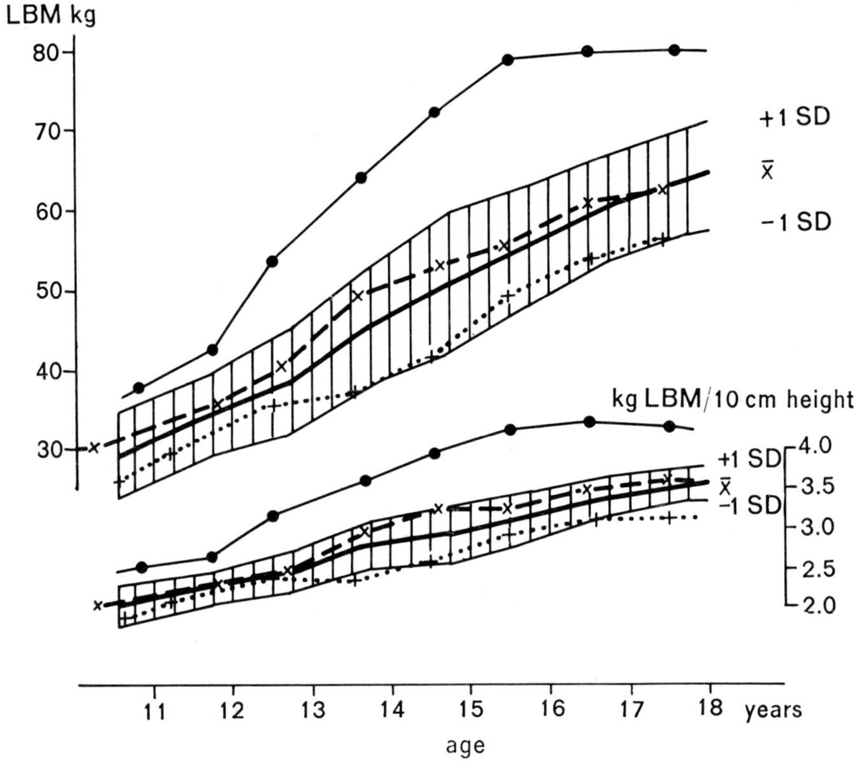

Fig. 59. Changes in LBM of three boys in relation to age on the background of developmental grid for LBM (mean absolute values in kg ± 1 SD) gained in 41 boys from 10.7 up to 17.7 years of age — upper part; mean relative values, i.e. LBM/10 cm body height ± 1 SD — lower part of the figure) (Pařízková 1976).

these boys adhered approximately the same pattern of somatic development throughout the period of investigation. This was demonstrated not only by comparison of absolute values of LBM but also when eliminating the influence of height, i.e. when relating kg of LBM/10 cm of height (lower half of Fig. 59). In the accelerated boy after some time also the influence of regular exercise was manifested by a relatively accelerated increase of LBM (Pařízková 1975c, 1976).

The parallel trend of the greatest increments of height, body weight and LBM points to the *important influence of maturation of the organism on the development of body components* and organs: we therefore also analyzed the *relationship of bone age to height, weight, body composition* and *heart volume* in individual years of the study. The analysis was made by correlations; Fig. 60 demonstrated changes of these relations during adolescence. *Only body weight displayed a close significant relationship with bone age throughout the period of investigation from 10.7 to 17.7 years;*

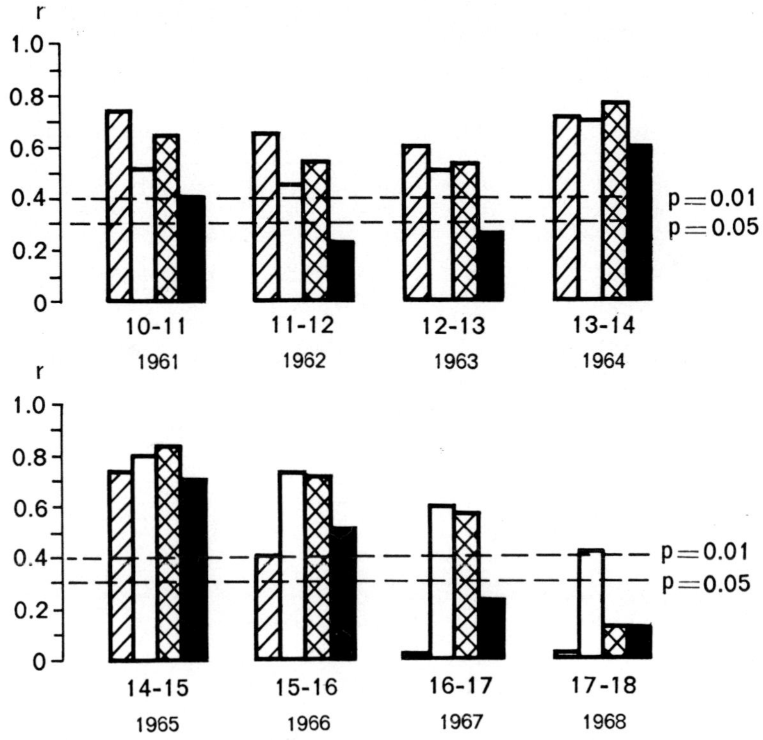

Fig. 60. Changes in the relationship (r) between values of height, weight, LBM and heart volume on the one hand, and bone age on the other hand measured longitudinally every year in 39 boys from 10.7 up to 17.7 years of age (Pařízková 1975c) (▨ = height; □ = weight; ⊠ = lean body mass; ■ = = heart volume).

the *correlation between height and bone age* disappeared *already between the 16th and 17th years.* The *loosest relationship with bone age* was that with the *heart volume* (Pařízková 1975c; Pařízková and Čermák 1975, in press) *which otherwise correlated most closely with LBM ($r = 0.490-0.842$)* (Čermák and Pařízková 1974, 1975); it *correlated significantly with bone age throughout the period of investigation except for the last year.* The period of the closest relations of height, body weight and LBM to bone age was between 13.7 and 14.7 years.

Longitudinal data on height (10.7–17.7 years) were used in our laboratory also for the *verification of the regression equations of Walker* (1974) and *tables of Bayley and Pinneau* (1952) for the prediction of height. As regards *means of the height* for the whole group the *results of both mentioned methods corresponded to the values of actual height* ($r = 0.6-0.9$), *and also mutually*. The analysis showed that in 60–70% boys before puberty the predicted values differed from the actual ones by not more

TABLE 40
Mean values ($\bar{x} \pm$ SD) of height, weight and body composition in 16 males followed up from 10.7 up to 23.7 years of age (1961—1974) (Pařízková 1976)

		1 1961	2 1962	3 1963	4 1964	5 1965	6 1966	7 1967	8 1968	14 1974
Height	$\bar{x}$	144.2	149.0	154.8	162.7	169.6	174.8	178.2	178.6	180.0
(cm)	SD	4.6	4.8	5.7	7.0	6.5	5.5	5.9	5.2	6.0
Weight	$\bar{x}$	36.6	39.8	44.3	50.3	57.7	64.0	67.3	70.7	77.3
(kg)	SD	3.9	4.6	5.8	7.4	8.0	6.5	5.8	6.2	9.4
Fat	$\bar{x}$	15.8	16.9	15.0	11.2	13.0	12.0	12.8	10.3	11.9
(%)	SD	3.9	7.0	5.3	3.6	4.9	4.6	4.2	5.7	6.2
LBM	$\bar{x}$	30.5	32.9	37.5	44.6	50.2	56.2	58.6	63.3	68.1
(kg)	SD	3.4	3.9	4.8	6.3	7.5	6.1	5.6	5.2	4.9

than 2.5 cm; after puberty this percentage increased considerably.—30–40% boys achieved marginal values of body height in both the positive and negative sense. In some of them a fluctuation of the speed of the bone maturation, i.e. consecutive acceleration and retardation occurred, and also the results of the prediction when using both mentioned methods varied markedly.—*Individual prediction of height was least reliable during puberty*, the beginning of which is individually different; for this reason in this period the evaluation of bone age was mostly important. The above mentioned analysis showed that *in approximately two thirds of boys it is possible to predict the development of height with satisfactory precision*, e.g. for the selection of certain somatotypes for special sport disciplines, etc. (Ulbrichová, in press).

Somatic development proceeded after the age of 17.7 years. After the subsequent six years, i.e. at the age of 23.7 we were again able to measure only 16 boys (Table 40). Height, weight and LBM increased significantly. The percentage of body fat declined up to the 4th year of the investigation; then varied insignificantly, i.e. changes in different subjects differed. The number of subjects did not render an analysis of physical activity possible.

6. Influence of physical activity on stability of somatotype in boys during adolescence

The technique of *somatotyping* has been estabilished as useful for *describing total body form.* Sheldon et al. (1954) have claimed that the somatotype is genetically determined and does not alter throughout life. However, this claim has been questioned by several investigators and adaptations of Sheldon's earlier somatotype methods have been made. Because the somatotype rating depends on the assumption underlying different rating methods, results of studies can be in conflict. Where, however, ratings have been allowed to vary for the individual, as is appropriate in growth studies, changes in somatotypes of children and adults have been observed. With respect to the influence of physical activity, the Medford boys growth study showed that outstanding athletes who were assumed to have more physical training and activity, showed a greater mesomorphy and lower endomorphy than non-athletes. Ross and Day (1972) found that in competitive skiers (boys and girls aged 6 to 14) the most successful were more ectomesomorphic than the least successful, however, the direct effect of physical activity on these results was not investigated. Studies on young and old men undergoing physical training have shown that somatotypes change significantly, but longitudinal studies are needed to assess the influence of physical activity on somatotype in growing children.

The purposes of this part of the study were to examine the stability of somatotypes in the above-mentioned group of boys followed for eight years, and to determine the effects of different physical activity levels on somatotypes. 39 boys followed up longitudinally (*see* Fig. 52–60, Table 36–40) were analyzed. The somatotypes were assessed by Heath-Carter anthropometric somatotype method (Carter and Heath 1971).

The somatotype distribution of the boys was plotted for each year on a somatochart; the somatoplots at 10.7 and 17.7 years were chosen for comparative analysis (Fig. 61a,b). The subjects were grouped according to their somatotype component dominance, and a contingency test was applied to test the significance of the differences in the distributions at the two ages. The obtained X^2 was not significant, indicating no differences in somatochart distribution among the two years. *The mean somatotype for the total group at the two age points was* $2^1/_2 - 4 - 3^1/_2$.

Next we examined the *changes in the individual somatotype components for the total group and the activity sub-groups.* For the total group, the boys at ages 10.7, 11.7, 13.7 and 17.7 were more endomorphic than they were at ages 14.7 and 15.7. While the mesomorphic were more so at 17.7 than they were at 15.7 and less ectomorphic at 17.7 than at 13.7, 14.7 and 15.7. *When analyzed according to activity group, the high and low activity group means showed no differences in the components during 11.7 to 17.7 years,* however, the moderate activity group showed some differences in all three components, and therefore seems to be the group which contribute most to the overall group differences observed earlier.

The previous results based on the group distributions and values produced *little evidence for marked change in the boys' somatotypes.* Next, we examined the *individual patterns of the boys' somatotypes.* First the relationship between the individual component ratings from year to year were examined by calculating the Pearson product moment correlation coefficients. In general, the correlations are highest for mesomorphy, next highest for ectomorphy, and lowest for endomorphy.

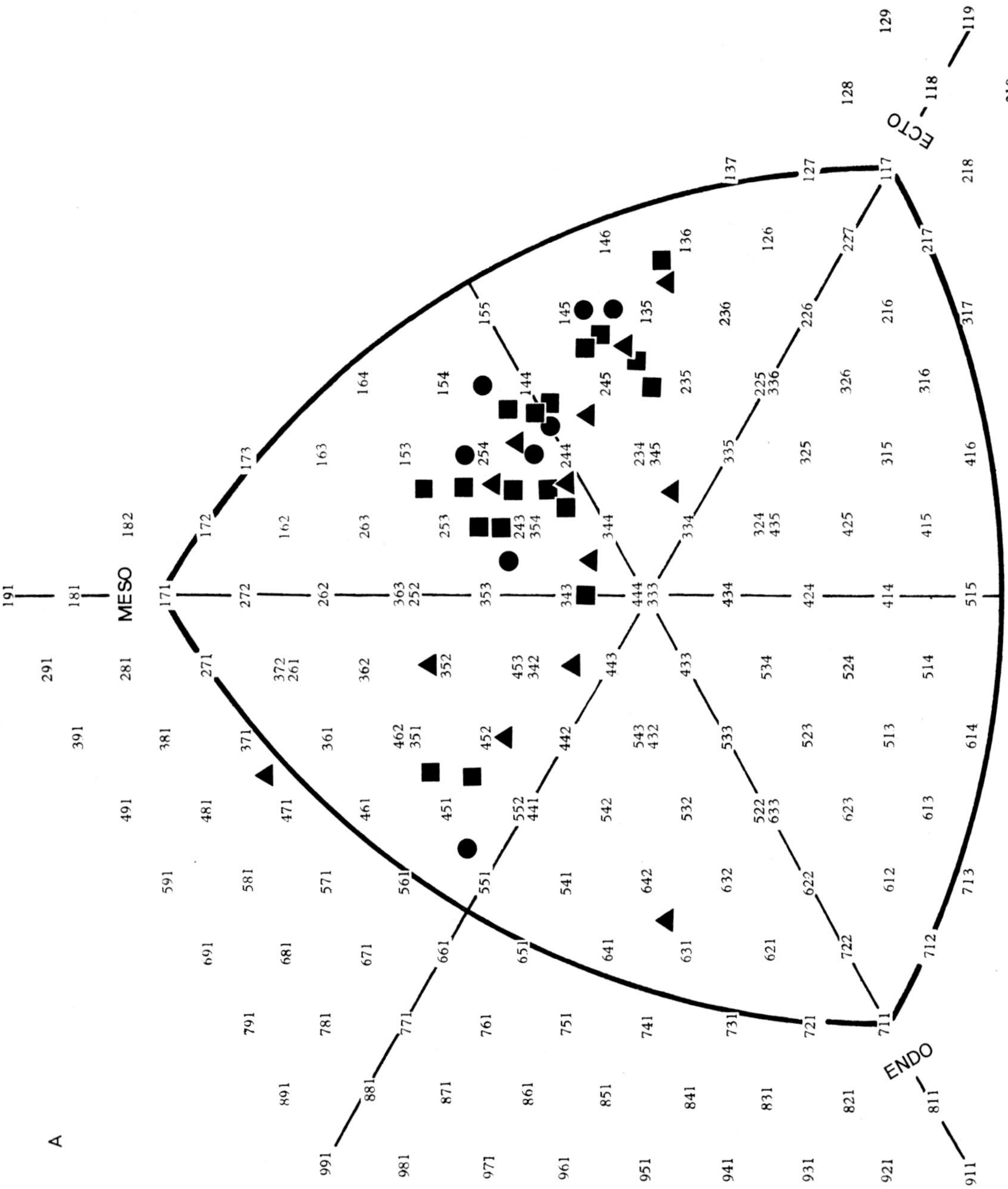
A
MESO
ECTO
ENDO

B

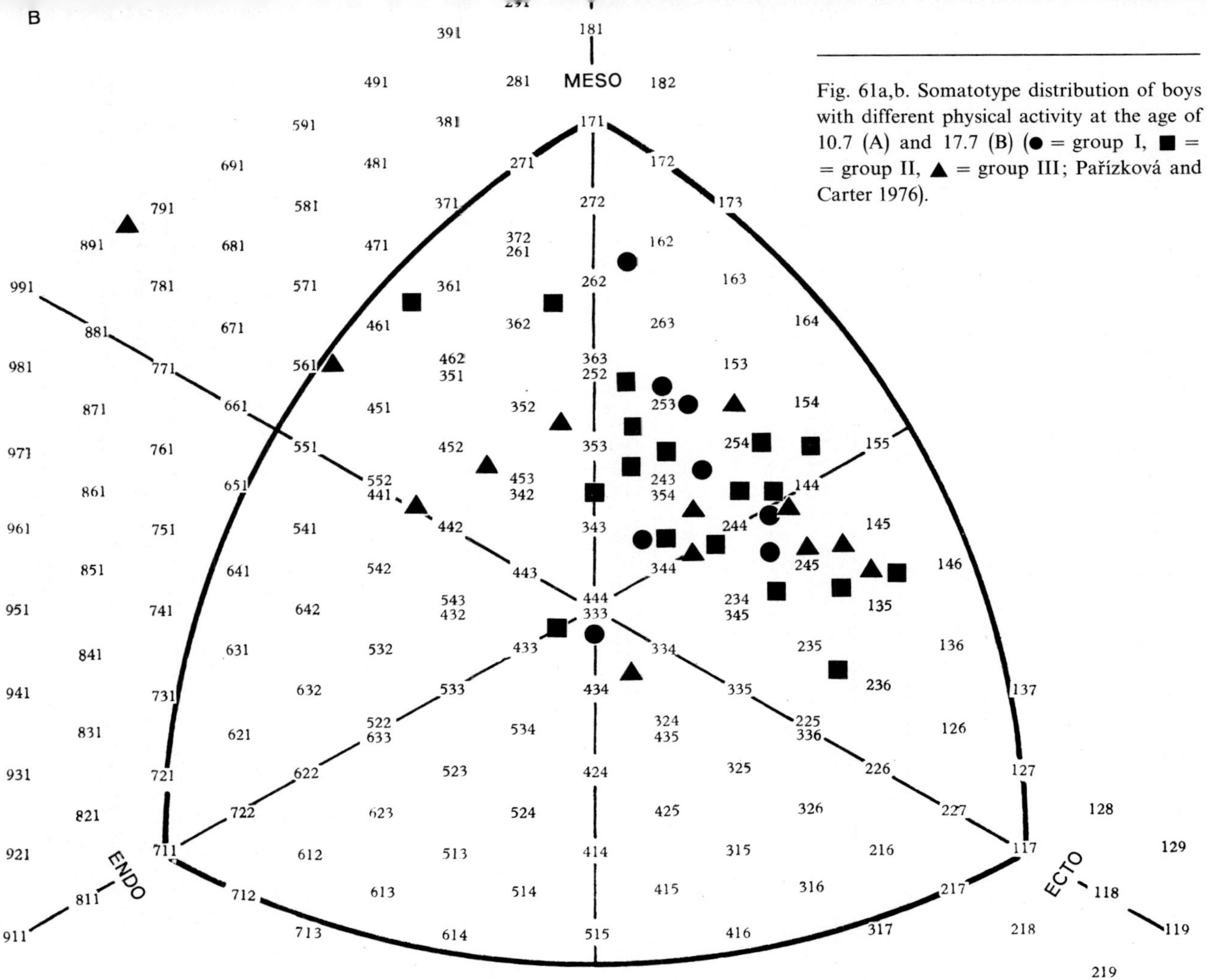

Fig. 61a,b. Somatotype distribution of boys with different physical activity at the age of 10.7 (A) and 17.7 (B) (● = group I, ■ = = group II, ▲ = group III; Pařízková and Carter 1976).

TABLE 41.

Summary of differences among somatotype component means for boys followed up longitudinally from 10.7 up to 17.7 years of age (Pařízková and Carter 1976)

Group									F-ratio[2]
				Endomorphy					
Total (n = 39)	15	16	17	13	12	11	18	14	9.09*
Group 1 (n = 8)	15	16	13	12	11	17	14	18	1.41
Group 2 (n = 18)	15	16	13	17	12	11	18	14	6.67*
Group 3 (n = 13)	15	17	16	13	11	18	12	14	3.03*
				Mesomorphy					
Total (n = 39)	16	15	17	12	14	13	11	18	7.08*
Group 1 (n = 8)	16	17	12	13	14	11	15	18	0.94
Group 2 (n = 18)	15	16	17	12	14	13	11	18	5.09*
Group 3 (n = 13)	12	17	16	15	14	11	13	18	2.58
				Ectomorphy					
Total (n = 39)	18	11	17	12	13	16	15	14	5.19*
Group 1 (n = 8)	18	17	11	13	16	15	12	14	1.28
Group 2 (n = 18)	18	11	12	17	13	16	15	14	6.23*
Group 3 (n = 13)	18	11	12	13	17	14	15	16	0.44

[1]) Difference according to the Newman-Keuls Multiple Range test. Means for each year ordered left to right from low to high. Years underlined by a common line do not differ, years not underlined by a common line do differ.

[2]) Those F-ratios with an asterisk are significant at the 0.01 level of confidence.

These results correspond to previous conclusions on body composition. The relationships are highest for adjacent years, and drop as the difference between years increase. To reach a common variance of 81 percent, the correlation coefficient would have to equal 0.90. Only ten of the 84 correlations equalled or exceeded this value. While these values for common variance are moderately high, the remainder were, of course, lower, and in terms of somatotype rating prediction there is *considerable common variance unaccounted for between the somatotypes in most years for all components,* indicating that good prediction is still a risky procedure from year to year for this sample. Prediction over spans of four years or greater, and particularly, within the maximum growth change years, appears to be fairly poor for all three components, with common variance of 50 per cent or less for many comparisons (Pařízková and Carter 1976).

The individual somatotypes of all 39 boys were plotted on a somatochart for each of the 8 years. The frequency and magnitude of the changes according to somatotype component were analyzed. *All 39 subjects had changes of at least one unit in one or more components during the eight years.* As with the intercorrelations, there was *greater stability (or fewer rating changes) between adjacent years than for comparisons four and eight years apart* (Table 41).

When somatotype change is examined as a whole, the longitudinal plots show that *some subjects are relatively stable with little change in component dominance or magnitude,* but on the other hand, *some subjects showed marked change* in magnitude even between adjacent years and in component dominance.

Probably the most outstanding characteristic of the analysis is the *contrast between the group statistics and the individual patterns,* which *implies partly also to body composition* and *skinfolds.* The means for the total group and sub-groups on individual components and in their somatotype distribution show relatively little change, however, examination of individual patterns over the eight years indicate that the individuals show considerable change. Apparently, the individual changes are in random directions, thereby cancelling each other out in group analysis (Pařízková and Carter 1976).

Most of the differences between the means of the somatotype components seem to be attributable to group 2, the moderate activity group; while groups 1 and 3 are more stable from 11 to 18 years. The effect of different activity levels on these results is unclear. *The apparently greater endomorphy of the low activity group might be explained in terms of the lower physical activity of the group,* which *agrees with the body composition analysis* (Pařízková 1970b,c, 1971b, 1972h) and maximal oxygen uptake analysis (Šprynarová 1974). However, the mesomorphy of both the high and low activity groups were virtually identical throughout the eight years, and the moderate activity group had lower mesomorphy. One might expect the high activity group would have greater mesomorphy because of the hypertrophy effect of exercise and that the low activity group would have lower mesomorphy because of the lack of stimulus for the hypertrophy effect. The indications from this data are that *variation in growth variables affects somatotype more than the exercise variables,* and possibly indicate the difficulty of using such broad classifications of activity levels. Perhaps more precise monitoring of physical activity would produce different results. This was, however, hardly possible in volunteers who were mostly not interested in becoming top athletes.

Within the limitations of this study, we conclude that the analysis supports the hypothesis that *changes occur in somatotypes of boys age 10.7 to 17.7,* that the evidence of the influence of physical activity on somatotypes in boys is inconclusive, and that further studies are needed on the influence of physical activity on the somatotypes of adolescent boys. Measurements of *body composition and aerobic capacity nevertheless showed the impact of exercise in adolescent boys more markedly* (*see* Fig. 54, 55 and Table 36) and characterized thus better the results of adaptation to regular exercise.

7. Body build and body composition in girl gymnasts and of non-training girls

At the onset of puberty a significant differentiation of body composition and subcutaneous fat in boys and girls takes place. We also investigated therefore the influence of adaptation to long-term sports training in girl-gymnasts whom we had the opportunity of following-up for a number of years starting at the age of 12–13 years. The first comparison in the course of six months was made in a major group, members of youth sports school (n = 32), along with a control group of girls not engaged in training (n = 45), shortly before summer training camps. During the stay in this camp (Fig. 62) the height and body weight of the gymnasts increased

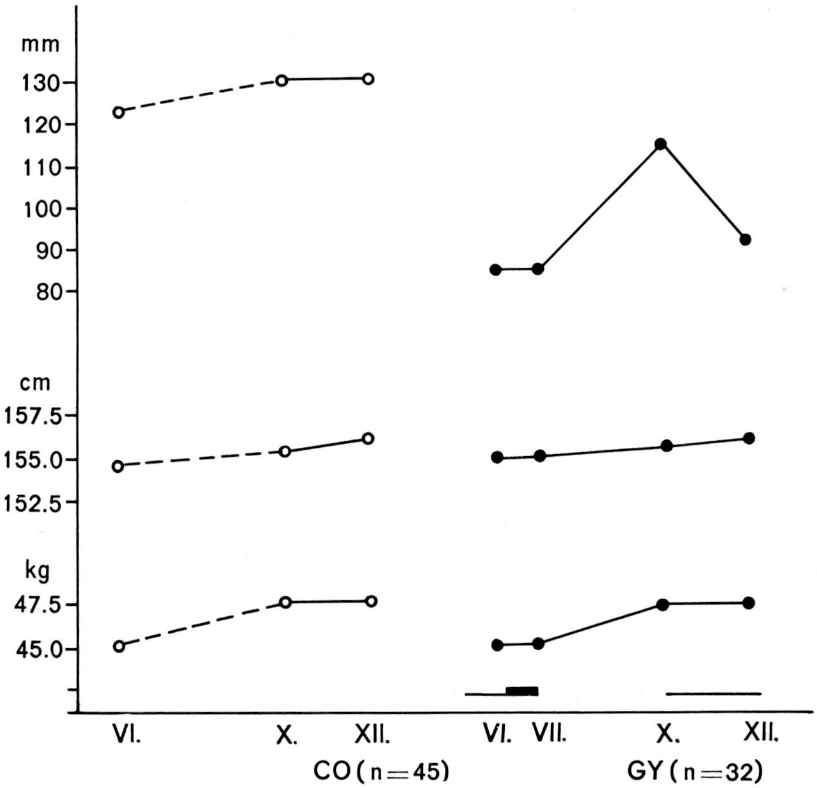

Fig. 62. Comparison of the development of weight (kg), height (cm) and sum of ten skinfold thicknesses (mm) in untrained, control girls (Co) and trained 12–13 years old gymnasts (Gy) during periods of different training intensity (bottom right: up to VI. — normal training during the school year; VI.–VII. — increased intensity of training during special summer camp; VII.–X. interruption of training; X.–XII. — normal training during the school year; Pařízková 1959b).

slightly, while the thickness of ten skinfolds, an indicator of adiposity, did not change. During the period after the camp when systematic training was for some time discontinued the weight as well as subcutaneous adipose tissue increased markedly. After training was taken up again from October to December weight and height increased again slightly, while the skinfold thickness declined significantly. Weight increments had during different periods a different composition as regards the ratio of LBM and fat. In girls of the control group where these changes in the amount of physical activity were lacking all investigated indicators increased gradually (Fig. 62) (Pařízková 1959a, 1960b).

From the group of gymnasts originally examined only the minority persevered in training for the entire five-year period. At the end of this period we again compared

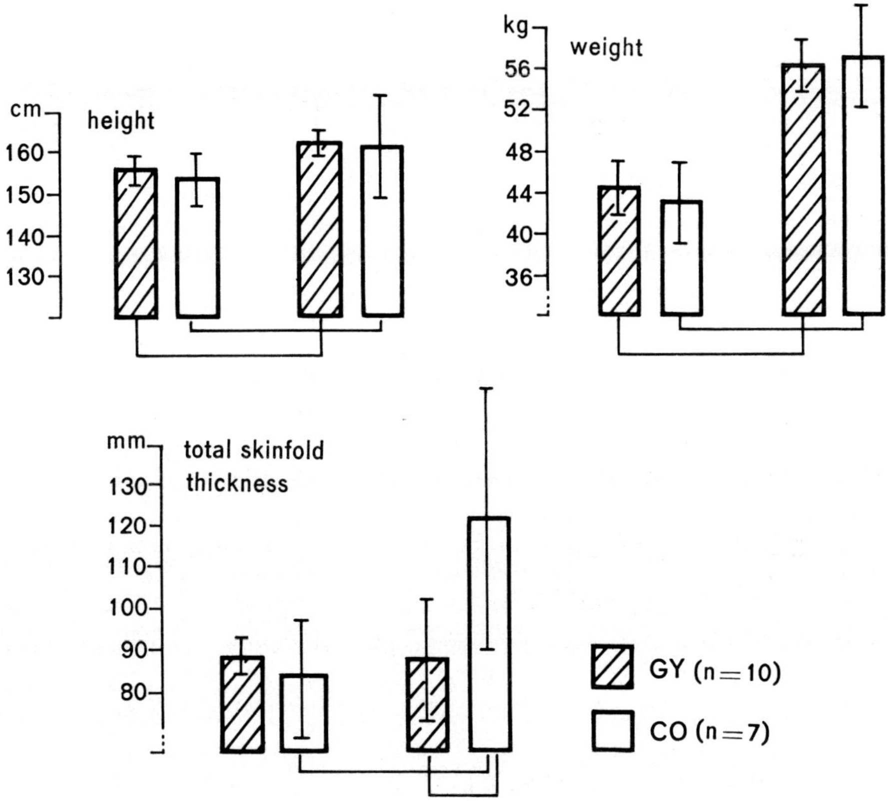

Fig. 63. Comparison of the changes of height (cm), weight (kg) and subcutaneous fat (sum of ten skinfolds — mm) in untrained, control girls (white columns) and girl-gymnasts (hatched columns) before and after five-year period of training (12–17 years; $\bar{x}$ + SD) (Pařízková 1963a).

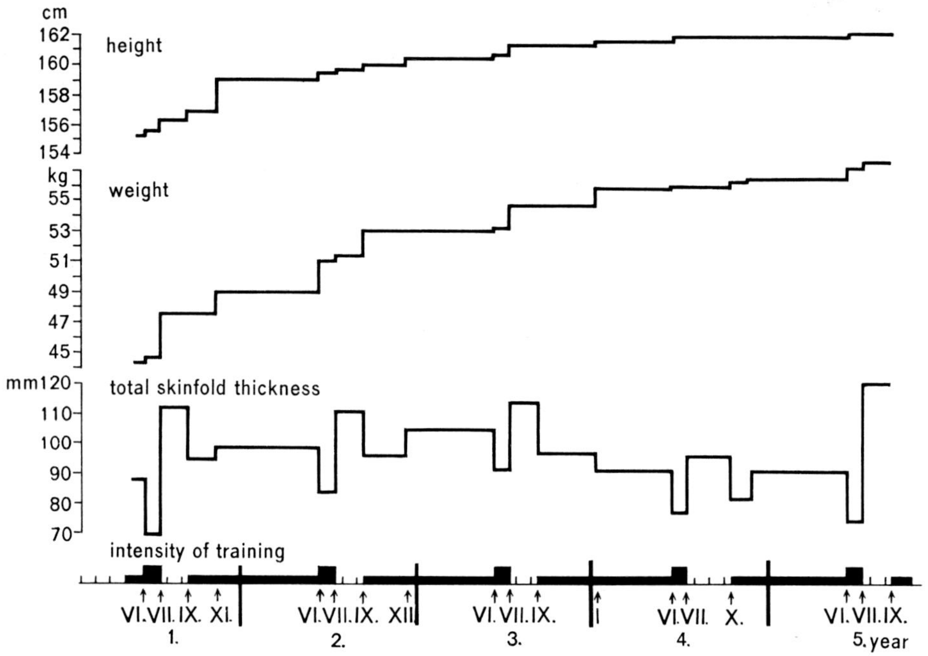

Fig. 64. Changes of height (cm), weight (kg) and subcutaneous fat (sum of ten skinfolds — mm) in a group of regularly training girl-gymnasts (n = 11) during five year period of varying intensity of training (bottom) (Pařízková 1963a, 1965).

height, weight and thickness of ten skinfolds in those who trained throughout the period of investigation and those who gave up training after a short time. *Height and body weight had the same trend in both groups, the subcutaneous fat remained unaltered in the gymnasts while it increased significantly in the girls not engaged in training* (Pařízková 1963a) (Fig. 63).

Changes during individual years in the gymnasts are illustrated in more detail in Fig. 64: *the skinfold thickness varied, depending on the actual level of physical activity.* During the period of more intense training body fat declined, when training was discontinued it increased more markedly and in the course of the year during a normal and constant level of exercise body fat did not change significantly, although body weight increased permanently (Pařízková 1962a,b, 1963a). *The weight increments had obviously a quite different composition*, similar to these in boys with a different intensity of physical activity (*see* Fig. 56).

It was possible for two years only also to check changes in body composition in ten gymnasts by means of densitometry (Fig. 65); the results were in agreement with the concurrent assessment of skinfold thicknesses (Pařízková 1963a, 1965). *The percentage of depot fat declined significantly during training of high intensity* (summer

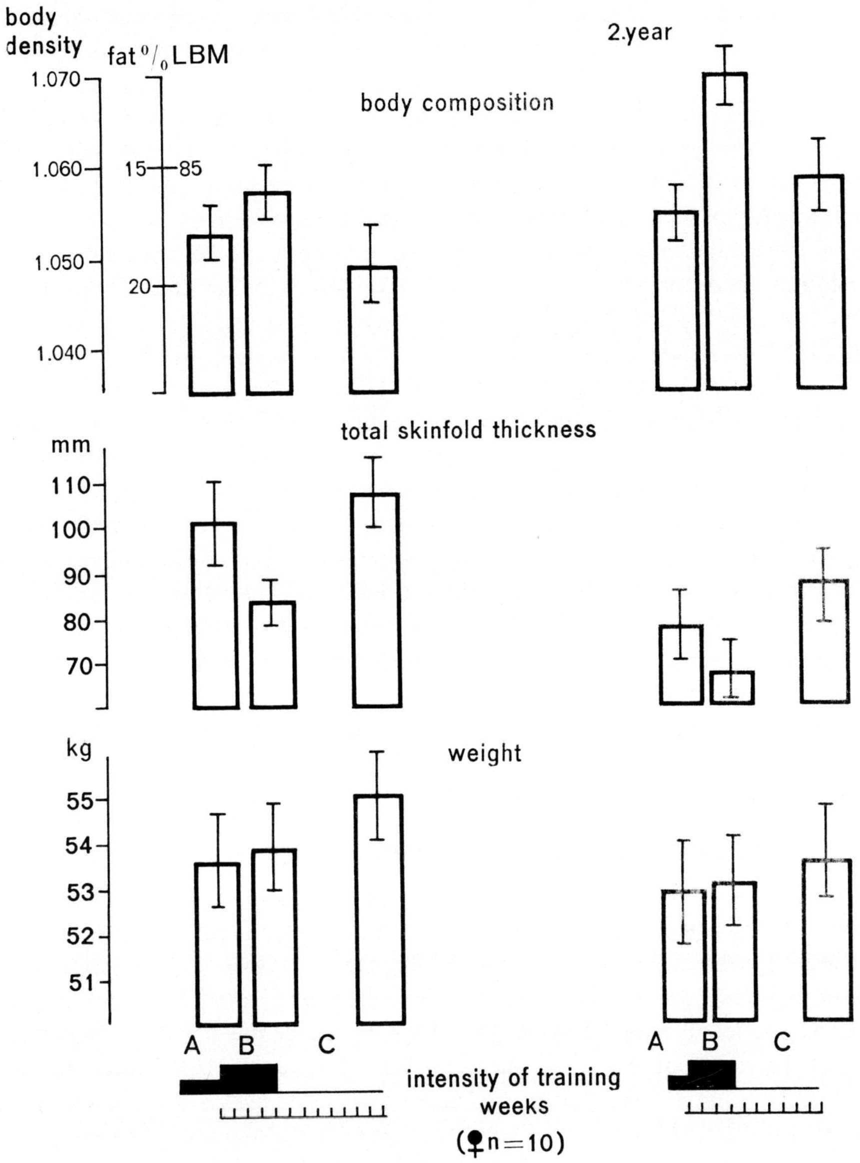

Fig. 65. Changes in weight (kg), sum of ten skinfolds (mm) and body composition (percentage of fat, body density) in a group of 10 girl-gymnasts during two-year period of fluctuating intensity of training- at the end of the school year (normal mean intensity of training — A), after special summer camp with increased intensity of training (B) and finally after period of completely interrupted training (C; $\bar{x} \pm$ SE) (Pařízková 1963a, Pařízková and Poupa 1963).

camp) *when LBM increased by more than corresponded to the weight increment,* and *increased when training was discontinued* and the weight increment was mainly due to deposition of fat. Analysis of weight changes in growing gymnasts, however, did not reveal a reduction of LBM when exercise was restricted (Pařízková 1960b, 1965). Although it is not possible to compare in detail the activity of boys and girls in the above studies in view of different sports they practised and different periods of investigations, the conclusions as regards body composition and its dependence on the intensity of the regime of physical exercise are in agreement.

Developmental changes of the organism in adolescents take obviously a much more complicated course than can be revealed by mere investigations of body weight. *In different stages of growth both basic components, LBM and fat, participate in the increase of body weight in a variable manner and in a different way before and after puberty in boys and girls.* Another factor is obviously the *level of energy turnover in the organism; when the caloric output is high during intense exercise, despite a high caloric intake fat deposition is substantially restricted* (*see* Fig. 36 and Table 18) *and LBM increases to a greater extent. Its increments may be even higher than* the *weight increments due to a concurrent reduction of fat.* The *reverse is true during relative inactivity, in particular when it follows after a period of adaptation to highly increased muscular activity.* An adequate and balanced regime of physical activity is from this aspect an essential prerequisite for harmonious development—preferably in the form of organized sports training and especially in large towns where there is little opportunity for spontaneous exercise.

8. Comparison of the development of body composition in girls and boys engaged in swimming training

We had the opportunity to compare changes in body composition simultaneously in boys and girls attending swimming classes for a period of four years. At the onset of the investigation at the age of 12 years between the boys (n = 12) and girls (n = 12) the *usual significant sexual differences in LBM and fat were lacking* (*see* Fig. 9, Fig. 66). The same applies to height and weight which moreover did not differ from mean values of the child population of this age group. *The ratio of LBM* was, however, *already higher than in non-training children of similar age during the first year of the study* (*see* Fig. 9). LBM in the boys was the same as in the above-mentioned group I in the second year of the investigation (*see* Table 33 – 34 and Fig. 52 – 56) who also were engaged in intensive training (track-and-field athletics, basket-ball). This finding implies that even at the onset of our investigation the children in the sports school had a different body composition compared with the normal child population. This is due to selection of gifted children who had already previously some training in swimming.

In the third year of the investigation significant differences developed in height, body weight and body composition between boys and girls (Fig. 66). *The percentage*

Fig. 65. Mean values ($\bar{x} \pm SD$) of height, weight, body composition, absolute and relative values of maximal oxygen uptake (ml; ml//kg weight or kg LBM) in boy- and girl-swimmers followed up longitudinally in four years (12–15 years of age; Pařízková 1972g; Šprynarová and Pařízková 1974). 1974).

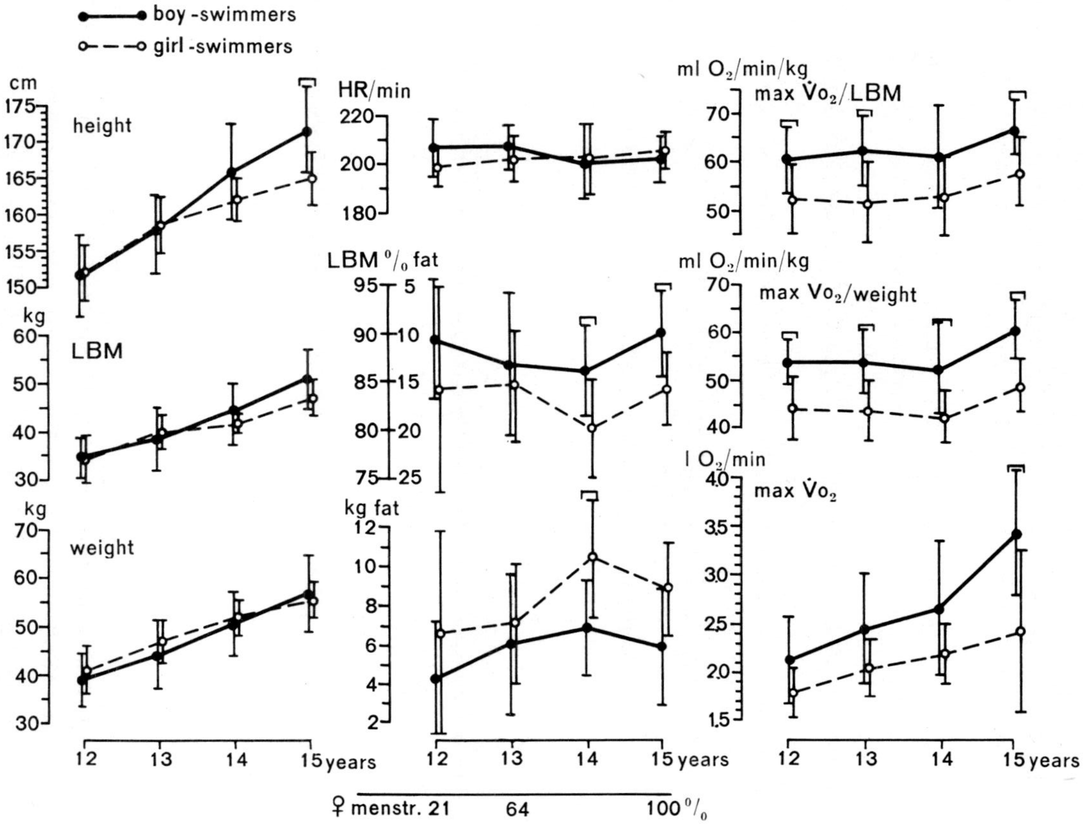

of fat was lower in boys as well as girls compared with the normal population. The body fat ratio in the boy swimmers was similar to that in the boys of group I of like age (Fig. 52 – 55 and Table 33 – 34). Although different sports were involved, the effect exerted on body composition was very much the same. In the course of our investigation, however, no very significant changes took place—an *increased ratio of LBM at the expense of fat was maintained by continuous training at a relatively constant level* (Pařízková 1972g, Šprynarová et al. 1975). In girls body fat did not increase as is usually the case in adolescent girls not engaged in training (Pařízková 1961a, 1962a, 1963a etc.). In the last year the absolute amount of LBM in kg in boy swimmers was significantly lower than in training boys of group I (*see* Fig. 54) who however at that age were somewhat taller and heavier (*see* Fig. 52 and 53).

As regards *body build,* we found significant *sexual differences*—the *relative width of the pelvis* (expressed in per cent of height) *was greater in girls* (16.1) already at the onset of the investigation than in boys (15.6). The relative width of the pelvis expressed in per cent of the breadth of the shoulders (biacromial) differed significantly by sex in the last year (girls 77.1; boys 71.5). These differences in body build develop generally in the course of puberty. *In girls along with a higher body fat ratio the typical figure with wider pelvic measurements develops and this development is not particularly affected by swimming training of the intensity recorded in our observation.* A typical body build, i.e. relatively narrow biiliocristal diameter (in relation to the biacromial width) are found e.g. in top gymnasts with a low body fat ratio during adolescence as well as in adult life (Pařízková 1974a).

The number of menstruating girls at the onset and at the end of the investigation is given in the lower portion of the figure (not investigated during the third year of the survey). Comparison with the normal population revealed a *slight acceleration of the onset of menarche in swimmers* (Pařízková 1975c). The onset of menarche did not show in our girls followed longitudinally by densitometry any marked relationship to weight and body composition as described by Frisch et al. (1973).

The *development of aerobic capacity* also displayed marked sexual differences which were most marked when the max O_2 consumption was related not only to body weight (Fig. 66) but also to LBM. In *absolute values sexual differences were found only in the last year of the investigation.*—Compared with the normal non-trained population, the *relative values of aerobic capacity were raised in boys as well as girls,* and compared with the longitudinal study of boys the data in swimmers are in good agreement with data obtained in boys of group I with highest physical load (*see* Table 36). As ensues from the comparison, swimmers of both sexes differ from the normal population from the onset, which is obviously (similarly as in morphological indicators) due to the selection of these children attending the sports school (Šprynarová et al. 1975).

In boy swimmers changes in the heart volume by the above mentioned method were also assessed (p. 138). Fig. 67 illustrates the development of changes in the heart volume/kg body weight in boys with the highest and lowest physical activity (practically identical with group I and IV investigated for five years—*see* Table 33 and 34). Although in the first year of the investigation the values of height and weight did not differ, *absolute and relative heart volume already differed in the first years. Swimmers and boys from group I did not differ* significantly but *boys from the inactive group IV had a significantly smaller heart volume.* This was particularly marked when evaluating relative increments of heart volume in relation to body weight (Fig. 67) (Čermák 1973). Similar conclusions are obtained when the heart volume is related to LBM.

9. Relationship between development of body weight, body composition and functional development

In general it may be concluded, based on the above investigations that during prepuberty and puberty adaptation to an increased load leads to a restricted formation of body fat, an increased development of LBM, while at the same time the aerobic capacity of the organism increases, both of which are attributes of greater fitness and better performance. We analyzed also the relationship of LBM and fat (relative and absolute) and various indicators of fitness, using different types of tests.

We compared obese and asthenic subjects during standard exercise of an optimal character on a bicycle ergometer which represented one sixth of the maximal load (according to Janda 1959) which is closest to the type of everyday work-load. In obese girls the O_2 consumption on the bicycle ergometer was by 56% higher and during the step test by 36.4% higher than in asthenic girls. The oxygen pulse was in girls with average weight by 45.8% higher on the bicycle ergometer and by 23.7% during the step test as compared with asthenic girls. In boys the differences between groups with different weight were similar (Vamberová et al. 1971). *The energy spent on relatively similar work was thus higher in heavier or obese subjects.*

Further analysis of somatic and functional indicators obtained in a longitudinal study of boys of groups I–IV (*see* p. 126) revealed a great variability of body composition as well as aerobic capacity which was, however, within the range of normal values. We selected therefore two groups of boys that did not differ significantly in height and weight, but already had, however, at the age of 10.7 a smaller (8.3% and 2.98 kg fat, n = 5) or greater (20.7% and 8.32 kg fat, n = 6) amount of body fat. Lean body mass did not differ significantly. The differences in body composition described were maintained by these boys up to the age of 17.7 years (8.5 and 17.2%, i.e. 5.5 and 12.0 kg body fat). The values of body fat did not exceed in that case the borderline of asthenia or obesity. Height and body weight in both selected groups of boys was within the normal range. As mentioned before, in these groups the oxygen consumption was compared during a standard and maximum load on a treadmill (Šprynarová 1974).

The maximum values of oxygen consumption were equal in both groups. During a medium load significant differences in the oxygen consumption per kg LBM were found at the ages of 12.7 and 13.7 years. *The difference between groups with a different body fat ratio and similar LBM was,* however, manifested by the fact that

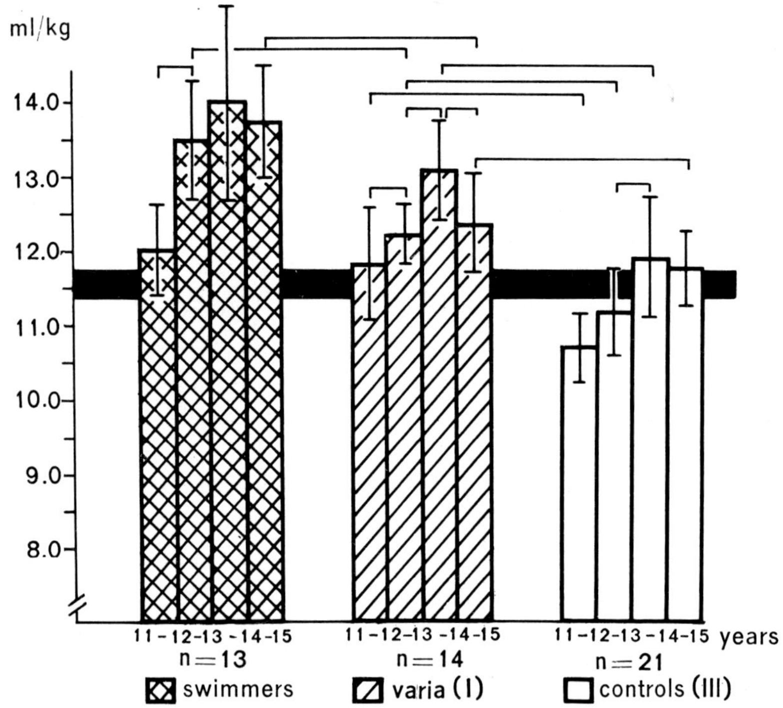

Fig. 67. Per cent increase (+ %) in relative heart volume (ml/kg weight) in boy-swimmers (*see* Fig. 66), trained boys (group I — *see* p. 138) and untrained control boys (group III or IV) of the same age measured repeatedly from 11th to 14th year of age (11.7–14.7 years: Čermák 1973).

the *maximum oxygen consumption was attained by some of the boys with a higher body fat ratio at a lower speed, after covering a shorter distance* on the treadmill *or after a shorter duration of the maximum load.* For instance at the age of 14.7 years in boys with a body fat ratio of 8.0 (± 1.7)% the maximal oxygen consumption (3250 ± 532 ml/min) was reached at a rate of 16.2 (±0.2) km/hour, while in boys with a body fat ratio of 18.8 (±3.6) % the maximal oxygen consumption (3451 ± ± 229 ml/min) was reached at a rate of 15.3 (±0.8) km/hour. The organism with a smaller body fat ratio is obviously able to attain at the same level of maximal aerobic processes (in absolute values as well as in relation to LBM) a greater speed during the maximum load than the organism which uses a larger amount of energy to carry its own weight, i.e. a larger amount of depot fat (Šprynarová and Pařízková 1972). *Although the indicators of aerobic capacity used to characterize fitness are equal, individuals with a different body fat ratio differ as regards actual working performance; the performance is uneconomic as more of the energy must be spent on useless work. These differences are well manifested already within the range of normal body composition.* At an age when the difference in the body fat ratio between the two groups of boys was no longer significant, the difference in speed etc. also disappeared (Šprynarová and Pařízková 1972).

These differences between individual subjects with different body composition appear only at the end of puberty; although even at the age of 10.7 and 11.7 years there were significant differences in the body fat ratio of the above two groups, we did not demonstrate any differences in the speed, duration and load, etc. at which the maximal oxygen consumption was reached. This is in keeping with previous findings that only at the age of 12.7 years is there a closer relationship between maximal oxygen consumption and LBM rather than total body weight (*see* Table 35), i.e. there is a closer relationship between body composition and aerobic capacity (Šprynarová and Pařízková 1972).

Differences in the response of vegetative functions to load are obviously due to a different final loading of the LBM by the work performed as well as by the load of body fat on LBM which causes a greater energy requirement for almost any physical activity. The greater energy requirement could be considered a compensating factor in the total energy expenditure (i.e. the greater energy expenditure for practically the same activity should adjust the final energy balance), *if it did not lead to restricted spontaneous physical activity, which in view of the greater energy requirement during physical activity is observed in subjects with a higher body fat ratio.* This was proved e.g. by Mayer (1968); the fitness of the organism deteriorates further by reduction of physical activity.

During the present accelerated somatic development of youth under oecological conditions of advanced industrial countries an increase of almost all mean values of somatic development is observed—height, body weight, longitudinal and circumferential measurements along with a higher body fat ratio (Pařízková 1972b, 1973b). *It is justifiable to ask whether this accelerated increase of body mass apparent from the secular trend of development* (although not solely accounted for by body fat) *is desirable for the harmonious development of the organism, in particular with regard to general functional capacity, physical fitness and perspective health status during adult life and old age.* This question has already been asked by some authors e.g. McCance and Widdowson (1962) and others (Widdowson 1962, Karsayevskaya 1964 etc.). Extensive surveys of physical fitness in advanced industrial countries lead to the *assumption that acceleration of somatic development due to more favourable living conditions proceeds more rapidly than the acceleration of functional development which due to the contemporary living pattern (hypokinesia) is relatively retarded* (Guminskiy et al. 1972, Gladysheva et al. 1974).

10. Body composition and fitness of youth in relation to socio-economic conditions

We had the opportunity of elucidating certain aspects of this problem in a study conducted in a sample of the youth in a developing African country—Tunisia. This country holds, however, among other developing countries a special position because the living conditions are on a relatively higher level than in other African and Asian countries and part of the population in larger towns (at least in some social strata) has a standard close to that in developed industrial countries. Cases of extreme malnutrition and serious health damage are very rare. The investigation comprised even in the relatively small sample due to local conditions a very wide range of children with substantially different social and economic characteristics which could not be found in our country.

We examined a total of 293 boys and girls aged 11 and 12 years. These children were a representative sample (i.e. 10 %) from the first and second class of a lycée in the capital and also a group of boys of equal age from a municipal school. As regards somatic development we assessed all indicators included in the Human Adaptability Section of the International Biological Programme (Weiner and Laurie 1969) supplemented by some other indicators used traditionally in our laboratory, incl. 10 skinfolds measured by means of our own and a Harpenden caliper. The body composition was calculated by means of nomograms and tables (*see* Fig. 10a,b and Table 8). Along with the above parameters indicators of functional development were also assessed — muscular strength of seven muscle groups, the latent period of contraction and relaxation using the dynamometric method. The level of strength is assessed from the maximum value of tension in kiloponds which the examined muscle group develops under isometric conditions in a standard position; for measurements an electric dynamometer was used (Sukop 1966, Merhautová and Pařízková 1971, 1973). The performance of the cardiovascular apparatus was evaluated by means of the step test modified by Čermák (1969). Furthermore we investigated the vital capacity, forced expiration (ml/0.5 s) and performance in some sports disciplines (Merhautová and Pařízková 1971, 1973a,b).

Comparison of boys and girls revealed *typical sexual differences:* at the age of 11 *boys* had, *as compared with girls a greater muscular strength*, they were *more efficient in disciplines requiring speed* (50 m run), they had *better results of the step test* and a *shorter reaction time during muscular contraction.* The girls who were a year older had greater circumferential measurements and widths along with a higher percentage of body fat the latter being as high as values recorded for the adult Czech female population (Pařízková and Merhautová 1970, 1971). *Sexual maturation was more rapid in girls* (evaluated by the secondary sex characteristics—Tanner 1962): e.g. 28 % of the girls had already reached the 3rd grade of sexual maturation while only 6 % of the boys belonged that group. *Individuals with an accelerated sexual development differed significantly from children with a slower sexual maturation in morphological as well as functional characteristics.* The trend of both these deviations was not identical in the two sexes. As a whole the developmental characteristics and nature of sexual differences in Tunisian boys and girls did not differ from similar changes during pubertal development found in developed industrial countries—*in girls with higher grade of sexual maturation an accelerated somatic development was found* (in particular *increased ratio of body* fat), *in boys greater development as regards functional indicators. The accelerated somatic development and larger body dimensions in particular in girls did not imply an advantage from the functional aspect: indicators of physical fitness were on a lower level in girls* (Merhautová and Pařízková 1971, 1973a,b).

The *effect of socio-economic conditions* was also investigated in a group of 160 healthy boys from the capital of Tunis.

Boys from group T_1 (age 11.7 years, n = 30) were pupils of a municipal school and belonged as regards social indicators to poorer strata of the population with very modest but adequate living conditions (according to Centre International de l'Enfance—CIE—category IV). In addition we examined 29 pupils of a lycée (T_2, 11.7 years) and another 100 pupils of the lycée who were one year older (T, 12.5 years). The latter two groups belonged to privileged social strata with a considerably higher living standard (IInd category according to CIE). The results of the examination were compared with data obtained in Czech boys of similar age with a corresponding living standard as group T and from a similar type of Prague school (C, n = 28, 11.7 years; C, n = 29, 12.6 years).

The heights and weights were highest in the Czech boys (Fig. 68). *The Tunisian boys from the poor population strata* (T_1) *were significantly shorter and lighter not only compared with Czech boys but also compared with Tunisian boys of similar age* (T_2). The lenght of the lower extremities (Table 42) was significantly greater in Czech boys aged 11 and 12 years. Boys of group T_1 had significantly the shortest extremities, compared with all the remaining groups. The differences in height were thus due in particular to shorter lower extremities which was also apparent from comparison of the sitting height. The chest circumference and breadth of the shoulders was again lowest in group T_1, as were the pelvic measurements (biiliocristal and bitrochanteric diameters) and the circumferential measurements of the extremities. In general the *body build of Tunisian boys of similar social standard differed from Czech boys by a trend towards wider measurements of the trunk and shorter extremities* (Table 42) (Pařízková et al. 1972a, 1974c).

The robustness of the skeleton evaluated from the breadth of the wrist and bicondylar femur did not differ in any of the groups (Table 42). *The percentage of LBM and fat was also the same in all groups* (Fig. 69). A significant difference from this aspect was found in absolute values of LBM; *boys from group* T_1 *had the smallest LBM in kg.*

The results of anthropometric investigations thus seem to indicate a retarded and inferior somatic development among Tunisian boys from poorer strata. The functional examination, however, does not support this conclusion. The absolute values of muscular strength were in most instances highest in group T_1 (statistically significant difference in the strength of the extensors of the elbow—Table 43), or at least they did not differ from values assessed in other Tunisian and Czech boys. *The differences in strength were manifested even more markedly when calculated per kg body weight* (Table 43): the *majority of values was significantly highest in boys of group* T_1 *as compared with Tunisian boys of equal age* (T) *as well as with boys a year older* (T). The same applies when strength is calculated per kg LBM (Merhautová and Pařízková 1971, 1973a,b).

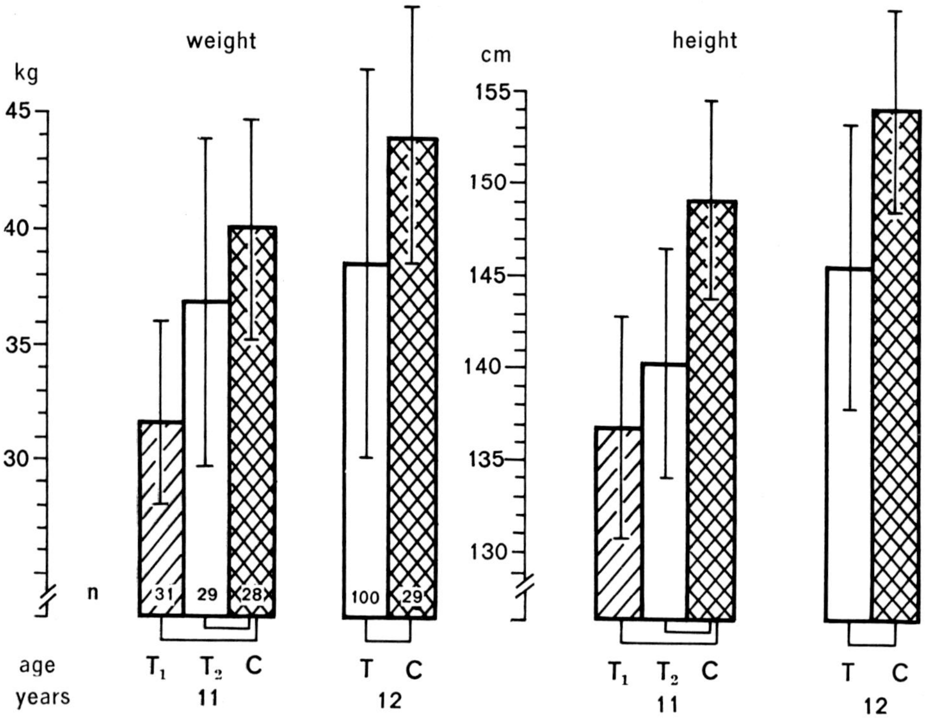

Fig. 68. Comparison of mean values ($\bar{x} \pm SD$) of height and weight in groups of Tunisian (T_1 = boys from poor families; T_2 = boys from well-off families) and Czech boys (C) at the age of 11 and 12 years (Pařízková and Merhautová 1970, 1971).

The step test also revealed the most favourable results in boys of group T_1. E.g. the *increase of pulse rate during work and the recovery period and the step test index suggest the greater fitness in group* T_1 (Table 44). These boys performed the work mostly in a true steady state, while this was not the case in the other groups of Tunisian boys. *Analysis of the work economy reveals also the most favourable results in group* T_1. One of the reasons is obviously the amount of work performed in relation to the size of the organism. *The results of the step test correlated negatively with body fat and positively with LBM* (Table 45): *the organism with a smaller fat load performs the same work more easily and economically, the demands on the circulation are not as high* (Pařízková and Merhautová 1970, 1971, 1973).

Also other comparisons with the results of functional tests assembled in Czech children indicate that although their body weight is higher, *Czech boys have similar results* of functional examinations which implies that *the size of the organism is not the decisive factor for the functional level.* The shortest Tunisian boys (T_1) had from the aspect of functional development the best results in almost all indicators assessed (Pařízková and Merhautová 1970, 1973).

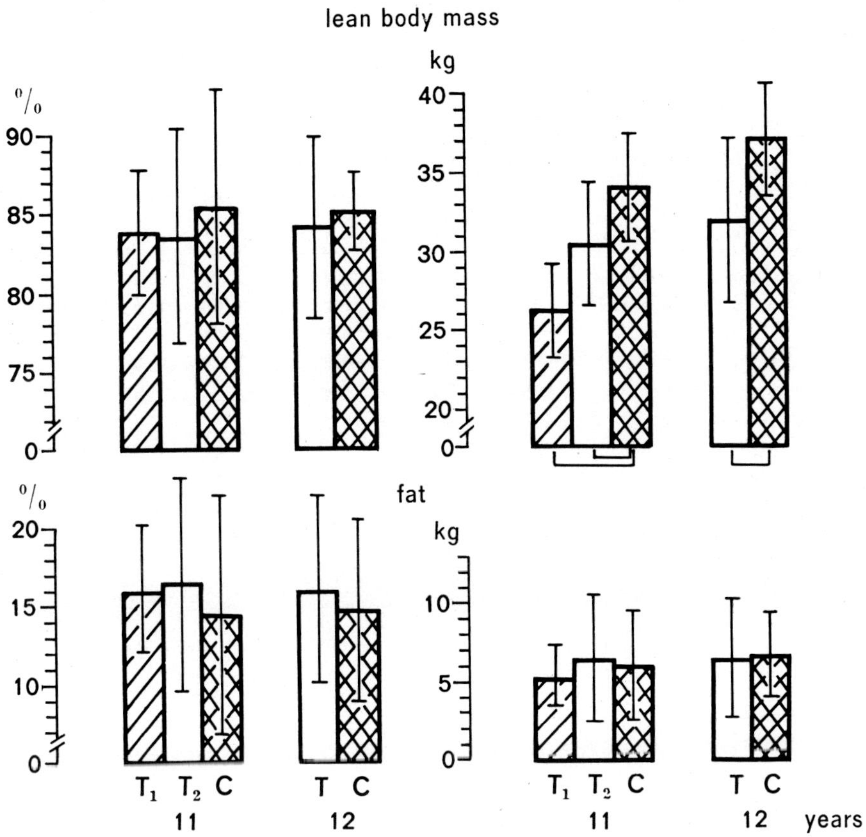

Fig. 69. Comparison of mean value ($\bar{x} \pm$ SD) of relative (%) and absolute amount of lean body mass and depot fat in groups of boys (for explanation see Fig. 68) (Pařízková and Merhautová 1970, 1973).

Similar conclusions were also reached in other comparisons of functional examinations, e.g. the *vital capacity, maximum voluntary ventilation, forced expiration.* Values obtained in group T_1 did not differ from group T_2 and when calculated in relative figures (i.e. per kg body weight and LBM) they were substantially higher. *The results in sports disciplines were also better in boys of group* T_1 *than* T_2 (Table 46) (Pařízková and Merhautová 1970, 1973).

The above results confirm moreover that *weight and height are not the decisive indicators for evaluating the child's development. Lower values need not always imply developmental retardation but may be the manifestation of adaptation to different nutritional and hygienic conditions at an early age* (Stini 1969, Frisancho et al. 1973 etc.) *and be associated with a satisfactory or even better functional status.* In experimental investigations in Tunisia even lower absolute values of LBM were not associated with a poorer functional development. Indeed the contrary was the case.

TABLE 42.
Mean values ($\bar{x} \pm SD$) of anthropometric measurements in Tunisian and Czech boys aged 11—12 years (Pařízková and Merhautová 1970, 1973)

Age — years	11						12			
	T_1		T_2		C		T		C	
	$\bar{x}$	SD	$\bar{x}$	SD	$\bar{x}$	SD	$\bar{x}$	SD	$\bar{x}$	SD
Length of lower extremities	82.8	3.4	86.3	4.2	91.3	4.4	88.9	5.8	95.2	4.3
Chest circumf. (inspirium)	70.8	3.4	75.4	5.8	75.3	3.7	76.6	6.2	77.6	4.1
Biacromial diameter	29.8	1.8	30.8	1.5	30.2	1.9	31.3	1.9	32.6	1.5
Chest (transverse)	22.1	2.2	22.7	2.5	21.0	1.4	22.9	2.0	22.3	1.4
Chest (anteroposterior)	15.3	1.1	15.8	1.0	14.9	1.1	15.9	1.3	16.3	1.3
Biiliocristal diameter	21.7	1.3	22.9	1.5	22.1	1.4	23.0	1.8	22.3	1.5
Bitrochanteric diameter	23.4	1.9	25.1	1.5	24.8	1.6	25.7	1.9	26.7	1.7
Wrist breadth	4.49	0.20	4.60	0.27	4.78	0.37	4.68	1.04	5.05	0.34
Bicondylar femur	8.22	0.40	8.49	0.46	8.68	0.50	8.61	0.65	9.15	0.48

TABLE 43.
Mean values ($\bar{x} \pm SD$) of muscle strength in absolute (kp) and relative values (kp/kg body weight) in Tunisian boys aged 11 and 12 years (Merhautová and Pařízková 1973a, 1971).

	Absolute values (kp)						Relative values (kp/kg body weight)					
Age (years)	11				12		11				12	
	T_1		T_2		T		T_1		T_2		T	
	$\bar{x}$	SD	$\bar{x}$	SD	$\bar{x}$	SD	$\bar{x}$	SD	$\bar{x}$	SD	$\bar{x}$	SD
Extensors of the trunk	61.4	11.3	58.1	9.8	61.9	12.0	1.97	0.35	1.60	0.29	1.65	0.33
Hand grip	15.8	3.6	16.7	3.3	19.4	4.7	0.51	0.20	0.46	0.14	0.51	0.10
Flexors of the elbow joint	20.1	4.4	18.4	3.6	20.2	4.7	0.64	0.13	0.51	0.13	0.54	0.12
Extensors of the elbow joint	14.1	2.2	12.8	2.2	13.6	2.6	0.45	0.09	0.36	0.08	0.36	0.08
Flexors of the knee joint	15.8	3.9	15.8	2.2	15.8	3.2	0.54	0.15	0.43	0.10	0.42	0.09
Extensors of the knee joint	29.3	3.9	28.2	4.4	30.9	5.7	0.91	0.20	0.78	0.10	0.42	0.09
Plantar flexors	39.4	9.1	39.6	10.1	42.2	11.4	1.27	0.29	1.10	0.33	1.20	0.37

TABLE 44.
Mean results ($\bar{x} \pm$ SD) of step test in Tunisian boys aged 11—12 years (Pařízková and Merhautová 1970, 1971)

Age (years)	11				12	
	$\bar{x}$	SD	$\bar{x}$	SD	$\bar{x}$	SD
Increase in pulse frequency during step test	346.1	53.7	370.0	86.9	361.3	43.9
Increase in pulse frequency during recovery period*	54.6	25.8	64.9	43.5	64.4	33.0
Index**	118.9	13.4	111.1	15.8	109.7	17.1

* Increase in pulse frequency during recovery period = pulse frequency during 5 minutes of recovery — rest pulse frequency during 5 minutes

** Step-test index $= \dfrac{\text{lasting of step test in seconds}}{\text{PF in 2nd, 3rd and 5th min of recovery}} \times 100$ (PF = pulse frequency)

The question remains whether the more slender children maintain this advantage during subsequent growth and adult life (this would be difficult to evaluate in view of the participation of other factors which are involved in subsequent years). In any case these findings *make us reflect whether trends aiming at a steady increase of body mass starting with birth weight* (Karsayevskaya 1964 etc.) *and all other somatic parameters which in contemporary child care is an expression of the effort to attain an optimal development of the young generation* (Bunak 1968, Wolanski 1970) *is really correct*. Investigations of the secular trend of the development of height and weight (Matiegka 1933) shows a significant increase of height and weight every ten years (Tanner 1962, Prokopec 1961, Suchý 1971, Vlastovskiy 1963 etc.). *We do not yet know exactly how individual constituents participate in the increase of body mass; comparisons over one decade have shown already that body fat increases relatively more than the other body constituents* (Pařízková 1972b, 1973b). Finally it has not been investigated yet whether *the increase of weight and of the absolute amount of LBM implies a proportional development of all bodily organs—in particular the heart muscle*. This will have to be examined in detail; answers to these questions pertaining to the secular trend of the development are lacking so far. More detailed information on further associated phenomena of the accelerated development will provide a more reliable basis for the optimum harmonious action on the organism in actual oecological conditions. It is desirable to prevent inadequately considered and scientifically unfounded provisions (unbalanced diet, incorrect pattern of physical activity etc.), in particular in the earliest stages of growth, from leading to disproportionate somatic development associated with a relative and possibly also absolute deterioration of the functional status.

TABLE 45.
Correlation coefficients of the relationship between the amount of depot fat and lean body mass (LBM) and the results of step test in Tunisian boys (Pařízková and Merhautová 1971, 1973)

Age (years)	11	12
% Fat: increase in pulse frequency during recovery period	0.547	0.262
% Fat: step-test index	—0.465	—0.379
% LBM: increase in pulse frequency during recovery period	—0.517	—0.256
% LBM: step-test index	0.502	0.286

TABLE 46.
Characteristics of respiratory function and sport performance in Tunisian boys at the age of 11 and 12 years (Merhautová and Pařízková 1971, 1973a,b)

Age (years)	11				12	
	T_1		T_2		T	
	$\bar{x}$	SD	$\bar{x}$	SD	$\bar{x}$	SD
Vital capacity (ml)	1953	284	2050	241	2191	391
Vital capacity (ml/kg weight)	62		55		56	
Vital capacity (ml/kg LBM)	74		67		68	
Forced expiration (ml/0.5 s)	1245	286	1263	237	1361	288
50 m dash (s)	9.4	0.6	9.5	0.7	9.1	0.8
300 m run (s)	67.5	6.1	69.4	6.4	65.7	8.0
Broad jump (cm)	255.6	29.8	226.0	41.1	265.7	48.0

These circumstances are during subsequent ontogenetic development a supporting factor which *promotes the development of pathogenic situations which may lead in their final stage to serious diseases* in particular of the *cardiovascular apparatus during later life.* Thus e.g. to the *danger of atherosclerosis nowadays attention is paid already in paediatrics* (Kannel and Dawber 1972, Mitchell et al. 1972, Wilmore and McNamara 1974, Fomon 1971, Fomon et al. 1969, etc.).—*Restricted physical activity* leading to *excessive adiposity* of the organism (associated frequently with hyperlipoproteinaemia etc.) and a *poorer performance of the cardiorespiratory apparatus* resulting in *reduced aerobic capacity* of the organism, is particularly marked in childhood. The most effective prevention of the above possible complaints thus should be started in the earliest stages of ontogenesis, using not only improved nutrition (Pike and Brown 1975) but also an optimum differentiated regime of physical activity as one of the basic protective means which is not only quite natural but also accessible to every normal subject.

IX. Consequences of adaptation to increased physical activity in obese children

Some selected problems pertaining to an uneven development of body composition and body weight were elucidated during investigations of groups of obese children examined in cross-sectional and longitudinal studies at a different age and in children with varying degrees of obesity.—The serious character of child obesity from the prognostic medical aspect is recently being discussed with increasing emphasis. Statistics indicate that overweight children account for cca 10–15% of the child population of Czechoslovakia (Ošancová et al. 1972, Ošancová and Hejda 1974 etc.). In adult and advanced age the proportion of overweight, obese people increases further. This trend is relatively constant in industrial countries (Tremolières 1971a,b etc.); in developing countries the number of obese children is much lower, but in social strata which have a similar standard as industrially developed countries the prevalence is, however, probably similar.

Extensive measurements have shown that the incidence of obesity increases with age; in preschool children marked obesity is an exception, and in younger school age it is more rare than later during prepubertal and pubertal age (Vamberová et al. 1964).

Some authors such as Bruch (1940), Mayer (1968, 1970) and others draw attention to the fact that overeating and excessive caloric intake in children are relatively rare. A frequent characteristic is, however, a reduced motor activity and lack of interest in physical exercise. Inactivity is thus not the consequence of obesity but as a rule precedes it. Even if the obese child participates in a game, or exercise, his activity is markedly lower than in a child with normal weight under the same conditions as has been proved by long-term cinematographic records (Mayer 1968). The conclusion is inescapable that a tendency to low spontaneous physical activity is genetically determined and strongly associated with certain body types (Mayer 1970). In the previous chapter we have mentioned the result of correlation analysis between the step test and body fat ratio and LBM resp. in the organism (*see* Table 45). The obese child gives a much greater load to his cardiovascular system during exercise and physical work. The energy output during the same activity is also higher in the organism which carries an excessive fat load as compared with normal individuals. *All physical activity is thus a much greater strain for the obese child.* This *reduces the pleasure of activity* and physical work and upsets the caloric balance, i.e. *there is a futher reduction of energy output.*

Recently papers were published which draw attention to possible factors in early ontogenesis which influence the number of fat cells in the organism and thus also possible predisposition for the development of obesity in later years when further indispensible factors are added (McCance and Widdowson 1962, Widdowson and McCance 1960, 1975, Hirsch and Knittle 1970). Even when there are also some reservations (Widdowson and Shaw 1973) this factor seems to play an important role. The example of newborn infants of mothers with metabolically not compensated diabetes and a high glycaemia indicate that the development of adipose tissue may be influenced already before birth, i.e. during the 8th and 9th month of pregnancy (chapter II) (Brook 1972). It is possible that also other circumstances which affect glycaemia of the mother (which need not necessarily be pathological) may affect the development of adipose tissue during this period. *The origin of obesity, however, cannot be explained by a single factor; its development is obviously influenced by the combined action of several factors in a complex chronological sequence during pre- and postnatal ontogenesis. Restricted physical activity* plays, however, *a very important role in the calorie balance and energy turnover* (Moody et al. 1969, Lincoln 1972 etc).

1. Somatic characteristics of obese children

Comparison of normal with obese children reveals not only a higher body weight as a result of excessive deposition of fat but also other marked somatic differences. In our investigations we followed up in particular children who attended out-patient clinics for obese children at the Paediatric Clinic of the Faculty of Hygiene, Charles University, where the children were subjected to a detailed clinical examination and where simple obesity was diagnosed. Children with more marked endocrine disorders, which were, however, very rare in this out-patient clinic were not included in our groups. Most of children followed up were of prepubertal age or adolescents; patients of younger school age were quite rare, and none in preschool age (Vamberová et al. 1964). The patients were diagnosed as simple hyperalimentary obesities, i.e. caused by absolute or relative overeating—the latter mostly due to inactivity. As regards *very low incidence of marked obesity in the preschool age* it *seems that overnutrition at 3 to 6 years results rather in generally increased body size starting with greater height, weight etc. than superfluous deposition of fat* (Pařízková 1973b). It is also a period when in normal children e.g. subcutaneous fat does not increase at all (Pařízková et al. 1974a, Pařízková 1975d) (see Fig. 49).

Fig. 70 compares groups of obese boys and girls aged 12–14 years. *The weight and ratio of body fat were significantly raised.* Another characteristic is the *typical*

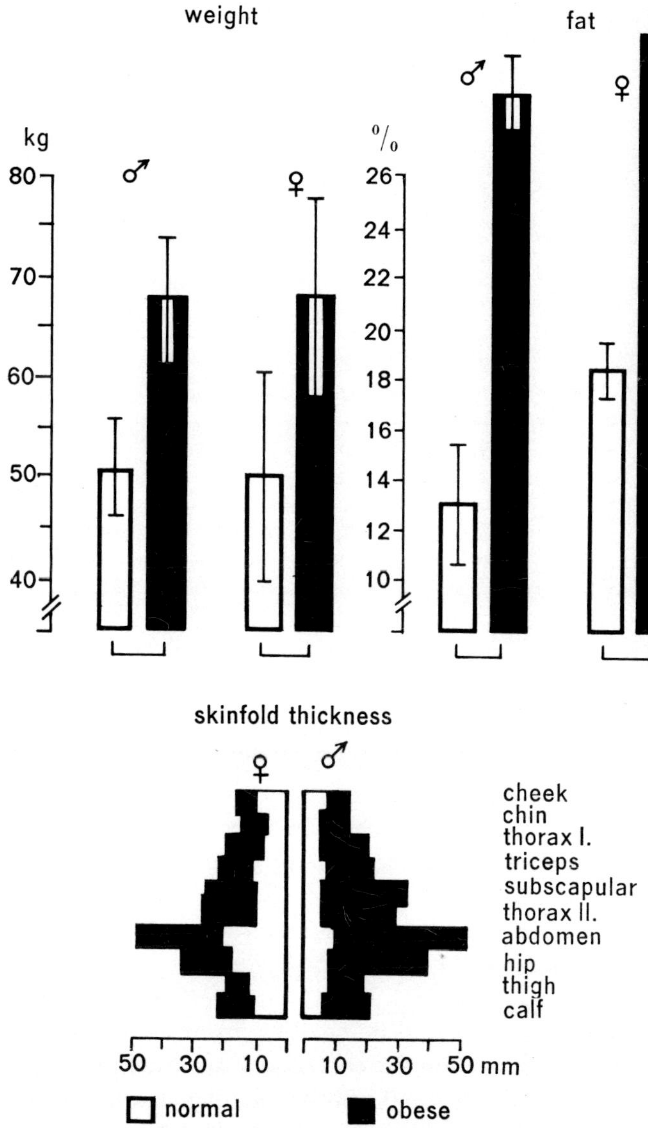

Fig. 70. Comparison of weight (kg), total (%) and subcutaneous fat (individual skinfold thicknesses — mm) in normal (white areas) and obese (white and black areas) boys and girls ($\bar{x} \pm SD$) (Pařízková 1960c, 1972c).

distribution of subcutaneous fat the amount of which is in both sexes increased to such high levels that it exceeds values recorded in much older subjects. The fat distribution is similar to that in older women. This applies to girls as well as boys (Pařízková 1960c,

TABLE 47.
Mean values ($\bar{x} \pm$ SD) of somatic indicators and body composition in obese and normal boys and girls aged 13–14 years (Pařízková 1970a).

			Height (cm)	Weight (kg)	% Fat	LBM (kg)	Biacrom. breadth (cm)	Biilio-crist. breadth (cm)	Chest circum-ference (cm)	Bicon-dylar femur (cm)
Boys	Normal	$\bar{x}$	161.8	50.4	12.5	43.9	34.4	22.8	78.6	9.6
		SD	6.3	6.7	5.9	5.1	1.6	1.8	3.3	0.3
	Obese	$\bar{x}$	161.2	68.9	29.5	48.6	33.8	27.7	88.3	10.1
		SD	2.1	6.9	3.2	5.0	1.4	1.0	5.5	0.9
Girls	Normal	$\bar{x}$	156.9	50.4	18.1	40.7	34.6	26.8	79.2	8.6
		SD	5.7	10.7	6.0	4.9	2.6	2.3	4.2	0.4
	Obese	$\bar{x}$	157.5	68.9	31.9	46.7	33.0	27.4	95.1	10.0
		SD	4.0	10.2	3.7	6.4	2.0	1.1	3.8	0.5

1961a, 1963c, 1965, 1968g, 1970b). Although sexual development and the onset of puberty in obese children did not differ from normal boys and girls, it was *not possible to prove sexual differences in the amount and distribution of subcutaneous fat, as is usually possible in normal youths of the same age.*

Comparison of further somatic parameters in other groups of obese boys and girls aged 13 – 14 years indicates differences in the weight, chest circumference and percentage of body fat (Table 47). However, also *the absolute amount of LBM is increased in both sexes.* In these severe obesities a generally robust constitution is found: along with a greater LBM we found also a *greater robusticity of the skeleton* (according to the bicondylar femur) and a *greater biiliocristal diameter in boys.* In this respect normal and obese girls do not differ having the same values of biiliocristal diameter as obese boys. Similar conclusions are reached when we compare relative dimensions of the pelvis, i.e. the biiliocristal diameter expressed in per cent of height or per cent of biacromial diameter. The width of the shoulders was however the same in obese and normal children. Here too, and much more markedly than in the normal population, the *relationship between body fat ratio and the width of the pelvis was manifested: the higher the fat content of the organism, the wider the pelvis and vice versa* (Table 47, Fig. 70) (Pařízková 1970a,b, 1972c). Even if we correct the width of the pelvis with regard to the layer of body fat, the difference in the biiliocristal diameter between normal and obese boys remains significant.

The circumferences are also markedly greater. When evaluating the bicondylar femur we must also consider the possible effect of subcutaneous fat, which cannot be eliminated at this site by measurement of skinfold thickness; evidence would have to be provided by X-ray. Forbes (1964), however, also found by measuring ^{40}K using a whole body counter in gross obesity a significant increase of LBM and greater robusticity of the organism. In view of these findings the greater robusticity of the skeleton of obese subjects is probable (Cheek 1968).

2. Heart volume in obese children

In a selected group of obese children the heart volume was also investigated, using the teleroentgenographic method in a recumbent position (Čermák et al. 1970) at the end of expiration; the heart volume was calculated by means of Musshoff's and Reindell's formula (1956); in a longitudinal survey of boys (*see* chapter VIII, Figs. 52–61 and 67, Table 37) it was found that in boys investigated from this aspect at the age between 12 and 15 years, there was a significant relationship between the heart volume and percentage of body fat (Čermák et al. 1970, Čermák 1969). This relationship was best demonstrated in groups with a wider variation in the percentage of body fat (Čermák and Pařízková 1974–5).

As compared with boys of the same age (i.e. 13 years) a *significantly higher volume of the heart was found in the obese not only in absolute values, but also relative to total body weight and lean body mass* (Table 48). Longitudinal measurements in obese boys showed, however, that three years later (i.e. at the age of 16 years) the heart volume had not increased further in spite of markedly increased height, weight, lean body mass and fat. In boys with milder obesity the volume of the heart did not change, in boys with severe obesity it decreased slightly in both absolute and relative values (i.e. per kg total and lean body weight—Čermák et al. 1970). Overloading by excess fat could cause the initial increase in heart volume, but sebsequent hypokinesia might lead later to underdevelopment of the heart (Pařízková 1972c).

TABLE 48.
Mean values ($\bar{x} \pm SD$) of anthropometric measurements, body composition and heart volume in normal and obese boys (Čermák, Tůma and Pařízková 1970)

	Normal		Obese	
n	29		30	
	$\bar{x}$	SD	$\bar{x}$	SD
Age (years)	13.0	0.0	13.1	1.0
Height (cm)	152.5	6.3	159.7	6.9
Weight (kg)	43.2	7.0	69.5	10.8
Lean body mass (kg)	36.5	3.5	45.5	9.3
Fat (%)	14.3	8.0	34.7	7.2
Heart volume (ml)	489.9	60.7	860.8	155.5

3. Economy of work in obese children

As has been mentioned, the *economy of work during a medium, optimal work load e.g. on a bicycle ergometer or during the step test was substantially poorer in obese children than in children with normal weight or underweight children.* This was manifested by a *raised pulse rate* and *higher O_2 consumption* when *performing the same work* (Vamberová et al. 1971).

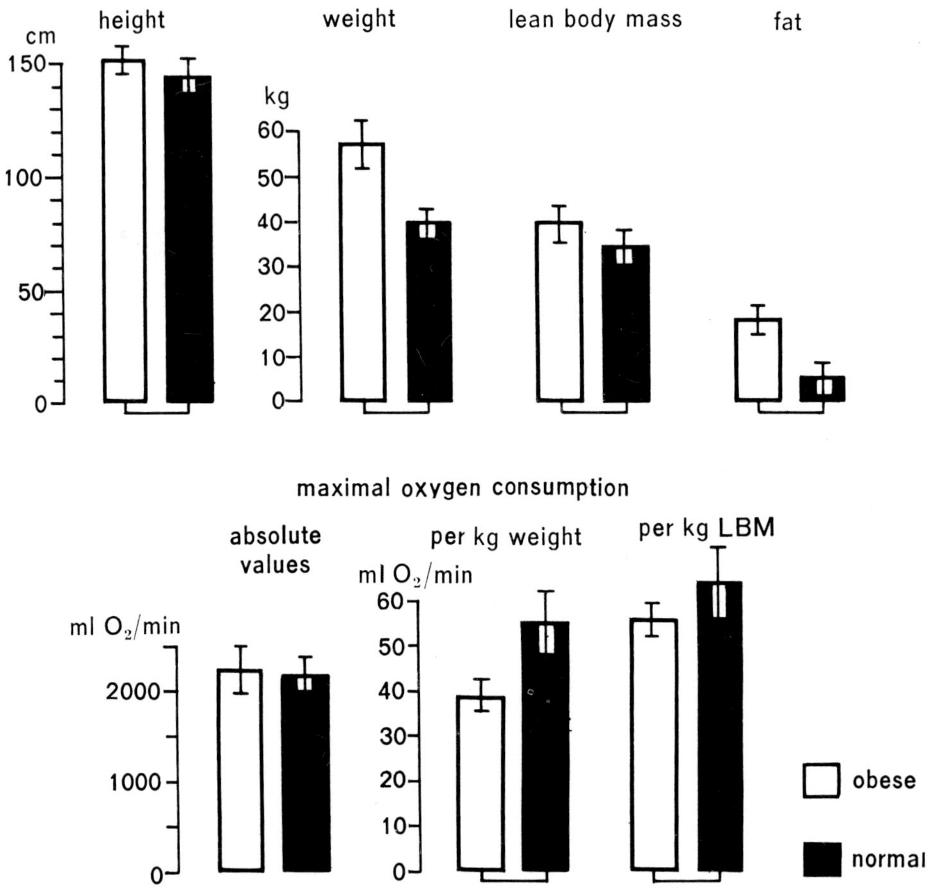

Fig. 71. Comparison of height (cm), total body weight, lean body mass and depot fat (kg — upper part) and of maximal O_2 uptake in absolute (ml O_2/min) and relative values (related to total and lean body weight — ml O_2/kg — lower part) in normal (black columns) and obese boys 11.7 years old (white columns; $\bar{x} \pm SE$; Pařízková and Šprynarová 1970).

The oxygen consumption, expressed in absolute values, during a maximum work-load on a treadmill was the same in obese and normal boys. In boys with a normal weight the maximal oxygen uptake (max O_2) *was reached on the treadmill at a higher speed than in obese boys. The relative values of maximal oxygen consumption calculated per body weight or LBM were in obese boys significantly lower than in boys of normal weight* (Fig. 71): *the aerobic capacity of obese subjects is thus lower,* much *more energy is used to move their own body and excess fat resp. The total performance* (we have in mind the total distance covered at a certain speed) *is significantly smaller when the maximal oxygen uptake is reached:* in obese boys it was reached at a speed of 11.1 km/hour, while in boys with normal body weight and a normal body fat ratio at a speed of 13.0 km/hour (Šprynarová and Pařízková 1962, 1965, Pařízková and Šprynarová 1970). This means that also in this type of functional examination the position for obese boys was markedly worse, although the maximum values of oxygen consumption in absolute values were the same.

From the functional aspect thus *obese children are characterized by a reduced economy of work, a relatively lower aerobic capacity* and *poorer performance.*

4. Effect of adaptation to a prolonged increased load on body composition and indicators of the lipid metabolism in blood

The importance of a high energy turnover and adequate calorie balance resulting also from a correct regime of exercise is manifested most markedly when the obese child changes its physical activity in a desirable way. This is why physical exercise and a general regime of increased physical activity are used as a remedy in the most physiological sense of the word.

A too sudden decrease of the caloric intake in adults can cause not only reduction of fat but also of LBM. This reduction can be *prevented by regular and sufficiently intense exercise in the course of treatment* (Rath and Slabochová 1964, Rath 1970). *In children reduction of the daily intake* to 1000 kcal causes *temporary slowing down or arrest of growth* (Vamberová 1961).

Although some authors such as Mayer (1968, 1970) recommend that during reducing therapy the arrest of weight increment should be ensured in such a way that the child gradually "reaches" its appropriate weight, it is not possible to avoid reducing treatment in cases of extreme obesity.

Weight reduction in a child, however, always implies an unnatural tendency during growth and it must be done very carefully to prevent, if possible, reduction of LBM. Increased exercise combined with an adequate and modified supply of calories is therefore much more useful during reduction than any low calorie diet alone; systematic checking of changes in body components helps to prevent impaired body composition.

In therapeutic recreational camps the following principle of treatment was applied: diet providing 1700 kcal per day with an elevated protein ratio and limited fat, carbohydrate and fluid intake (total daily intake 1500 ml) and regular physical exercise incl. all suitable sport disciplines, games, walks, dancing, etc. Physical exercise was supervised by special instructors and was under medical control. This treatment was supplemented by a programme the purpose of which was to teach the children correct dietary habits and exercise (Vamberová 1961). These summer holiday camps lasted usually seven weeks.

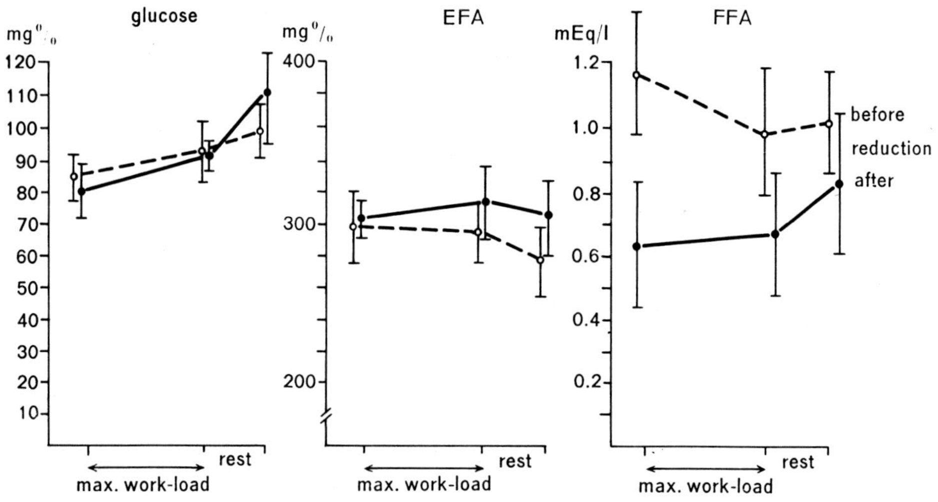

Fig. 72. Changes in blood levels of glucose (mg%), esterified (EFA) and non-esterified, free fatty acids (FFA) in obese boys 11.7 years old before and after reduction of weight and fat in a training summer camp ascertained before and after maximal work load on a treadmill, and after ten minutes recovery period (abscissa) (Pařízková et al. 1963, 1965).

As mentioned above, metabolic processes during a work are directed by a complicated interplay of nervous and humoro-endocrine systems (Métivier 1975). The metabolic response to these factors can be demonstrated in the blood what concerns also lipid metabolites—mainly free fatty acids and glycerol (Fritz 1961, Issekutz et al. 1965, 1966, Paul 1975 etc.). During a single load changes in FFA are also observed which indicate an increased mobilization and utilization of lipid metabolites—in particular fatty acids.

In view of changes in the body fat ratio after long-term adaptation to increased muscle work also a change in the response of indicators of fat metabolism in blood during a load may be assumed. We also investigated therefore, along with changes of the blood sugar level, changes of esterified fatty acids (EFA—Stern and Shapiro 1953) and nonesterified, free fatty acids (FFA) (Dole 1956) before and after maximal work loads on a treadmill and subsequently after 10 min rest, in obese boys before and after weight reduction.

The body weight of boys (n = 7, age = 11.8 years) declined after seven weeks in the summer camp by 11.4%, depot fat diminished from 17.5 to 12.2 kg. The percentage of LBM increased from 69.9 to 75.9. The blood sugar values at rest and

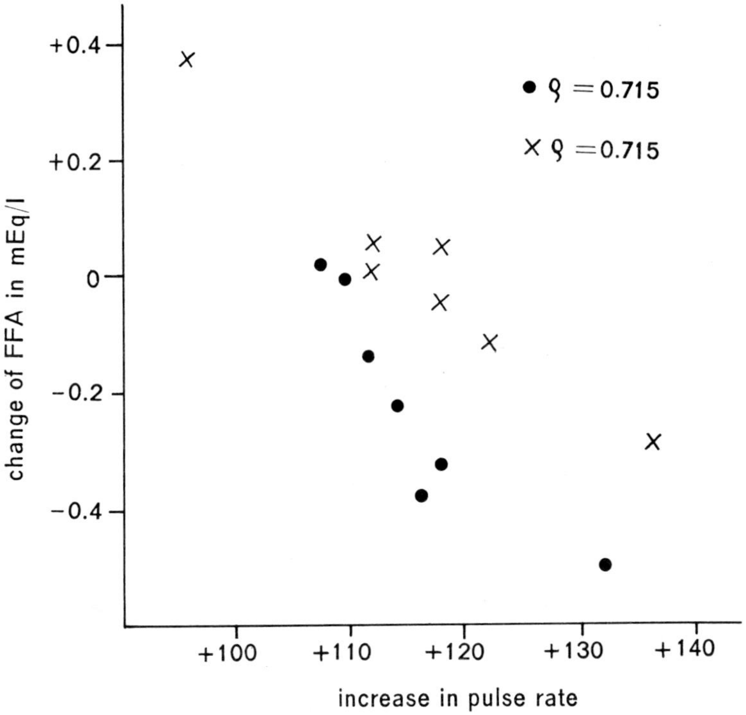

Fig. 73. Relationship between changes in the level of non-esterified, free fatty acids (FFA-ordinate; changes both in positive and negative direction) and the increase in pulse rate (abscissa) during maximal work load on a treadmill measured before (●) and after reduction of weight and fat (×) in summer training camp (Pařízková et al. 1965).

EFA did not change, nor did their response to a maximal load on a treadmill and the response after 10 min rest (Fig. 72). *The values of EFA at rest after weight reduction declined, however, to almost half their values. During the work-load the FFA level before weight reduction* (i.e. before the period of adaptation to increased muscular work) *declined significantly and after 10 minutes rest did not change further. After weight reduction the lower FFA levels remained during the maximal load at the same level and after the period of rest they increased significantly* (Fig. 72) (Pařízková et al. 1965, 1971b).

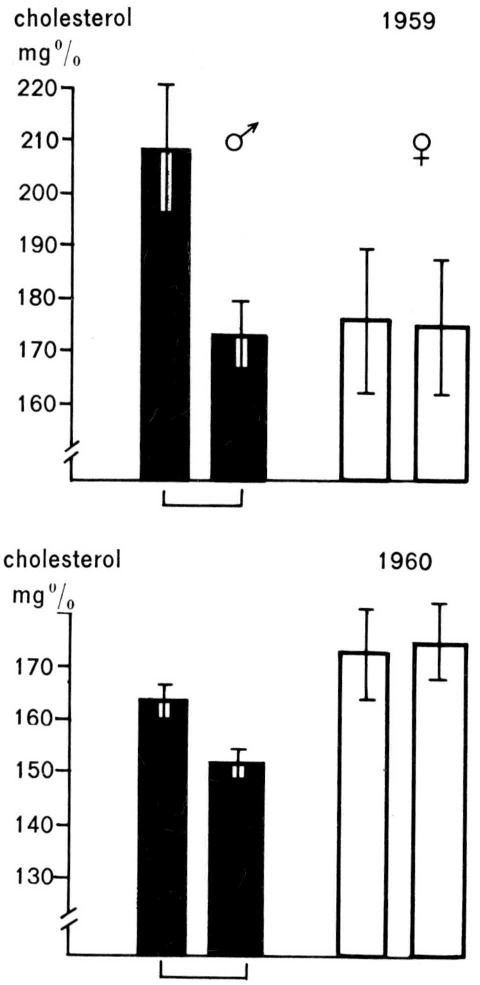

Fig. 74. Changes in blood cholesterol (mg %) in obese boys and girls before and after reduction of weight and fat in a special training summer camp in two successive years (Pařízková et al. 1963).

These changes of FFA after reduction can be explained either by a reduced uptake and utilization by the working muscles or conversely by a *more rapid and increased mobilization from fat depots.* The second possibility is more logical, in particular *with regard to the diminution of body fat.* Before weight reduction the FFA mobilization in the non-adapted organism is not sufficiently high. During work FFA are utilized but their adequate supply is not ensured. The level declines therefore and does not rise after the work is terminated. After reduction and the adaptation period to the load FFA obviously are mobilized to a greater extent (*see* example of experimental model of running animals—Fig. 37 and 38). Therefore the blood level does not decline and after termination of work it even rises. *Adaptation to increased muscular work thus* also *changes the metabolic activity of adipose tissue and its ability to release FFA promptly as a source of energy for muscular work;* this *finally* leads to *changes in the body fat ratio* (Pařízková et al. 1965, 1971b etc.).

The ability to mobilize and also obviously utilize FFA during a load is one of the associated features of adaptation to an increased load (Issekutz et al. 1965, Paul 1975). We analyzed further the relationship of increments of the heart rate during a maximal load with the concurrent drop of FFA. Spearman's rank coefficient revealed the significance of this relationship (Fig. 73): *the greater increment of the heart rate during the work load* (i.e. the poorer the fitness and adaptation to increased physical work), *the greater the decrement of FFA in blood during this load* (i.e. the obvious inability to mobilize FFA promptly as a source of energy) and vice versa. These findings are in agreement—*the organism adapted to the work load requires a smaller increase in the heart rate* and is at the same time *able to mobilize all sources of energy incl. FFA from adipose tissue* more effectively. Therefore after the stay in the camp and after reduction the shift of values in the direction towards lower increments of the heart rate and more favourable changes in the FFA level occur (Fig. 73). These relations are very readily demonstrated in obese children where within a short period both the physical fitness (characterized by aerobic capacity in relation to body weight, sport performance, etc.—Pařízková et al. 1965, 1971b) and quantitative and qualitative properties of adipose tissue change markedly. These findings are also in keeping with the conclusions of studies performed on adipose tissue of animals adapted to different loads (*see* Fig. 25, 37 and 38, Table 19).

Along with changes of FFA in the blood after weight reduction the *cholesterol level also changed.* In two groups of children, boys (n = 32) and girls (n = 35), we repeadly checked values at rest. *The decline was significant only in boys* and there was no relationship to the amount of reduced fat. In boys thus in this respect the response to reducing treatment was more marked and more favourable (Fig. 74) Pařízková et al. 1963).

5. Changes in the response of vegetative functions to a load in obese children after weight and fat reduction

Weight reduction resulting from diminution of body fat during the period of adaptation to increased activity was also manifested in other parameters characterizing the functional efficiency of the organism. In a group of 18 boys and 15 girls we demonstrated that *along with weight reduction* and *an increase in percent of LBM* (Table 49) *a reduced oxygen consumption during a standard load* of an optimal character (according to Janda 1959), worked out with regard to the initial weight also occurred. The reduction of oxygen consumption in boys was significant in absolute figures as well as in relation to body weight, LBM, kgm performance (Fig. 75). In girls the reduction was in some instances not significant. *Improvement was also apparent in ventilation and heart rate during the load, the vital capacity also increasing after reduction.* The height of the boys increased on average by 0.94 cm, in girls by 0.75 cm,

TABLE 49.
Changes in weight, relative LBM, absolute and relative values of oxygen uptake during standard work load and energy output in obese boys and girls before and after reduction in a special summer training camp (seven weeks) (Pařízková et al. 1962)

	Boys (n = 18)				Girls (n = 15)			
	Before reduction		After reduction		Before reduction		After reduction	
	$\bar{x}$	SE	$\bar{x}$	SE	$\bar{x}$	SE	$\bar{x}$	SE
Weight (kg)	65.75	3.26	58.52	2.82	70.33	2.85	63.13	2.35
LBM (%)	68.6	0.97	74.8	1.14	68.1	0.95	72.9	1.01
ml O_2/l min	770	30	570	30	730	50	620	80
ml O_2/l min/1 kg weight	11.6	0.2	9.7	0.4	10.2	2.0	9.7	2.0
ml O_2/l min/1 kg LBM	17.2	0.3	12.9	0.06	15.4	1.0	13.3	0.2
ml O_2/l min/1 kgm	2.8	0.11	2.2	0.08	2.90	0.19	2.11	0.14
ventilation/1 min abs. in l	15.74	0.59	13.26	0.60	15.48	0.65	15.09	0.77
ventilation/1 kg LBM	0.34	0.01	0.29	0.00	0.34	0.02	0.33	0.01
Vital capacity	2942	105	3073	115	2640	124.8	2838	133.8

i.e. the regime with smaller dietary restriction (see above) and an intense load of physical exercise did not impair growth (Pařízková and Vamberová 1967).

The *more favourable response of boys*, compared with girls, may be related to a different adaptability of vegetative functions (which is apparent at the onset of puberty). The increase of the body fat ratio implies during puberty in particular a greater abnormality in boys than in girls with regard to their normal body composition during this developmental period (*see* Fig. 9) (Pařízková 1959b, 1961a, 1962a, 1963a etc.). This too may be the reason why the relief of this abnormality leads to a more marked response in boys.

Miller and Blyth (1955) proved in adult men that an organism with a higher fat content consumes during the same medium load significantly more oxygen in relation to LBM than an organism with a low body fat ratio. A similar difference was found in our children after fat reduction where a reduction of energy output when performing the same work was observed (Pařízková et al. 1962, 1971b).

Adaptation to increased activity led thus to significant differences in body composition as well as to better performance. When analyzing changes in oxygen consumption it is difficult to differentiate between what should be ascribed to a more economical course of the functions of the adapted organism and what is due to reduction of fat and an increased ratio of LBM. These changes run parallel and are an integral part of the adaptative consequences of increased muscular work. In subjects who had originally a high body fat ratio the increase of the ratio of LBM will be finally manifested in work economy more markedly than e.g. in trained athletes where the body fat ratio is very low and where improvement of performance takes place mainly in other systems.

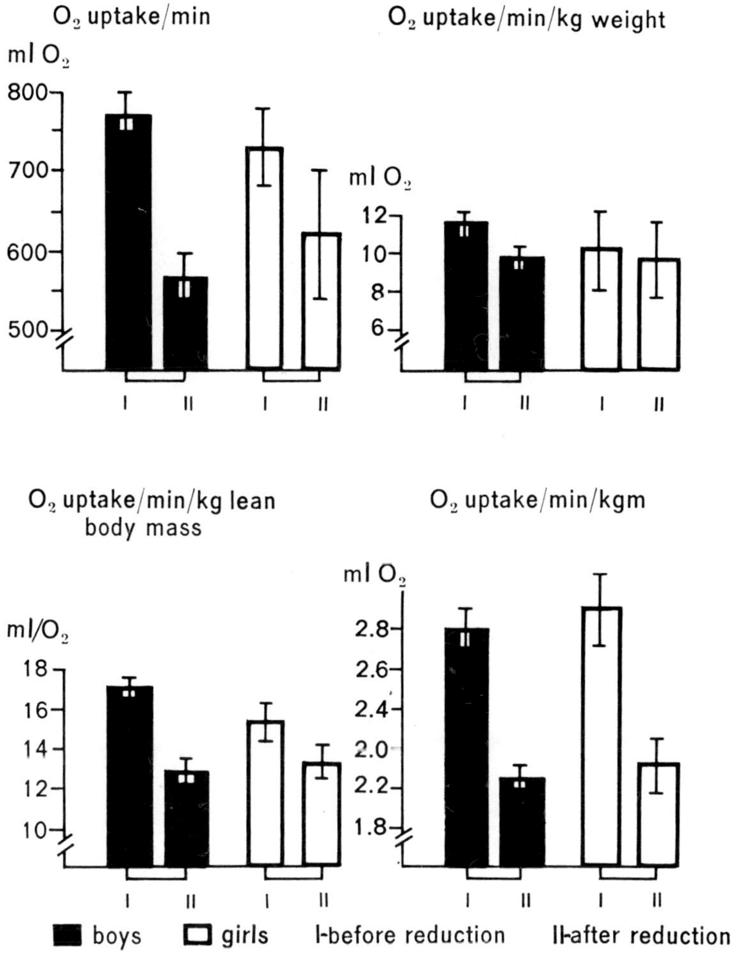

Fig. 75. Changes in O_2 uptake during submaximal, standard work load on a bicycle ergometer in obese boys (black columns) and obese girls (white columns) before (I) and after (II) reduction of weight and fat in a special training summer camp; given both in absolute values (ml O_2/min) and relative values (ml O_2/min/kg weight; ml O_2/min/kg lean body weight; ml O_2/min/kgm; $\bar{x} \pm$ SE; Pařízková et al. 1961, 1962, 1971b).

The results of investigations of oxygen consumption, heart rate, caloric output for work etc. in relation to changes in body composition after reducing therapy were moreover confirmed in a four-year longitudinal study in selected, extremely obese children (n = 8) who were followed up for prolonged periods in the outpatient clinic of the Medical Faculty of Hygiene, Charles University. These children participated four times in reducing therapy at recreational summer camps. They formed a very homogeneous group as regards age and degree of obesity. The height of the boys (n = 4) was at the onset of the investigation, i.e. when their mean age was 11.8 years in the 75th percentile of Tanner's growth grid (Tanner et al. 1966) and shifted to the area of the 90th percentile. During the last two years growth became slower and shifted to the zone of the 50th percentile (Fig. 76). The body weight was extremely elevated and after every summer camp a significant drop was recorded. *After return to normal living conditions in the course of the school year, however, as a result of inadequate adherence to therapy the condition deteriorated and the body weight before the next summer camp was higher than before the previous one.* This happened throughout the four years. Comparison of the absolute amount of LBM revealed again raised values in obese children compared with normally developed boys of the same age (Fig. 77). After the first and second summer camp the

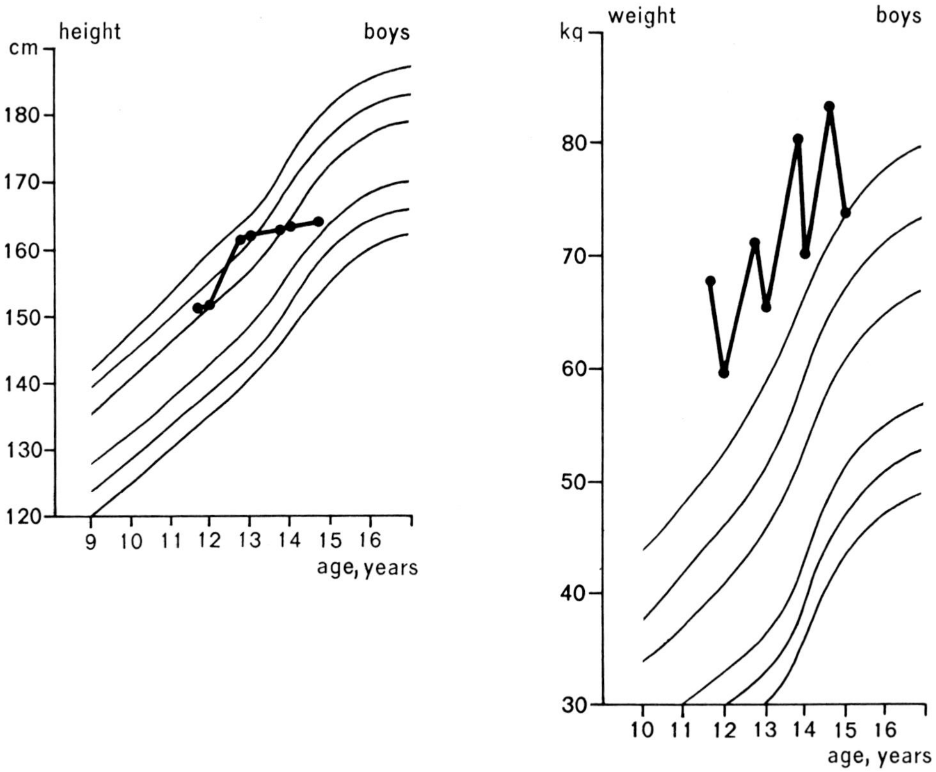

Fig. 76. Changes in height (left) and weight (right) in a group of obese boys during a four-year period during which four special training summer camps were attended; presented on the background of Kapalín's growth grid (1967) (Pařízková et al. 1971b).

absolute amount of LBM remained the same, and during the subsequent two years it diminished. *The percentage of fat declined significantly but increased again during the school year along with the body weight.* It is, however, important to draw attention to the fact that the *percentage of fat did not increase in any instance to such an extent as to exceed the values recorded during the previous year.* The resulting trend after four years was for the percentage of fat to decline slightly (as in normal boys of similar age—*see* Fig. 9 and 55) but it persisted in the zone of excessive values.

The oxygen consumption and the pulse rate, during a medium load of an optimum character also declined in all instances significantly *after weight reduction* in the summer camp (Fig. 78) *although the performance expressed in kgm after weight reduction was the same or even higher.* The greatest drop of oxygen consumption occurred after the first camp which was obviously due to an excessive oxygen consumption during the very first estimation in obese children (hyperventilation etc.).

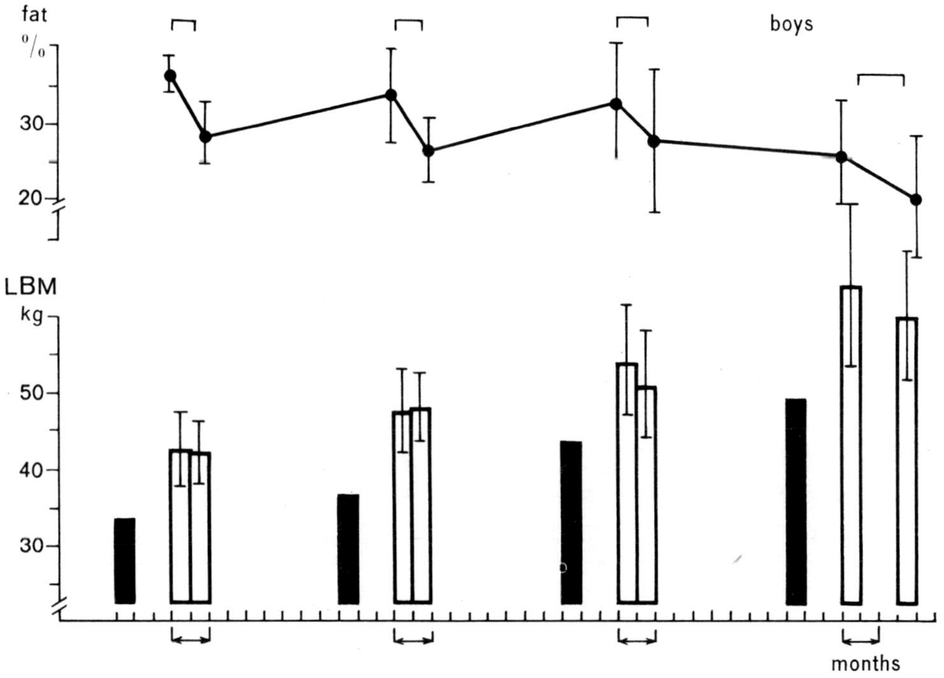

Fig. 77. Changes in per cent depot fat (%, upper part) and kg lean body mass (lower part) followed up during various stages of reducing therapy. Abscissa — months; special summer training camps indicated by arrows. Black columns — normal boys of the same age; white columns — obese boys before and after reduction; $\bar{x} \perp$ SD (for explanation *see* Fig. 76) (Pařízková 1972c, Pařízková et al. 1971b).

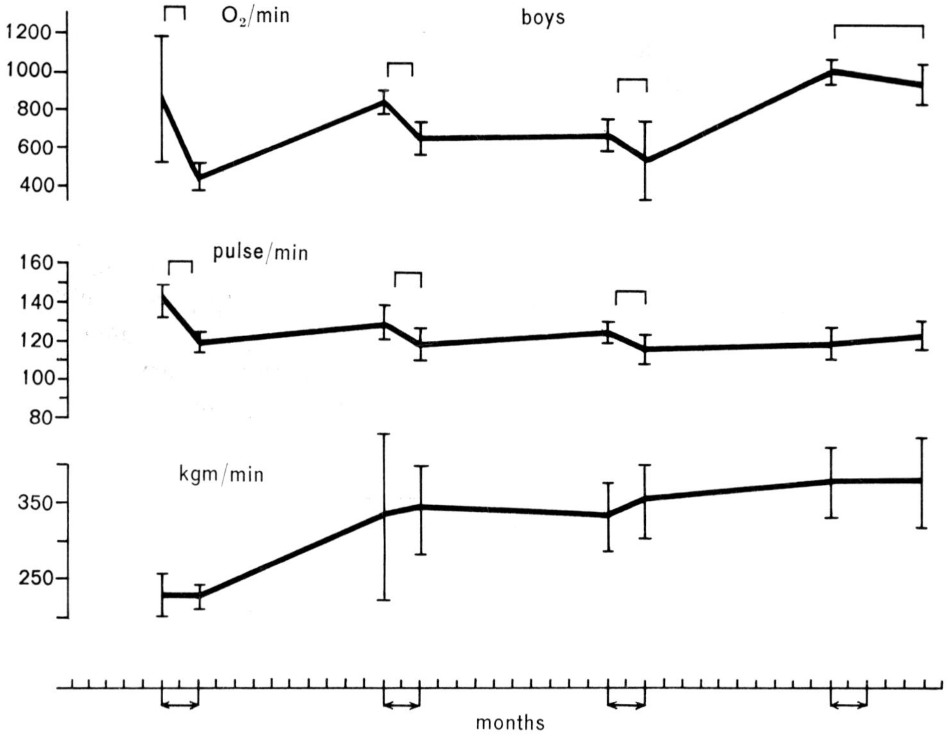

Fig. 78. Changes in O_2 uptake (ml O_2/min), pulse rate and the performance (kgm) during standard work load of optimal character on a bicycle ergometer in a group of obese boys followed during various periods of reducing treatment (four years). Abscissa — months; special summer training camps indicated by arrows, $\bar{x} \pm SD$ (for explanation *see* Fig. 76, 77) (Pařízková 1972c, Pařízková et al. 1971b).

The oxygen consumption during this load in relation to body weight and LBM declined significantly except for the last years. The improved economy of work during a medium load after reduction of excessive fat as a result of adaptation to an increased load was thus regularly manifested in the same children during growth (Pařízková 1972c,e).

Along with this group of boys a group of *girls* selected in the same way and followed up for an equal length of time was also investigated. In view of the criteria applied and the long-term follow-up their number was limited (n = 4). *Changes in body weight, body composition, oxygen consumption, pulse rate etc. were almost equal* (Pařízková 1972c,e), the results are therefore not presented.

As apparent from the presented data, *reduction of excessive fat by the above reducing therapy involving exercise* gives the *most favourable results in the early stages of growth, in particular before the full development of clinical puberty*. In later years, after a longer period of obesity, the results of weight reduction are relatively smaller and along with weight reduction a slight reduction of LBM also occurs. Although the LBM is higher than in normal children, its diminution does not seem to be a desirable effect. A conclusive opinion on this phenomenon will be expressed only after the data will be supplemented by functional examinations e.g. of the aerobic capacity, performance of the children, etc. If regular exercise is started in the very initial stages of obesity before puberty, the results of weight reduction are more marked and are achieved more readily and more rapidly (Pařízková and Vamberová 1967).

The *return of body weight* to the previous level and maintenance of a persistently raised ratio of body fat even after prolonged reducing treatment indicates that *exercise improves the condition but does not lead to quite normal values of body composition.* As soon as the conditions of treatment are not respected, the amount of fat increases markedly. It seems that the *types of obesity mentioned* already have a very well *defined metabolic stereotype which cannot be altered permanently by the applied procedure* because it has developed as a result of the action of various factors in earlier stages of life. These factors are mostly of a nutritional character as demonstrated in experimental animals e.g. during weaning (Knittle and Hirsch 1968), or when changing the diet of the lactating mother (Knittle et al. 1972) which results in greater cellularity and weight of the epididymal fat pads. Similar impact have also changes in the physical activity regime in early life (Oscai et al. 1974). An organism manipulated differently during early stages of ontogeny has first of all different degree of adipose tissue cellularity. In an organism with hypercellular adipose tissue resulting from early nutritional manipulations etc. the influence of further essential factors (absolute and relative overfeeding, hypokinesia etc.) especially during certain critical periods of growth can cause excessive deposition of fat more readily than in another organism under similar conditions. As follows fat in such a case is reduced only with difficulty and whenever the reducing regime is not respected, the adipose tissue returns almost to its level before treatment (*see* Fig. 77). Permanence of adipose tissue hypercellularity even after marked degrees of weight loss was confirmed by several authors (Salans et al. 1974, Knittle 1975) which renders repeated increase in weight and fatness possible.

The best response in these summer camps was obtained in younger children with a lower grade of obesity. In a considerable number the body composition almost approached normal values and this was maintained during subsequent growth (Pařízková and Vamberová 1967).

6. Changes of anthropometric indicators after repeated reductions of body fat during growth of obese children

In another selected group of obese boys (n = 7) and girls (n = 9) we studied along with changes of body composition in a longitudinal investigation the width of the trunk and extremities and the circumference of the chest during three consecutive years (i.e. between 11 – 13 years). *Height, weight and LBM in kg increased in boys and girls. The percentage of fat declined,* while the *absolute amount of fat remained the same* (Fig. 79). The width of the shoulders increased in both sexes, the bicondylar humerus in boys only, the biiliocristal diameter in girls only. The chest circumferences during inspiration increased in both sexes along with the vital capacity. The chest circumference during expiration did not change (Fig. 79).

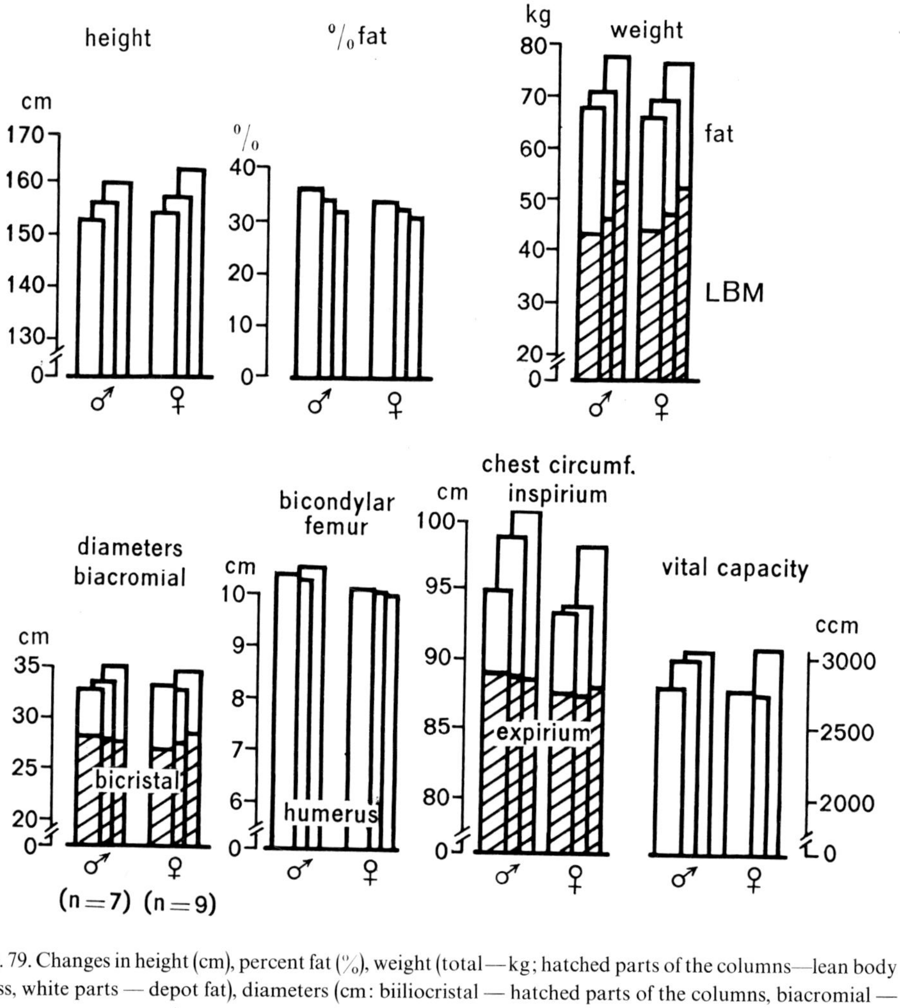

Fig. 79. Changes in height (cm), percent fat (%), weight (total—kg; hatched parts of the columns—lean body mass, white parts — depot fat), diameters (cm: biiliocristal — hatched parts of the columns, biacromial — hatched and white parts) bicondylar femur and humerus, chest circumference (hatched parts of the columns — values measured during expiration; hatched and white parts — values during inspiration) and of vital capacity in obese boys and girls from 12 to 14 years. Measured always before special summer training camps during a three-year period (Pařízková 1970a).

The sudden drop in body weight resulting from reduction of excess fat achieved by the described treatment in summer camps and at the clinic did not therefore affect the growth or other indicators of skeletal development (widths) which differed markedly depending on sex (increased robusticity of the skeleton and increase in width of shoulders i.e. biacromial in boys and increase in pelvic breadth i.e. biiliocristal diameter in girls). The chest circumference during inspiration and the vital capacity indicate further development of the respiratory apparatus, while the unaltered value of the chest circumference during expiration obviously does not imply stagnation: the increased values of this circumference are masked by simultaneous reduction of the adipose tissue ratio (Fig. 79) (Pařízková 1970a).

7. Conditions for the maintenance of reduction of body fat during repeated treatment

Figs. 76 and 77 revealed a significant reversibility of results of reducing therapy as regards total body weight as well as body composition, caused by lack of adherence to the principles of the reducing regimen, in particular from the aspect of physical activity. The easy return almost to the initial state indicates the participation of internal factors, as well as of external ones which condition further hypertrophy of fat cells (and possibly also their hyperplasia). In young children we cannot assume, even if the family and environment are cooperative, the necessary discipline in adherence to the principles of the reducing regimen and maintenance of the therapeutic results and an ever improving body composition resp.

Some exceptional cases, however, showed that in principle it is possible. We are quoting the case of a boy F.S. who started treatment somewhat later than the other children (age 15 years) and though extremely obese reached almost normal weight.

Except for several cases of obesity there were no serious diseases in the family history of this boy. The boy himself was in a satisfactory clinical condition, and suffered from no endocrine abnormality, although he had the highest body weight which was treated in our groups in the way described (Table 50). His body weight was already elevated at birth, but starting at the age when F.S. attained the height of 140 cm his body weight increased—without any apparent reason more than before. From his appearance there was a certain suspicion of Fröhlich's syndrome.

Even after the first summer camp there was a significant decline in body weight and body fat and in the course of the year his condition did not deteriorate, as in the other children and his body weight and body fat declined further. Next improvement was recorded during the subsequent summer camp and next school year (Table 50). In this boy, however, discipline and adherence to therapeutic principles was perfect with regard to dict and physical activity. In the initial stages of treatment changes of body density also suggested losses of LBM. In this case of extreme obesity this phenomenon can also be explained by a loss of body fluids

TABLE 50.
Changes in height, weight and fat in an obese boy F.S. during two years reducing treatment (diet, exercise) (Pařízková and Vamberová 1967)

	Height (cm)	Weight (kg)	Fat (%)
5. 2. 1960	168.5	126.2	43.5
2. 7. 1960	171.0	102.7	35.0
26. 8. 1960	171.0	89.0	33.0
10. 7. 1961	171.0	91.5	27.5
31. 8. 1961	172.0	78.4	16.0
7. 2. 1962	175.0	77.5	15.0

which could when calculating density in terms of body fat distort LBM values. Certain losses of LBM during such a marked decrease of body weight (almost 40% of the initial values), however, are not improbable, in particular in an adolescent boy. In view of the improved functional condition (which corresponded to the above mentioned changes in oxygen consumption during a standard load, sports performance etc.) these changes could not be evaluated as adverse. At the end of the two-year period the percentage of fat in F.S. was only little raised as compared with normal values (*see* Fig. 9) (Pařízková and Vamberová 1967).

8. Changes in the aerobic capacity after weight reduction in obese boys

Adaptation to an increased activity associated with an increased ratio of LBM and reduction of body fat affects also in obese children the aerobic capacity of the organism characterized by a maximal oxygen consumption (Šprynarová and Pařízková 1965). Changes in the aerobic capacity in obese children after weight reduction have not been investigated so far; we therefore examined from this aspect two groups of boys before and after reduction of body weight and body fat using the treatment described above. The first group was tested after their stay in the summer camp with the regimen mentioned above while the second group underwent reducing treatment during the school year in a special spa institution where in addition to the treatment described baths, massage and showers were also used.

When the latter treatment was used in a selected group of boys (n = 5) aged 14.5 years *body weight and body fat declined, the percentage of LBM increased significantly*, but the absolute amount of LBM did not change significantly (Fig. 80). *The maximal oxygen uptake did not change either, but in relation to weight it increased significantly*, while in relation to LBM it remained unaltered along with the same values of pulse frequency and maximum O_2 pulse. *The maximal oxygen uptake after reduction was*, however, *attained after a longer run at a greater speed than before*

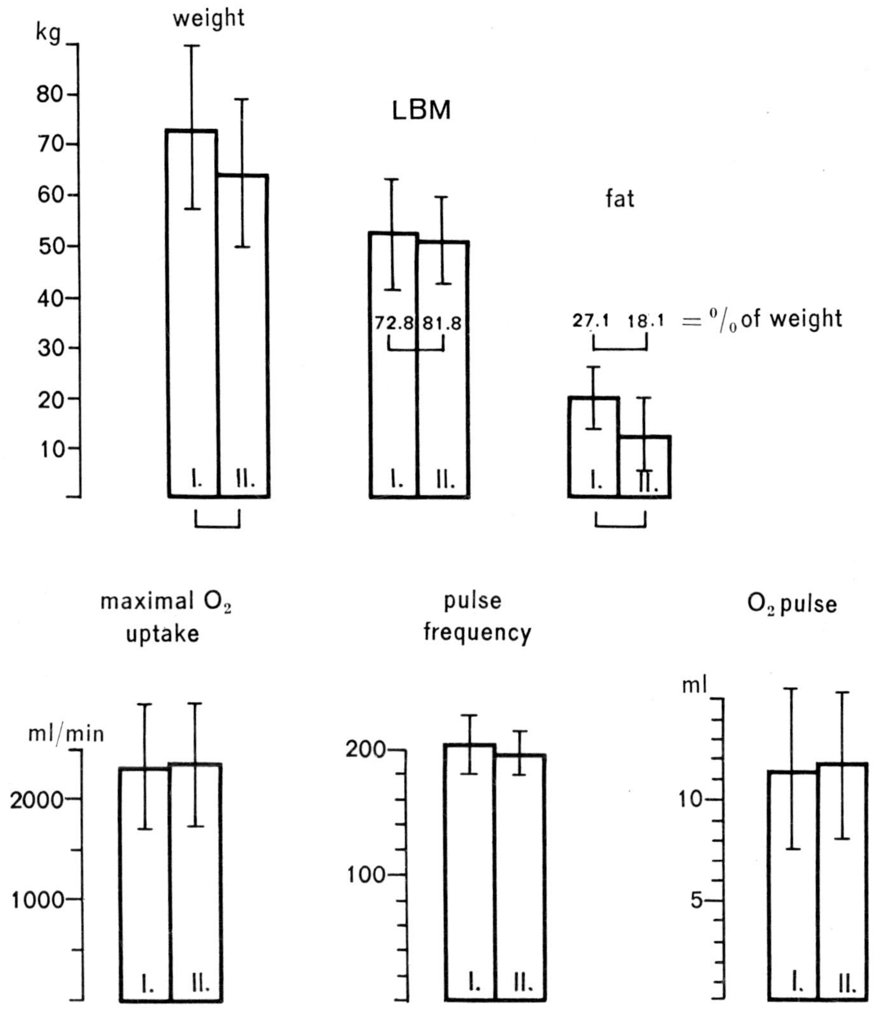

Fig. 80. Changes in weight, lean body mass and fat (kg — upper part) and of maximal O_2 uptake (ml/min), pulse rate and O_2 pulse (ml — lower part) in a group of 5 obese boys before (I.) and after (II.) reduction of weight and fat during special spa treatment lasting two months; $\bar{x} \pm SD$ (age 14.5 years) (Pařízková 1973b).

weight reduction, i.e. under conditions of the same aerobic capacity a better performance was achieved (Pařízková et al. 1971b).

After the usual summer camp treatment in the other group of seven obese boys in addition to the usual changes of body weight and body fat a *small but significant drop in the amount of LBM was observed* (Fig. 81). *A significant drop in the maximal absolute oxygen consumption was also recorded.* Again this *reduced maximal oxygen*

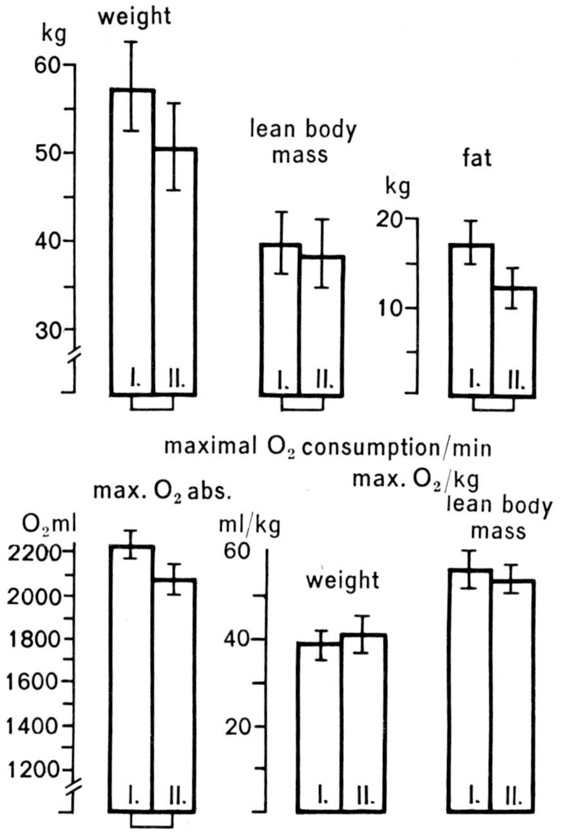

Fig. 81. Changes in weight, lean body mass (LBM) and depot fat (kg — upper part) and of maximal O_2 uptake in absolute values (ml O_2/min) and related to total and lean body weight (ml O_2/min/kg — lower part) in a group of 7 obese boys 11.7 years before (I.) and after (II.) special summer training camp ($\bar{x} \pm$ SE) (Šprynarová and Pařízková 1965).

uptake was, however, *achieved after a longer run on a treadmill at a higher rate* (during the initial measurement the total duration of the run was 3.7 min at a rate of 11.1 km/hour, pulse 200/min; after reduction the run lasted 4.5 min at a rate of 11.7 km/hour, pulse 195/min). *The maximal oxygen consumption in relation to body weight and LBM remained unaltered. Correlation analysis revealed that changes in oxygen consumption correlated only with changes of LBM* and not with the total body weight and body fat. Spearman's rank coefficient of maximal oxygen consumption with weight before weight reduction was 0.750, after weight reduction 0.929, with LBM 0.750 and 0.964. As apparent, in children the aerobic capacity is, as in adults, particularly related to LBM (Buskirk and Taylor 1957). The effect of weight reduction and concurrent changes of body composition was manifested in its functional aspects particularly in that the maximal oxygen consumption was attained after prolonged running at a greater speed, and was achieved more economically after reduction of body fat (Šprynarová and Pařízková 1965, Pařízková and Šprynarová 1970).

In view of the drop in maximal oxygen consumption and reduction of LBM it is necessary to consider in the second trial the possible impairment of respiratory and circulatory functions as a result of the sudden weight reduction which was excessive in the short period. However, *the aerobic capacity required for the movement per unit of body weight and LBM did not change nor did the maximal oxygen pulse.* On these grounds we may conclude that changes in the maximal oxygen consumption were related to changes in LBM; in view of the other findings (better performance, unaltered relative values of maximal oxygen consumption, etc.) we cannot consider the reduction of LBM observed as harmful. Last but not least, we must take into account that obese children have a significantly greater LBM than children with normal body weight (*see* Table 47 and Fig. 77); even after weight reduction the investigated group of boys had a greater LBM than boys of similar age with normal body weight.

In obese children after weight reduction various indicators of fitness were assessed repeatedly, e.g. *muscular strength* of the hand by dynamometry, *performance in different sport disciplines* (running various distances, swimming, climbing etc.). *Weight reduction and decrease in the percentage of body fat* was associated in the great majority of cases with *improved performance* (Wells et al. 1962, Jokl 1964).

The results of treatment by increased physical activity and diet thus influence not only body composition but also the aerobic capacity and performance of the organism in a positive sense. Analyses of mutual relations between LBM and maximal oxygen consumption in obese subjects before and after weight reduction indicate a significant parallelism and mutual relationship of these functional and morphological characteristics when adaptation to an increased load are influenced. *The development of the ability to supply tissues with adequate amounts of oxygen during muscular work is an indispensible prerequisite for increased fat utilization which is the basis of diminution of depot fat* as an adaptive consequence in response to a load (Pařízková 1971b, 1972c,g).

9. Consequences of reduction treatment of child obesity in adult age

Repeated measurements of the same children after one or more years have proved that the results of our therapeutic regime were only of a temporary character; most of the children, as previously mentioned, put on excess weight and fat again as if to "catch up" with a certain programmed weight and depot fat curve (Pařízková 1972c). This is apparent e.g. from Fig. 76 and 77. Only very few children were able to maintain

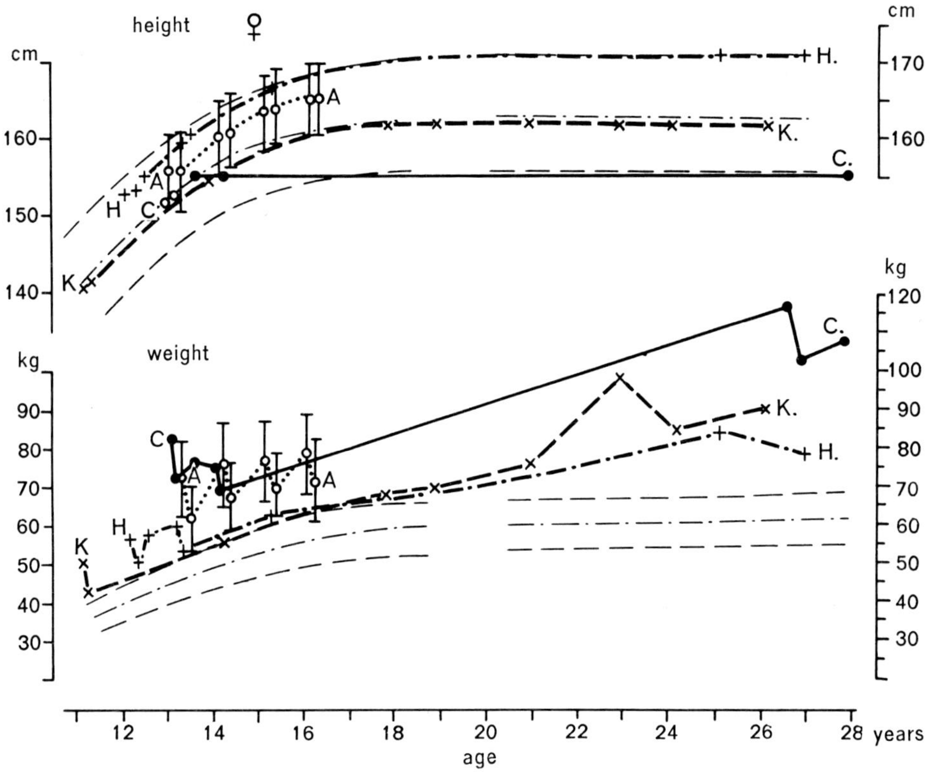

Fig. 82. Changes in height and weight in obese females (H., K., C.) followed up longitudinally over a period of several years (presented on the background of national weight and height standards (Kapalín 1967; Hejda and Hátle 1960, Pařízková 1975a). A = average values for a group of five girls ($\bar{x} \pm SD$) followed up only four years before and after summer camps.

their new weight level, or even to decrease it further under home conditions (e.g. Table 50) (Pařízková and Vamberová 1967).

As a great effort is needed to achieve lasting improvement in obese children, selected subjects were invited by personal letters for control examination 14 – 15 years after their first visit to the out-patient department. Around fifty subjects were chosen who attended the out-patient department during prolonged periods of at least several years, and also participated in the summer training camps. Unfortunately, only some of these subjects could be found after so many years, and moreover only a small proportion answered our invitation (at least by providing information on their height and weight) or were subjected to examination. Of those from the original group who responded or were measured in adult life none had normal weight.

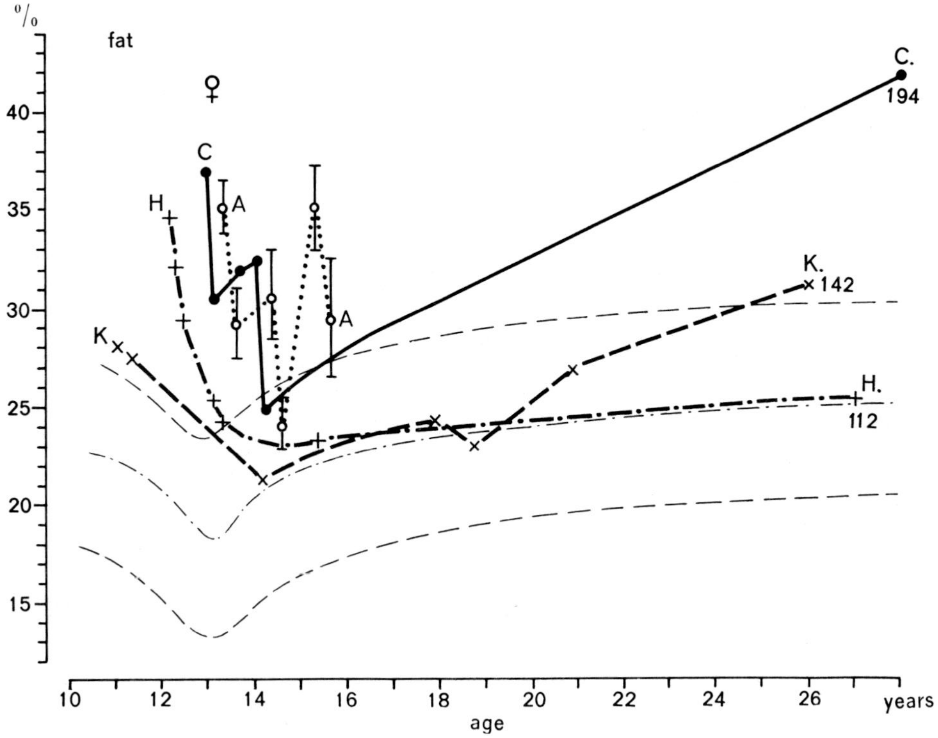

Fig. 83. Changes in proportion of depot fat in obese females (H., K., C.; group A — for explanation *see* Fig. 82) presented on the background of standards for body composition (Pařízková 1963a, 1968g, 1971b). Numbers at the right side — relative weights according to Broca's index.

Generally, the women were more willing to come and participate in our experiments, while the men mostly did not answer.

From those who finally could be measured (approximately 12 – 15 %) it was not possible to form groups according to age and sex, onset of obesity or effect of the reducing treatment etc. Therefore, only several individual cases were selected for presentation.—In Fig. 82 longitudinal data on the changes in height and weight during 14 – 15 years are given in several obese females (Pařízková 1975a).

Subject K. started the reducing treatment (i.e. diet and exercise) quite early at the age of 11 years; as regards family-history her father was overweight (115 kg/170 cm). K. started to put on excess weight before school age without obvious reason. Outpatient treatment had slight success but after the summer reducing camps her weight and fat loss was remarkable (Fig. 82 and 83). Lean body mass was markedly greater than in normal girls. During adolescence the development of body composition was close to normal (Fig. 83). K. was engaged in sports and did not diet. But after interruption of sports activity, marriage and childbirth her weight again increased excessively. She succeeded in losing some weight but still remained more overweight than before the first treatment.

The highest degree of overweight and ratio of body fat was found in subject C. Again both parents were overweight (father 96 kg/170 cm; mother 72 kg/162 cm), but two brothers were normal. C. was born as the third child (birth weight 2500 g/46 cm), and up to the age of 4 years she was very thin. At the age of 9 years she developed severe otitis media and started to gain weight (as much as 15 kg per year). Menstruation started early (9 years), growth in height ceased at the age of 13–14 years (Fig. 82). Roentgenographs showed early closing of the epiphyseal openings. C. was treated in the out-patient department for several years, and participated in three summer camps (Fig. 82 and 83 shows the results of two of them), which always had significantly favourable results. Nevertheless, after returning home weight and fat increased markedly, and her final state as an adult is disastrous. She has a normally developed child. In 1973 she underwent reducing treatment by means of thyroid preparations and Phenmetrazine as the reducing diet alone did not help. After this treatment her weight increased again but nevertheless, no marked endocrinological etc. distrubance was found.

Only subject H. displayed slightly better results. In spite of an unfavourable family-history (father 90 kg/170 cm, died at the age of 54 years of diabetes mellitus; mother 85 kg/159 cm; both brothers also overweight) she was obese from the age of 6 years after tonsillectomy. Her birth weight was 3500 g/50 cm, and her development in early childhood normal. She started to menstruate at the age of 13.5 years and attained higher values of body height (Fig. 82). She began with out-patient reducing treatment at the age of 9 years, and participated later in six summer camps. As apparent from Figures 82 and 83, she improved significantly. During adult life she put on weight up to 85 kg, but reduced by diet and exercise without medical assistance. She was not yet married when examined as an adult and her constitution was rather robust with lean body mass raised as is obvious from the higher body weight (Fig. 82) but nearly normal percentage of depot fat (Fig. 83).

Only one male in adult life, who was treated repeatedly in the out-patient department and summer camps was suitable for presentation for the above mentioned reasons. Parents of K. were slightly overweight; his birth-weight and development during childhood was normal. He was always taller than other boys of his age. At the age of 8–9 years he began to put on weight more rapidly and started to visit the out-patient department regularly, and also participated in two summer camps. The improvement in weight and body fat was marked (Fig. 84 and 85). During adolescence he was quite normal and did not visit the out-patient department again. But at the age of 21 years he had an accident and an operation of his shoulder joint, and after interruption of a more active life his weight increased markedly.

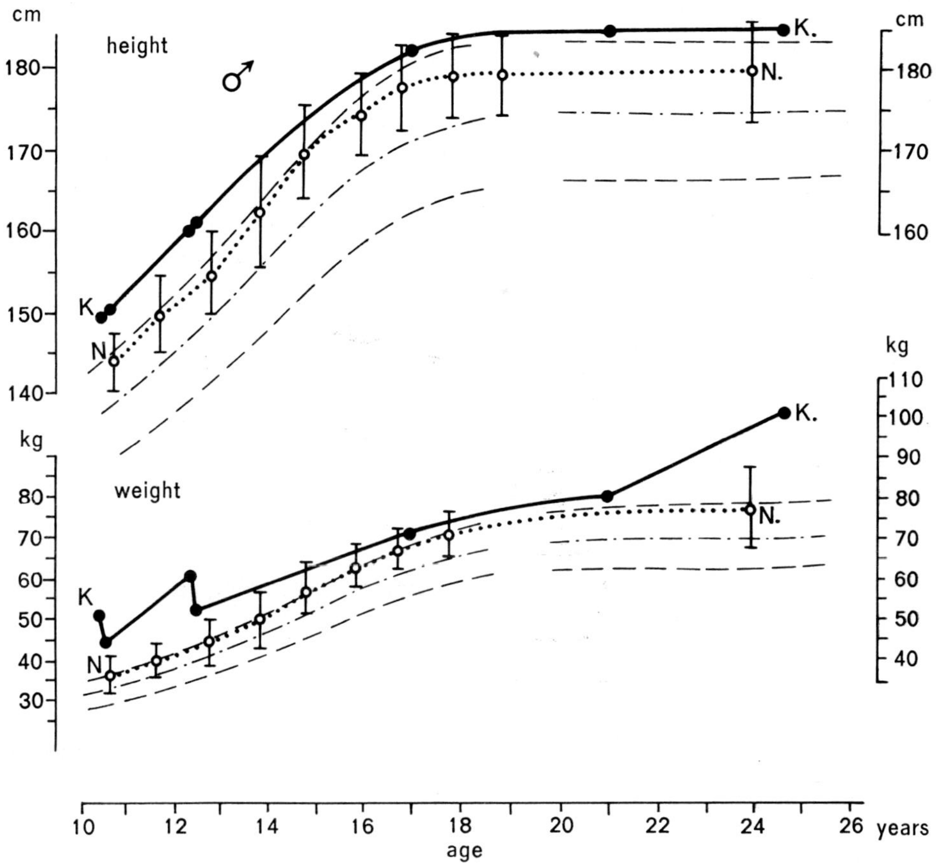

Fig. 84. Changes in height and weight in obese male K. followed up longitudinally. N = mean values for a group of 16 normal males followed longitudinally from 10.7 up to 23.6 years; presented on the background of national standards (for explanation *see* Fig. 82) (Pařízková 1975a).

He attained 116% of relative weight and his body fat is significantly higher as compared with standard values for the Czech population (Pařízková 1959b, 1962a, 1963a, 1974c, 1975a etc.). Comparison with a group of normal boys who were followed up as controls (also longitudinally), from the age of 10.7 to 23.7 years, shows a substantial deviation from the development of body weight and body composition (Fig. 84 and 85).

When comparing the previously mentioned subjects, we can find that a more marked increase in body weight appeared always after an illness etc., which involved inter alia relative immobilization in bed. But most children are occasionally ill and only sometimes obesity develops; obviously further causes play a part in the

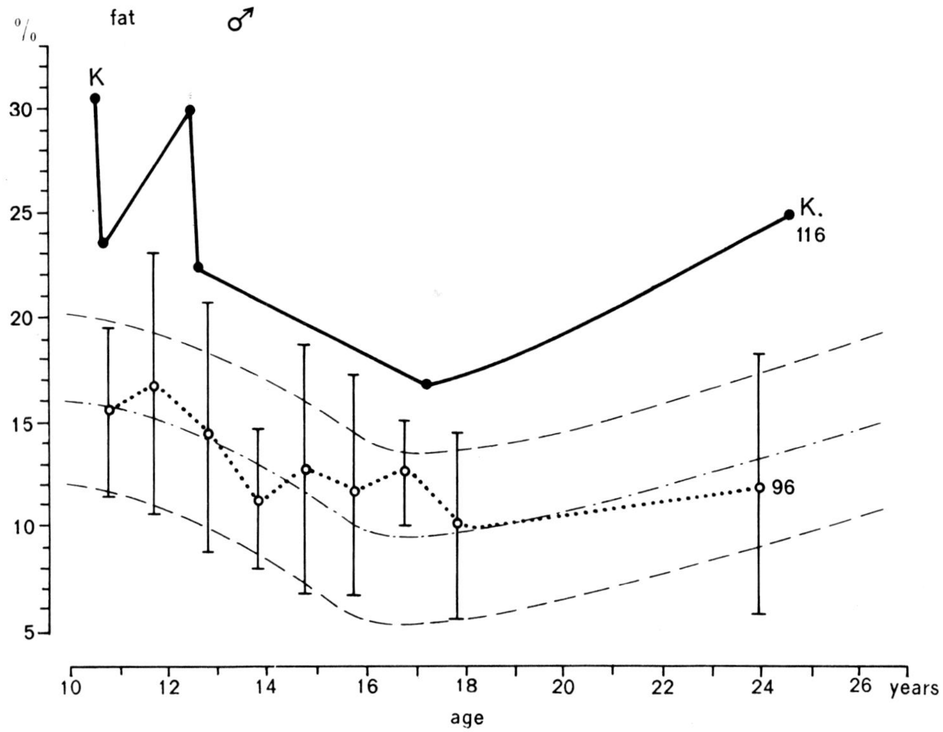

Fig. 85. Changes in proportion of depot fat in obese male K. followed up longitudinally. N = mean values for a group of 16 normal boys presented on the background of standards for body composition (Pařízková 1963a, 1968g, 1971b). Numbers at the right side — relative weights according to Broca's index.

onset of obesity, which may have latently existed before excess deposition of fat appeared.

As follows from the above mentioned cases, severe child obesities did not display long-lasting improvement in adult life as a result of regime therapy by means of diet and exercise. This kind of treatment is successful only when continued without any interruption and this is difficult, especially with regard to desirable physical activity in big cities. This was also apparent from the information about other participants in summer camps. Experience gained from the above subjects further confirms that the sooner the onset (especially before puberty) and the longer the initial reducing therapy, the more successful are its results. Therefore, an exact control of development of body composition during growth combined with an optimal diet and a proper regime of physical activity maintained even in adult life, is an important part in prevention of obesity.

X. Body composition and body build of champion athletes in relation to fitness and performance

In adult life and particularly at the end of the second and during the third decade, the most marked changes in body composition can be achieved (*see* Fig. 35), due to the highest possible intensity of work load. Under contemporary oecological conditions in industrial, advanced countries the influence of physical load at work does not play such an important role. Wirths (1975) e.g. showed that nearly 70% of workers, including housewives, in Western Germany can be classified as light workers (75 kcal/hour, or 315 kJ/hour), about 20% as moderate workers (75–150 kcal/hour, or 630 kJ/hour), and only about 10% as heavy or very heavy workers (150–200 or more/kcal/hour, or 840 kJ/hour). People living under different oecological, nutritional and working conditions have a different physical fitness, morbidity and mortality (Suzuki 1975).

An example of adaptation par excellence to an intensive load is that of champion athletes. The possibility to investigate LBM in relation to other somatic and functional parameters in top athletes gives a special opportunity to elucidate the role of body composition, in particular the importance of LBM and its relative and absolute size in relation to body fat for different sport disciplines from the aspect of the specific nature of the performance, and also the relationship of LBM and aerobic capacity in different athletes.

Physical prerequisites play an important role in sport performance, although recently it has been maintained that a decisive role in champion sports is played by functional and psychological factors. The *somatic factors* playing a part are mainly of *genetic and constitutional character, plus those which develop during training as a consequence of adaptation to a certain type of sport activity,* their importance differing for various disciplines.

The typology of sports was studied by various authors (e.g. Cureton 1951, Grimm 1960, Tanner 1964, Correnti and Zauli 1964, Novotný 1962, Chtetsov et al. 1967, Tittel and Wutscherk 1972, Malina et al. 1971, Carter 1970, deGaray et al. 1974,

Milicer 1973 etc.). The characteristic of people engaged in various sports was based mainly on classical anthropometric indicators. The aspect of body composition i.e. evaluation of the relative and absolute amount of LBM has been investigated more rarely so far in this connection (Behnke et al. 1942, 1966, Chtetsov et al. 1967, Khanina and Chagovetz 1954, Pařízková 1963a, 1965, 1972d, 1973a, 1974a, Zhdanova and Pařízková 1962, Novak et al. 1968, Šprynarová and Pařízková 1969, 1971, Lutovinova et al. 1964, Behnke and Wilmore 1974, Wilmore and Haskell 1972, Malkovská 1971, Piechaczek 1975, etc.).

1. Characteristics of body build and composition of champion athletes

Along with basic somatometric indicators we assessed the body composition in 93 athletes (members of representative teams of the Czechoslovakia or at least members of the top performance groups) and compared it with regard to body build, LBM and body fat with 30 men of similar age from the normal population.

The oldest athletes in our group comprised skiers and athletes (Table 51). The tallest athletes included swimmers, long distance runners and volley ball players, the shortest ones weight lifters and gymnasts. Body weight was not in agreement

TABLE 51.
Mean values ($\bar{x} \pm SD$) of anthropometric measurements in different champion athletes and control untrained men (Pařízková 1972d).

Groups		1	2	3	4	5	6	7	8	9	10
n		7	6	13	12	9	15	8	9	14	30
Age (years)	$\bar{x}$	17.60	25.70	17.19	17.73	23.12	21.14	18.34	24.68	24.94	18.2
	SD	0.93	3.00	0.97	0.72	1.91	2.20	0.77	3.19	3.37	0.9
Height (cm)	$\bar{x}$	181.7	176.2	180.4	172.4	177.0	182.0	170.5	173.1	166.2	176.7
	SD	5.5	6.5	4.9	8.0	5.5	4.9	8.0	8.9	7.0	5.9
Weight (kg)	$\bar{x}$	95.4	—	91.9	—	93.6	95.9	92.6	—	89.1	91.9
	SD	3.6		2.2		2.5	2.8	4.6		2.6	3.0
Biacromial (cm)	$\bar{x}$	39.2	—	39.4	—	41.2	—	39.5	—	37.9	40.4
	SD	3.7		1.8		1.7		2.1		10.4	1.9
Biiliocristal (cm)	$\bar{x}$	26.5	—	28.8	—	29.6	29.3	25.3	—	27.9	28.6
	SD	2.8		1.3		1.8	1.6	2.3		2.1	1.4

(1 — long-distance runners; 2 — skiers; 3 — volley-ball players; 4 — hockey players; 5 — canoeists; 6 — swimmers; 7 — gymnasts; 8 — wrestlers; 9 — weight-lifters; 10 — control untrained men)

with this classification—the highest weight was recorded in swimmers, followed by weight lifters.

The highest percentage of LBM was found in long distance runners, the lowest in swimmers. The highest absolute amount of LBM was recorded in wrestlers, the lowest in volley-ball players, hockey players and gymnasts. The highest absolute amount of body fat was found in swimmers, in weight lifters and non-trained people (Fig. 86). The lowest relative weight corresponds to the highest percentage of LBM; the highest relative weight was found in heavy athletes, i.e. wrestlers and weight lifters. The order of athletes according to Quetelet's index (original as well as calculated by substituting weight by kg of LBM) was almost identical (Fig. 86). The smallest amount of fat per 1 kg LBM was found in long distance runners, wrestlers, gymnasts, the greatest amount of fat in weight lifters, normal young men not engaged in systematic sport activity and in particular in swimmers (Pařízková 1972d).

Selected anthropometric indicators could not be investigated in all athletes. The sitting height was highest in long distance runners and swimmers which corresponds to the order of height. The biacromial diameter did not differ, *the smallest biiliocristal diameter was found in gymnasts who differed in this respect from all other sportsmen* (Table 51). *The relative dimensions* which *characterize the body build* differentiated most markedly the group of *weight lifters with the relatively widest shoulders* and *long distance runners with the relatively narrowest shoulders.* The *relatively widest pelvis* (biiliocristal diameter in relation to their height) was found in *weight lifters,* the *smallest in long distance runners* and *gymnasts.*

The above data indicate that the *athletes* examined *differed in their somatometric indicators from several aspects.* They include above all the *absolute size of different parameters*—height, weight etc., then *mutual relations of these indicators which express the proportionality of the figure and body build,* and finally *body composition.* Different properties which play a marked role in different sports vary and are combined in different ways. In some we may assume that they are *mainly of a genetic and constitutional character,* i.e. certain physical types which have prerequisite morphological characteristics for performance of a certain kind usually select special sport discipline. E.g. running and volley-ball are more suitable for tall people with relatively long extremities, relatively narrow shoulders and pelvis which characterize the linear type. In gymnastics or weight lifting, on the other hand, performance is facilitated by a short stature with relatively short extremities and relatively broader shoulders. In some sports special body build does not seem to play such an important role—e.g. skiers, hockey players, canoeists who do not differ from men in the normal population (Pařízková 1972d).

The *body composition* differentiates these athletes in a different way. The *highest percentage of LBM* was found in *long distance runners together with a marked linear type,* but also in *gymnasts* and *fighters.* In those sportsmen there is the smallest amount of fat per kg LBM. This is most probably due to the *nature of the above sports* which involve *moving one's own body weight* which is rendered more difficult by excessive amounts of fat (Pařízková 1972d). In skiers, volley-ball players, hockey

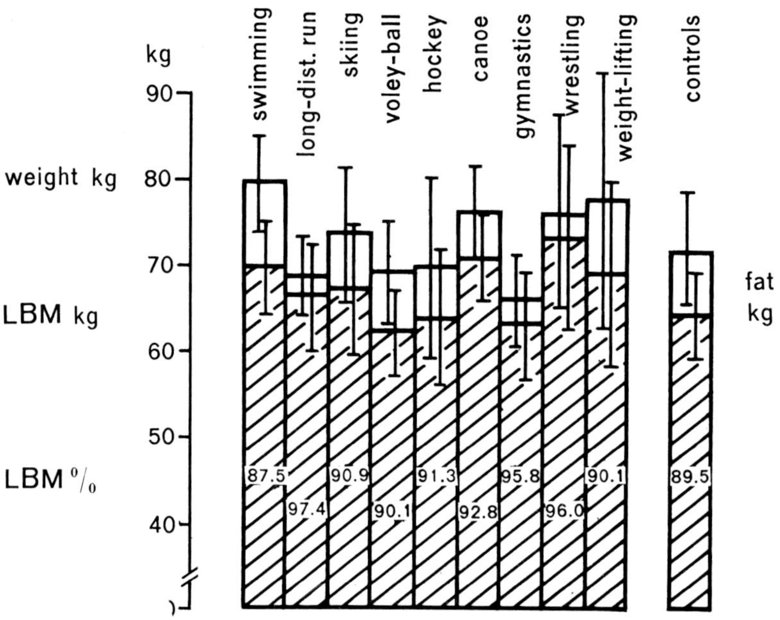

		swimming	long-dist. run	skiing	voley-ball	hockey	canoe	gymnastics	wrestling	weight-lifting	controls
height cm	x̄	182.0	181.7	176.2	180.4	172.4	177.9	170.5	173.1	166.3	176.7
	SD	4.9	5.0	6.5	4.9	8.0	5.5	8.0	8.9	7.0	5.9
relative weight %	x̄	97.0	83.6	97.1	85.9	96.2	97.7	94.0	104.1	115.5	93.5
Quetelet index (kg weight/10 cm height)	x̄	4.3	3.7	4.2	3.8	4.0	4.2	3.8	4.4	4.6	4.0
kg LBM/10 cm height	x̄	3.8	3.6	3.8	3.4	3.7	3.9	3.7	4.2	4.1	3.6

Fig. 86. Comparison of weight (kg), lean body mass (kg— hatched parts of the columns), relative weights — (%, according to Broca's index), Quetelet's index (weight/10 cm height) and our index (LBM/10 cm height) in nine groups of champion athletes compared with controls (x̄ ± SD) (Pařízková 1972d).

players functional factors play a more important role than somatic prerequisites—either neuromuscular coordination or aerobic capacity (which is relatively low e.g. in gymnasts—Čermák et al. 1967).

In *static sports (e.g. weight lifting) the ratio of body fat is high,* the *largest amount of body fat* was recorded in *swimmers* which is in keeping with data of Grimm (1960) and others. In swimmers the largest amount of fat is combined with the greatest height (advantage of long levers for swimming) and body weight (*see* Table 51) and one of the largest amounts of LBM (*see* Fig. 86). The increased amount of body fat obviously does not hinder the performance of weight lifting; during swimming (which differs as regards the medium where it is performed—elimination of gravitation, different thermoregulation, etc.) fat may play moreover a positive part because it promotes buoyancy and insulation which prevents loss of energy (Pařízková and Šprynarová 1972, Pařízková 1972d). As apparent body composition in champion athletes is not determined only by energy requirements (which during contemporary training are high in all instances) but also by the nature of the sports performance and specific adaptive changes of the organism with regard to needs.

Absolute and relative values of the biiliocristal diameter in champion athletes are also related to body fat. A lower body fat ratio together with lower values of the biiliocristal diameter are found e.g. in long distance runners or gymnasts; on the other hand, a higher body fat ratio and higher values of the biiliocristal diameter are found in swimmers and in particular in weight lifters who have a broader pelvis in relation to their height (Pařízková 1972d, 1974a).

2. Lean body mass in relation to functional characteristics in champion athletes

In youths and adults evidence was provided that the development of LBM does parallel the development of aerobic capacity. In different disciplines at a top level we may, however, in this respect, anticipate a considerable differentiation due to the specific features of the sports investigated (Šprynarová and Pařízková 1969, 1971).

Several other selected groups of athletes (runners, skiers, swimmers, weight lifters) were also examined during a maximal load on a treadmill and the relationship between body composition and aerobic capacity was investigated (Šprynarová and Pařízková 1971).

In athletes the oxygen consumption was assessed first during a 10-minute run on a treadmill at a rate of 8 km/hour. After 5 min rest the oxygen consumption during a graded load was assessed, i.e. by increasing the rate every minute by 0.5 km/hour, the initial rate being 12 km/hour, till the feeling of subjective exhaustion was reached (slope—weight lifters O; runners and skiers—5%; swimmers—3%) (Šprynarová 1966, Šprynarová and Pařízková 1971).

In this closer selection skiers were oldest, swimmers were again heaviest and tallest. The lowest weight was recorded in runners, weight lifters were shortest (Table 52). The highest ratio of lean body mass was found in runners, the largest amount of fat in weight lifters and swimmers. The results were in agreement with the conclusions of previous investigations (Pařízková 1972d).

The highest ventilation in litres was recorded in skiers along with the highest respiration rate, the highest maximal oxygen consumption, the lowest pulse rate and highest oxygen pulse. Swimmers and runners did not differ from skiers (Table 52).

TABLE 52.
Mean values ($\bar{x} \pm$ SD) of height, weight, body composition, ventilation, pulse rate, absolute and relative values of maximal oxygen consumption (Šprynarová and Pařízková 1971)

	Weight-lifters		Swimmers		Runners		Skiers	
n	14		13		10		9	
	$\bar{x}$	SD	$\bar{x}$	SD	$\bar{x}$	SD	$\bar{x}$	SD
Age (years)	24.9	3.4	21.8	2.2	22.5	5.0	25.9	2.8
Height (cm)	166.3	7.8	182.2	4.0	177.3	5.0	176.6	6.5
Weight (kg)	77.1	14.9	79.1	4.7	64.5	5.0	74.8	5.9
Lean body mass (%)	90.1	5.1	91.5	2.9	93.7	1.8	92.5	1.9
Lean body mass (kg)	69.0	10.5	72.3	4.5	60.4	4.3	68.8	5.5
Fat (kg)	8.1	5.7	6.7	2.3	4.1	1.4	5.6	1.5
Ventilation (l/min BTPS)	112.7	10.3	133.4	24.7	142.6	14.2	149.0	14.8
Pulse frequency	193.2	7.8	191.7	7.6	190.9	5.4	185.6	10.9
Max O_2 (l/min)	3.29	0.33	4.50	0.36	4.13	0.27	4.66	0.44
Max O_2 pulse (ml/min)	17.3	1.9	23.6	1.7	22.0	1.3	26.0	3.6
Max O_2/kg weight	43.6	5.9	56.9	2.9	64.1	2.3	62.4	5.4
Max O_2/kg lean body mass	48.4	5.8	62.2	3.6	68.4	2.5	67.8	5.6

Weight lifters were in all indicators of aerobic capacity last. For this sport discipline apparently the aerobic capacity is not decisive for performance and therefore training in weight lifting does not promote substantially the development of maximal oxygen consumption. Values of maximal oxygen consumption in relation to body weight do not differ from mean values obtained in untrained men of the Norwegian population (Harmansen and Wachtlová 1971) and other groups of untrained men (e.g. Bottin et al. 1968). *Runners and skiers have the highest values of maximal oxygen consumption in relation to body weight and LBM* (Šprynarová and Pařízková 1971).

Analysis of the relationship between maximal oxygen consumption and LBM revealed in weight lifters a significant correlation between the maximal oxygen consumption and body weight ($r = 0.710$) and LBM resp. (0.581). In the same group a correlation was demonstrated between oxygen pulse and weight ($r = 0.732$) and LBM resp. (0.644). Only in runners were similar relations demonstrated between the maximal oxygen consumption and LBM ($r = 0.721$) and maximal oxygen pulse and weight ($r = 0.721$) or LBM (0.770). In the remaining groups these relations were not significant (Šprynarová and Pařízková 1971).

These examples indicate that in runners the development of LBM is very closely related to the aerobic capacity of the organism. The absence of these relations in skiers is surprising. As has been already mentioned it did not prove possible in these athletes to demonstrate a defined constitutional type nor relationship between the aerobic capacity and LBM. In this sport, however, along with other factors performance depends in an important way on the technique of skiing which results from a high standard of neuromuscular coordination, somatic factors being secondary. In the group of weight lifters where training does not increase the maximal oxygen consumption the relationship between weight and LBM on the one hand and maximal oxygen consumption and maximal oxygen pulse resp. on the other hand was manifested very convincingly, obviously also as a result of the greatest variation of body mass (body weight categories). The same can also be shown in normal population groups: the aerobic capacity not influenced by other factors (e.g. training) depends in particular on the amount of tissue which consumes most of the oxygen during a maximal load (Šprynarová and Pařízková 1971).

As apparent *also in champion athletes* there is in some instance a *close relationship between the development of the aerobic capacity and body composition:* e.g. *in runners* where *training leads to a high aerobic capacity deposition of fat is very limited, the percentage of LBM being very high.* On the other hand, in *weight lifters with a relatively low aerobic capacity the amount of body fat is high.* These relationships vary, however, in different disciplines in view of the specific characteristics of sports.—The most extreme example of fat athletes are Japanese sumo-wrestlers (which is a static sport discipline), who in addition to great amount of LBM and high body fat content (which reaches values usual in really obese subjects, in spite of relatively low age—Suzuki et al. 1961) are moreover characterized by impaired glucose tolerance and high insulin levels; these latter deviations are parallel with the degree of obesity (Kuzuya et al. 1975).

In another trial in addition to body composition and aerobic capacity in two different groups (I—runners + cyclists, II—gymnasts) the size of the heart, blood red cell and plasma volumes and haemoglobin (Hb) were examined (Čermák et al. 1967). The athletes of both groups were of similar age (17 – 18 years). From the somatic aspect we found that group I was taller and had relatively longer extremities. The body weight was the same in both groups but the relative weight significantly higher in gymnasts. The sitting height, biacromial and biiliocristal diameter, the robustness of the skeleton (breadth of the wrist and bicondylar femur) were similar in both groups. There was no difference in body composition (Table 53). In this case too, the results are in agreement with the data of the formerly mentioned investigation—*intensive training in dynamic sports calling for endurance, and in gymnastics promotes the development of LBM at the expense of fat.*

Specific adaptation to a certain type of work load was manifested most markedly in functional indicators (Table 53). In *group I* the *heart volume was in absolute and relative values, i.e. in relation to body weight and LBM significantly greater, as were the total red cell volume, percentage and g of Hb and blood volume* (assessed by means of ^{131}I). Also *the maximal oxygen consumption and maximal oxygen pulse were higher in runners and cyclists (group I)* than in gymnasts (group II). *Intensive training in dynamic sports markedly promoted the development of the ability to release large amounts of energy aerobically* which was *not found in gymnasts* (Čermák et al. 1967).

The above data indicate the marked differences between the selected sports mentioned which pertain to functional characteristics (Seliger 1968), even in the absence

TABLE 53.
Mean values ($\bar{x} \pm SD$) of anthropometric measurements, body composition, skinfold thicknesses, absolute and relative heart volume, blood indicators, maximal oxygen uptake and oxygen pulse in groups of runners and cyclists (1, n = 7) and gymnasts (2, n = 8) (Čermák, Brousil and Pařízková 1967)

		Height	Weight	Relat. weight	Leg weight	Biacrom. diameter	Biiliocrist. diameter	Wrist breadth	Bicondylar femur
1	$\bar{x}$	181.7	68.4	83.6	109.5	39.2	26.5	5.8	9.9
	SD	5.0	4.2	4.0	3.9	3.7	2.8	1.0	1.2
2	$\bar{x}$	170.5	66.0	94.0	101.1	39.5	25.3	5.6	9.5
	SD	8.0	5.3	8.8	5.4	2.1	2.3	0.9	1.4

		Body composition				Skinfolds (mm) (Best)			
		LBM %	LBM kg	Fat %	Fat kg	Triceps	Sub-scapular	Abdomen	Sum of 10
1	$\bar{x}$	97.4	66.5	2.6	1.7	4.9	6.4	7.6	48.8
	SD	4.5	6.0	2.0	1.4	1.7	1.4	2.5	11.5
2	$\bar{x}$	95.8	63.2	4.2	2.8	5.6	7.9	8.5	57.4
	SD	4.4	6.0	3.8	2.5	1.2	1.5	2.1	8.0

		Heart vol. (ml)	Heart vol./weight	Heart vol./LBM kg	Haemato-crite %	Plasm. vol.	Eryth. vol.	Hb %	Hb g
1	$\bar{x}$	927.0	13.55	13.95	48.3	2661.0	2444.0	17.36	895.0
	SD	84.8	1.24	1.24	1.44	463.3	444.8	1.20	212.3
2	$\bar{x}$	738.5	11.67	11.67	42.0	2469.0	1793.9	15.70	667.5
	SD	107.4	1.14	1.29	6.8	475.4	361.2	1.29	75.7

		Blood vol. (ml)	Blood vol./weight	Blood vol./LBM	Hb/weight	Hb/LBM	Max. O_2 ml/min	Oxyg. pulse (ml/min)
1	$\bar{x}$	5105.4	74.5	76.7	13.02	13.39	4001.7	20.45
	SD	874.1	11.9	12.6	2.74	2.86	352.0	1.96
2	$\bar{x}$	4269.0	65.3	68.1	10.16	10.61	3393.7	17.8
	SD	475.4	10.7	10.1	1.31	1.39	338.0	1.3

of differences in body composition (percentage of LBM and fat). From the point of view of different sports it is necessary for an understanding of their specific features to use a wider spectrum of examinations testing different aspects of performance in their entire range. Also in champion athletes body composition can be considered in the group of morphological indicators as one of the most important signs, particularly when evaluated in conjunction with other indicators or as a reference standard (similar to body weight) for oxygen consumption during a work-load, muscle strength, etc.

3. Changes in body composition during Olympic training of gymnasts

Particularly in those sports where it is important to move one's body weight the development of LBM and restriction of fat depots in the organism play an important role. Gymnastics is an example of a sport in which body composition and weight has a great effect; repeated investigations revealed a minimal body fat ratio. Practical experience indicates that gymnasts "perceive" every increment of body fat in their performance. The ratio of LBM in champion athletes, in particular in the above mentioned sport discipline, is on a very high level. Despite this even here we can observe certain fluctuations of body composition during periods with different intensity of training in relation to preparation for important contests and discontinuation of training resp. (Pařízková 1966). The changes in body composition as compared with changes in youths engaged in gymnastics during the growth period have nevertheless somewhat different character (*see* Table 18 and Fig. 62–65).

In a longitudinal investigation we followed up a group of men (n = 7) and women (n = 8) from the national Olympic team of gymnasts during their final preparation before the Olympic games and after their termination. Height, body weight and percentage of LBM and fat, thickness of ten skinfolds were investigated during 36 weeks by the methods described above. *Intensive training shortly before the Olympic games did not influence the body weight of men or women* (Fig. 87). *The total and subcutaneous fat diminished while LBM increased. Discontinuation of intensive training after the games caused a significant increase of weight and in particular of body fat in women, while in men an increase of body fat without increase of body weight was noted which implies a reduction of LBM*. This second period, i.e. *discontinuation of intensive training* was *associated with a decline in condition and performance* (Pařízková 1963a, 1966, 1974a). We had no opportunity to check longitudinally the nitrogen balance which might be negative in this period.

The results indicate that significant *changes in body composition along with a reduced performance may occur even when the total body weight is unaltered.* In adults during a marked decline of intensity of physical exercise and work even under physiological conditions *a reduction of LBM may occur.* This phenomenon was not observed in normal youth: it seems that during growth "dystrophy" of LBM as a result of relative inactivity is prevented by the action of growth hormone. In adult athletes it is quite a regular phenomenon. It is most marked in champion athletes who discontinue training completely and do not compensate it by routine training. As revealed by the case-histories of some athletes who were followed up for prolonged

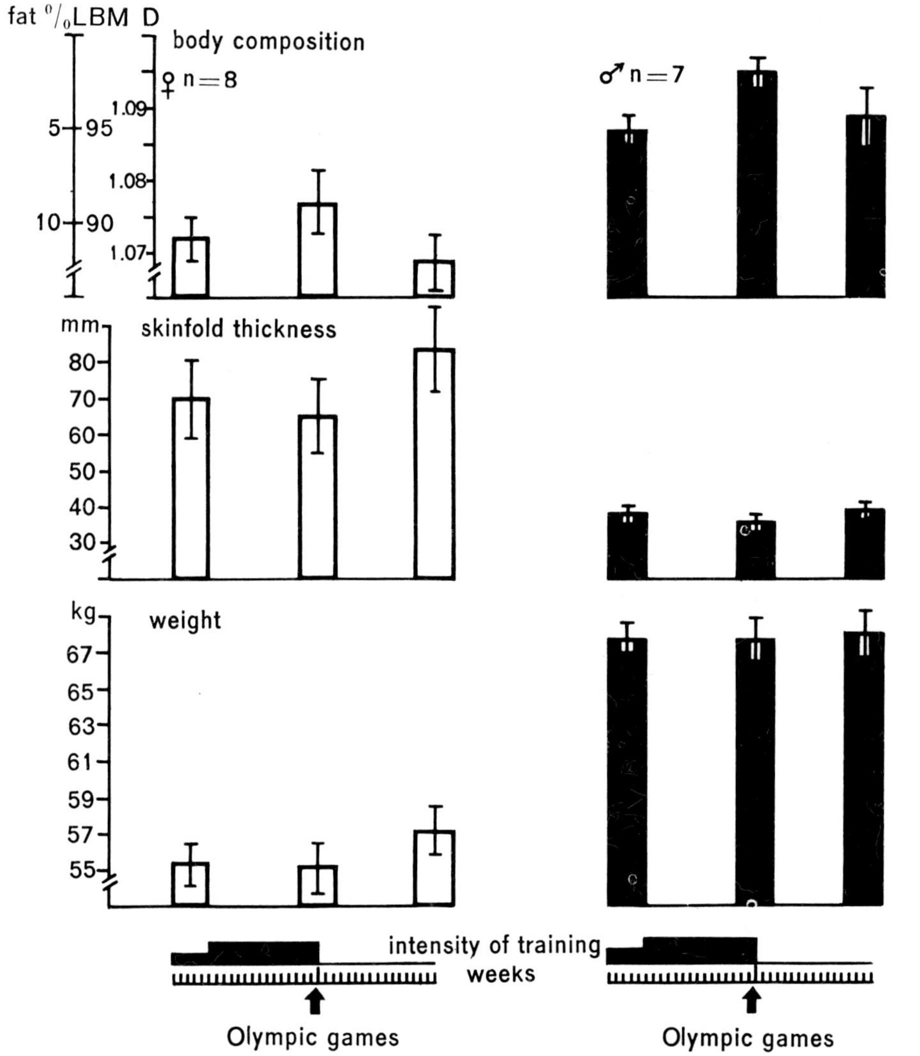

Fig. 87. Changes in percentage of body fat (%, or body density), skinfold thickness (mm) and total body weight (kg) in national Olympic team of gymnasts (left = women; right = men) ascertained before and after the period of top preparation for the Olympic games in Rome (1961), and after discontinuation of top training. Abscissa — weeks; intensity of training — bottom (for explanation *see* Fig. 36 and 65). Arrows indicate Olympic games (Pařízková 1963a, 1966).

periods under these conditions *the response to discontinued intensive training is not always the same; some individuals become fatter and put on fat more readily and reduce LBM,* in others this happens more slowly and only to a slighter extent.

As in the experimental model a marked individual variability is found in the response to discontinued load to which the organism has been adapted for a long time. Elucidation of these differences would call for a more detailed and more accurate follow up of differences in the energy output and input during different periods of training (or during its discontinuation) and individual peculiarities of the energy metabolism resp. in relation to other characteristics of the individual.

During the last 10–15 years a marked change in the physique of gymnasts, especially women, has been observed, along with the increase in the intensity of training and improvement of performance in gymnastics. The mean body weight decreased (both absolute and relative) which results in a *much more slender physique.* Best gymnasts have a *very narrow pelvis* especially when relating biiliocristal breadth to biacromial breadth. At the time of Olympic Games in Rome (1961) *the mean percentage of fat* in the Czechoslovak Olympic team of best women-gymnasts was *approximately 8%* (*see* Fig. 87), before the Olympic Games in Munich (1972) this value equalled *approximately 2%*, parallelled by much lower body weight. The same applied to Soviet gymnasts at that time (Pařízková 1974a). These data indicate a great increase in the demands of the champion sport as regards both selection of special physical type and intensity of training in gymnastics, started usually early in childhood. This situation reminds that of acrobats in circuses or ballet-dancers etc.

4. Body composition during excessive training

In one longitudinal study with rowers we have found, after initial amelioration of the morphological and functional characteristics during intensive training, a *slight decrease of lean body mass together with a decrease of maximal oxygen uptake as well as of strength of selected muscle groups in final periods of preparation for top competitions.* But even in this case sport *performance in rowing and strength of selected arm muscles increased further* (Čermák et al. 1975). These findings concerned only a *short period before competitions,* when the athletes are generally characterized by *top form in their narrow sport specialization, but at the same time also by increased sensitivity to the impact of various negative environmental stimuli* (infection, cold, psychic stress etc.) which can sometimes cause a failure during competitions.

The most marked decline of LBM is found in athletes during exhaustive training and illness resp. Long-term investigation of basket ball players and gymnasts by means of densitometry revealed e.g. that an athlete who had to discontinue training on account of a poor functional state and poor performance lost 1.5 kg body weight, incl. 0.2 kg LBM. A similar drop occurred during serious digestive trouble in a gymnast; the loss of weight—2kg—included 0.6 kg LBM (Zhdanova and Pařízková 1962).

Investigations of the body composition thus provide information on the fitness and degree of training from the morphological aspect and may draw attention to serious disorders which as a rule are also manifested very clearly in functional indicators, performance, etc.

Checking body composition after certain intervals makes it possible to evaluate the intensity of training: *long-term investigations revealed that a well adapted sportsman cannot discontinue* or *reduce training without putting on fat even when he restricts his dietary intake.* This is also in agreement with the results in our experimental model of trained, exercised laboratory animals (*see* p. 77). An increase in body weight may be masked by fasting or excessive sweating, the deposited fat, however, cannot be concealed when body composition is assessed.

On the other hand *during intensive training the body weight may increase while the body fat declines and thus the increment of LBM is greater than the increment of body weight.* An increase in body weight may lead to the idea that it should be reduced which in this case would cause an undesirable reduction of LBM and possibly poorer performance.

All the examples quoted were observed during examinations of selected champion athletes. The results cannot be documented in view of the great variability of the temporal course of individual cases with a different specialization. During long-term investigations of our representatives as well as rank and file sportsmen *checking of body composition proved useful as one of the means rendering it possible after a prolonged period to analyze somatic characteristics in relation to the intensity of training, fitness as well as the dietary regime* (Åstrand 1972a, Pokrovsky 1975, Rogozkin 1975 etc.) *and performance even without frequent control by the trainer* (Pařízková 1963a, 1965, 1966, 1968a,b, 1973a, 1974a). Skinfold measurements by means of a caliper are used as a regular examination in out patient departments for sports medicine in Czechoslovakia and supplement thus investigations of champion as well as rank and file athletes.

XI. Body composition, body build and fitness of elderly men with a different life-long regime of physical activity

Ageing of the organism is manifested among other things by a reduction of LBM (*see* Fig. 9). Involution of LBM is preceded by functional involution (Hollander 1970) which proceeds more rapidly than morphological involution, e.g. the aerobic capacity during ageing declines not only absolutely but also in relation to body weight and LBM (*see* Fig. 20 – 22); this also applies to the basal oxygen consumption (Behnke 1956, von Döbeln 1956). Regressive changes begin to appear as early as the third and fourth decade, they are very individual and depend on the health and functional status. It may therefore be assumed that these changes will be related, inter alia, to the degree of motor activity (*see* Fig. 35). Some pathological processes in old age are caused by senile hypoxia which can, however, be effectively compensated by a special regime of physical activity (Sirotinin 1972). The same applies to the regulation of cardiovascular activity (Arinchin 1972) and manifestations of atherothrombosis in old age (Wright 1972) etc.

Investigations of somatic changes in old age have so far been focused mainly on classical anthropometric indicators. Data on height and weight are most plentiful. However, only very rarely are more detailed characteristics from the medical, functional, nutritional aspect and the case-history of physical activity available. It is thus difficult to decide to what extent simple senile changes are involved and to what extent pathological factors participate in these changes.

Cross-sectional studies reveal a decline in height in old age (Trotter and Gleser 1951, Pett and Ogilvie 1956, Lee and Lasker 1958 etc.) which, however, was not confirmed by others (e.g. Hrdlička 1936). Longitudinal investigations of height were made by Büchi (1950), Damon and Stoudt (1963). Findings pertaining to body weight are also controversial: some authors describe a decline with advancing age (Pett and Ogilvie 1956), while others did not observe this decline (Lee and Lasker 1958). Other anthropometric indicators were studied more rarely (Nikityuk 1972).

The body composition in old age was investigated, but due to some methodological difficulties, initially only by means of whole body counters by assessing ^{40}K (Allen et al. 1960, Forbes and Hursh 1963 etc.). These studies confirmed a decline of LBM with age. Lee and Lasker (1958) did not reveal any changes in skinfold thickness in advanced age; Pett and Ogilvie (1956) on the other hand, described a decline in skinfold thicknesses, particularly in men. The senile changes described are thus controversial and obviously depend on the health, nutritional and professional status of the subjects investigated.

With regard to the conclusions on changes induced by a different regime of physical activity during ontogenesis the question arose whether and to what extent the body composition along with other indicators of the functional status can be influenced by life-long physical training or systematic physical training commenced at an advanced age. Therefore groups of old men with a different life-long regime were subjected to single and long-term investigations.

1. Body composition and body build in active and inactive men of advanced age

The first part of the investigation comprised a cross-sectional comparison of groups of 170 normal men aged 55 – 79 years.

All the selected men had sedentary occupations and were thus in this respect comparable. Before the trial they were subjected to a detailed clinical examination. Subjectively these men felt well, although in some of them symptoms of chronic diseases, common in old age were found (emphysema of the lungs, arteriosclerosis, etc.). All men with signs of serious disease were eliminated from the group. The group was subdivided by age (55—64 and 65—79 years) and by the amount of physical activity and participation in sport activities throughout life, i.e. for at least 35 years: A — active; C — control, inactive men. The group of active men comprised men who were engaged for at least 15 years in intensive sport activity and participated in contests (athletics, gymnastics, canoeism, equitation, skiing, football, tennis, etc.). The mean period during which they were engaged in intensive physical activity was 30 years, followed by at least 15 years of sports on a recreational basis. This group included also individuals who were engaged in sports on a recreational basis but very intensively, the mean period of sports activity being 46 years. All men participated at the time of the investigation in physical training in type and intensity suited for advanced age (Eiselt 1968, Kuta et al. 1964).

Comparison of the mean age of the groups revealed only slight differences (Table 54); in view of the advanced age these differences were not important for interpretation during further comparisons. The mean values of height, body weight, relative weight, sitting height, span of the arms, breadth of shoulders (biacromial) and of the pelvis (biiliocristal and bitrochanteric diameters), depth and circumference of chest did not differ by age or physical activity. The waist measured at the level of the navel was significantly smaller in the younger active men (group A) who had also a greater circumference of the forearm. The circumference of the thigh was greater in all active men of both age groups. The percentage of LBM and fat did not differ, the *absolute amount of LBM was,* however, *significantly greater in the group of younger active men than in the remaining groups* (Table 54). When comparing

TABLE 54.
Mean values (x̄ ± SD) of anthropometric measurements and body composition in active, trained (A) and control, inactive men (C) up to and above 65 years of age (Pařízková and Eiselt 1966)

	A (trained)				C (untrained)			
	Up to 65 years		Above 65 years		Up to 65 years		Above 65 years	
	x̄	SD	x̄	SD	x̄	SD	x̄	SD
n	40		40		35		55	
Age (years)	60.10	1.94	73.33	4.31	62.91	2.52	69.41	4.42
Weight (kg)	73.40	8.71	71.25	9.34	70.73	8.46	71.31	9.47
Height (cm)	170.79	5.55	169.70	7.33	168.91	6.36	168.94	5.35
Spread of the arms (cm)	174.63	6.07	176.26	8.43	173.78	7.95	174.73	5.94
Biacromial diameter (cm)	38.51	2.55	38.84	2.02	38.62	2.39	38,71	1.60
Biiliocristal diameter (cm)	27.95	1.49	28.67	2.31	27.82	1.90	28.61	1.57
Chest circumference (cm)	92.80	6.24	93.05	6.46	94.78	5.58	90.98	7.32
Abdomen circumference	83.56	7.28	85.90	30.17	87.45	6.94	88.75	11.78
Arm circumference	28.75	1.27	28.05	2.28	29.09	2.01	28.45	2.25
Forearm circumference	28.19	1.81	26.76	1.63	27.04	1.43	26.84	1.66
Thigh circumference	54.70	3.56	53.39	9.76	52.83	3.20	52.18	3.54
Fat (%)	18.8	6.8	19.5	6.3	20.9	5.3	22.2	5.0
Lean body mass (kg)	58.1	6.6	55.8	7.7	55.7	6.6	55.3	6.1

the older active and inactive men this difference was not found (Pařízková and Eiselt 1966).

From the aspect of relative measurements we found only a significant difference in the chest circumference during expiration expressed in relation to values to chest circumference during inspiration, which was higher *in active men.* This finding characterizes the *greater expansibility of the chest* (Pařízková and Eiselt 1966). A similar difference expressing the *better functional state of the arm musculature,* was found in the relative value obtained by expressing the arm circumference during relaxation in relation to the circumference of the arm during contraction.

The negative correlation between the percentage of LBM and body weight revealed that *during old age the higher the weight the smaller the percentage of LBM and thus the higher the ratio of body fat.* Body weight, the relative and absolute amount of LBM correlated significantly with the relative measurements of the pelvis expressed in values of height: the relative width of the pelvis increases with an increase in the total body weight due to an increase in both components, LBM and fat.

Cross-sectional data revealed no significant differences in the majority of somatic indicators. *With age only the circumferences of the forearm and thigh and the absolute amount of LBM declined.* These changes were, however, *significant only in active trained men;* it may be assumed that they were significant mainly *because the original values were higher as a result of adaptation to an increased load* (Pařízková and Eiselt 1966). We did not find differences in the skinfold thickness with advancing age which supports the explanation that the circumference of the extremities was reduced as a result of involution of muscle mass, i.e. LBM.

Systematic physical exercise in which the group of active men was engaged throughout life *led thus to a larger amount of LBM which implies delayed involution of LBM at that age, associated with higher values of thigh and forearm circumference* (which, however, was significant only in the age group under 65 years). Reduced relative values of chest circumference during expiration were also found suggesting a *delayed senile reduction of chest motility due to increased motor activity*. As these data were obtained in a cross-sectional study they must be interpretated very carefully because we do not know the initial somatic state of these men before they were engaged in physical activity. The results of other longitudinal studies conducted in younger subjects suggest nevertheless an influence of physical exercise.

2. Body composition in relation to aerobic capacity

In conjunction with changes of the LBM in older men with different physical activity we investigated also possible differences in the maximal metabolic activity of LBM, i.e. in the aerobic capacity expressed in relation to LBM. In selected groups of old men (active, engaged in sports, since the 7th decade—A_7, n = 34, and eighth decade—A_8, n = 20; inactive controls C_7, n = 48, C_8, n = 14). The maximal oxygen consumption was investigated during a graded load on a bicycle ergometer as described above—*see* p. 53). We compared the *maximal performance in watt* and *maximal oxygen consumption* (Fischer et al. 1965); *both indicators were significantly higher in active men.* Although in this smaller group the difference between the LBM of active and inactive men was not significant even in the seventh decade, *in active men the absolute maximal oxygen consumption as well as in relation to LBM was higher*. Moreover we found *in group C_8 significantly lower values than in C_7, while between A_8 and A_7 no differences were revealed* (Fig. 88).

The results indicate that *in men who are engaged throughout life in systematic exercise and sport training and have an intensive regime of physical activity the aerobic capacity and maximal metabolic activity of LBM are maintained in old age at a higher level corresponding to values recorded in inactive men approximately ten years younger* (Fischer et al. 1965). Similar values were also obtained by other authors (Åstrand 1972a, Shephard 1969 etc.).

3. Body composition in relation to muscular strength

Similar conclusions are also reached from results of measurement of muscular strength (Kuta et al. 1964, 1970), tested in the above group.

The muscular strength of flexors and extensors of the elbow was assessed by means of an electric dynamometer constructed on the tensometric principle. The strength of hand grip was measured by means of a Collins dynamometer.

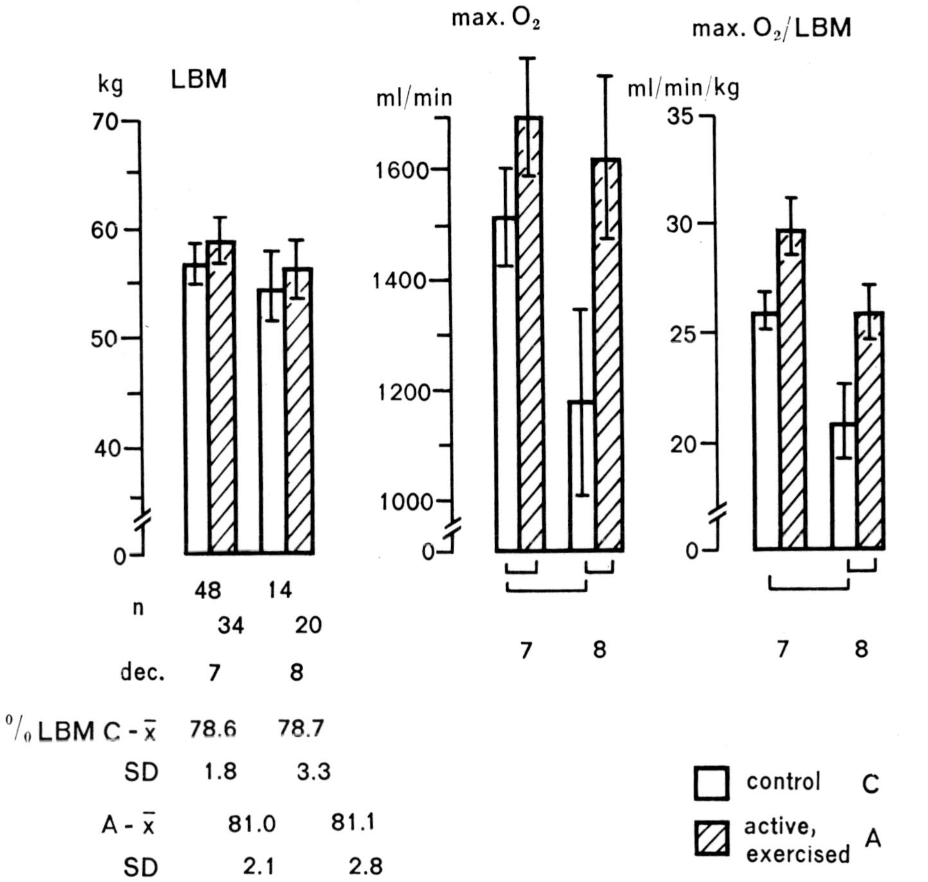

Fig. 88. Comparison of lean body mass (kg — above; numbers below = % lean body mass), maximal O_2 uptake in absolute values (ml O_2/min) and related to lean body mass (ml O_2/min/kg lean body mass) in a group of old men in the 7th and 8th decade of life with different life-long physical activity regime (white columns — control, inactive — C; hatched columns — active, trained — A; $\bar{x} \pm$ SD). (Fischer et al. 1965, Pařízková 1974c).

In the seventh decade the muscular strength was significantly greater in active trained men (Kuta et al. 1964, 1970). *Active men in the eighth decade had values significantly higher* (Table 55). Values for active men in the eighth decade did not differ significantly from values assessed in inactive men in the seventh decade, similarly as the aerobic capacity. Obviously more intense oxidative processes in the LBM also rendered a better performance as regards muscular strength possible. In the literature these data are so far unique (Sulkin 1972).

TABLE 55.
Mean values ($\bar{x} \pm SD$) of muscle strength (kp) in active, trained ($A_{7,8}$) and control, inactive men ($C_{7,8}$) in the seventh and eighth decade of life (Kuta, Pařízková and Eiselt 1964)

	A_7 (Trained)		C_7 (Untrained, controls)		A_8 (Trained)		C_8 (Untrained, controls)	
n	17		63		12		13	
	$\bar{x}$	SD	$\bar{x}$	SD	$\bar{x}$	SD	$\bar{x}$	SD
Hand grip (right hand)	47.0	7.9	43.6	7.6	40.4	5.1	38.1	4.7
Flexors of the elbow joint	27.2	3.5	22.8	4.4	24.3	2.8	22.4	2.9
Extensors of the elbow joint	16.2	2.9	14.6	0.6	13.5	3.5	12.7	2.2
Flexors of the knee joint	13.1	2.7	11.3	3.1	11.3	2.2	10.3	3.1
Extensors of the knee joint	29.8	6.2	25.4	6.0	24.0	2.6	21.3	5.7

TABLE 56.
Mean values ($\bar{x} \pm SD$) of performance in different sport disciplines in groups of active, trained ($A_{7,8}$) and control, inactive men ($C_{7,8}$) (Kuta, Pařízková and Eiselt 1964)

		A_7 (Trained)			C_7 (Untrained controls)	
Sport disciplines	n	$\bar{x}$	SD	n	$\bar{x}$	SD
Run 60 m (s)	35	11.3	1.5	37	13.1	1.8
Run 2000 m (s)	33	755.7	122.2	34	878.5	147.6
Broad jump (spot-cm)	35	181.7	23.0	37	166.5	23.9
Broad jump (run up-cm)	35	298.5	43.7	37	259.5	44.2
Putting the shot (spot-cm)	35	549.5	64.6	37	476.5	71.0
Putting the shot (dx) (leap-cm)	29	580.0	72.2	24	480.0	75.6

		A_8 (Trained)			C_8 (Untrained controls)	
Sport disciplines	n	$\bar{x}$	SD	n	$\bar{x}$	SD
Run 60 m (s)	28	15.0	2.7	17	14.9	2.3
Run 2000 m (s)	25	958.0	132.9	16	984.0	136.9
Broad jump (spot-cm)	28	159.5	32.5	17	142.5	28.6
Broad jump (run up-cm)	27	221.7	41.7	17	213.0	44.5
Putting the shot (dx) (spot-cm)	28	436.2	84.2	17	391.5	68.3
Putting the shot (leap-cm)	26	444.0	83.8	17	414.0	51.5

During the period between the seventh and eighth decade the muscular strength declined significantly. The decline as in morphological indicators, was relatively greater in active men. Changes in muscular strength and LBM had a very similar trend. There were also *significant relations between LBM and other somatic indicators* (in particular *circumferences of the extremities*) and *muscular strength*. The muscular strength of the right and left upper extremity correlated in age subgroups of active and inactive men with the arm circumference (r = 0.448 – 0.613). *LBM in kg correlated with the general strength*, i.e. *the sum of the hand grip, strength of flexors and extensors of the elbow and knee joint, more closely* (r = 0.430 – 0.629) *than with the total body weight* (r = 0.284 – 0.565). *The relations between somatic indicators and muscular strength were particularly marked in the seventh decade*. In the eighth decade they were not as a rule significant, particularly in active men. In our opinion this is due to the fact that the *functional involution proceeded even more rapidly and markedly than the morphological involution in active* compared to control men. In the seventh decade this was not so marked because during this period the majority of active men were still engaged in some sport, while in the eighth decade the activity was very low and involution was more marked due to the originally higher values in active men, A_8, as compared with inactive men, C_8. Therefore in the eighth decade the relationships between morphological indicators and muscular strength became more loosely related and were less closely approximated in active than in inactive men (Kuta et al. 1970).

4. Body composition in relation to sports performance

Sports performance was evaluated in selected disciplines which when viewed comprehensively rendered it possible to evaluate physical fitness at this age: covering *60 and 2000 m with alternate running and walking permitted, standing jump, flying jump and throwing a ball*. Table 56 shows *better performance in active men, the difference being significant only in the seventh decade. The more favourable results in active men were manifested in particular in those disciplines which call for technique and skill* (Kuta et al. 1964).

In different sport disciplines LBM was in the closest relationship to performance. A significant relationship was found between the *percentage of LBM and the results of the 60 and 2000 m run* (r = 0.447 – 0.607); the *higher the percentage of LBM, the better the results*. The absolute amount of LBM, contrary to muscular strength in kp, did not correlate with performance in the sport disciplines mentioned. This is, however, logical in view of the nature of the performance: the higher the ratio of LBM and the smaller the amount of body fat the better the results in running. The absolute amount of LBM does not matter. On the other hand, the higher the amount of LBM which is the effective body mass, the greater the total strength in kp.

Relations between performance in running etc. and LBM again become less close in the 8th decade obviously due to the different trend of functional and morphological involution. However, in the *7th and partly also in the 8th decade there is a delay in the senile decline of muscular strength as well as performance in men who throughout life were systematically engaged in physical training* (Kuta et al. 1964, 1970).

5. Density of the capillary network in skeletal muscle and body composition

In view of the differences mentioned in aerobic capacity, muscle strength and sports performance between active and inactive old men, we considered also the possiblity of delayed senile changes in other indicators. All the functional parameters mentioned are related in an important way with the supply of oxygen and other necessary metabolites to muscles which depends above all on the density of the blood vessels. Therefore we again compared the number of capillaries and muscle fibres from biopsy specimens of the quadriceps muscle with body composition and aerobic capacity in selected men in the eighth decade.

At this advanced age it was no longer possible to show significant differences between active and inactive men in body composition and the absolute maximal oxygen consumption in relation to LBM and oxygen pulse. This applied also to the number of capillaries and muscle fibres. The ratio capillaries: fibres was practically the same (Table 57). *Comparison between both groups with a similar group of younger men* (*see* Fig. 23) revealed that *active men did not differ from them* in *any significant way, while the inactive did.* The lack of difference between young men and active men of advanced age is obviously due to a great scatter of values of the ratio capil-

TABLE 57.
Mean values ($\bar{x} \pm SD$) of anthropometric measurements, body composition, absolute and relative maximal oxygen uptake, and characteristics of microstructure of skeletal muscle (Pařízková et al. 1971a)

Group	A (active, trained)		C (control, inactive)	
n	10		8	
	$\bar{x}$	SD	$\bar{x}$	SD
Age (years)	73.90	3.14	72.49	2.97
Height (cm)	167.5	2.8	169.2	3.9
Weight (kg)	67.3	6.4	69.3	9.6
LBM (%)	80.2	4.3	81.7	3.3
LBM (kg)	54.7	3.6	56.4	5.5
Fat (%)	19.8	3.6	18.3	3.3
Quetelet index, kg wt/10 cm ht	4.0	0.4	4.1	0.5
LBM kg/10 cm ht	3.2	0.3	3.3	0.3
Max O_2 uptake (ml/min)	1,393	282	1,181	538
Max pulse rate/min	140.0	21.5	133.8	15.4
O_2 pulse (ml/min)	10.1	2.0	9.3	1.4
Max O_2/kg wt/min	20.4	5.0	18.2	3.6
Max O_2/LBM kg/min	24.9	4.9	21.7	3.4
Capillaries/mm^2	362.4	134.9	314.7	99.2
Muscle fibres/mm^2	556.2	108.3	532.8	154.1
Capillary: fibre ratio	0.65	0.30	0.59	0.08
D/2	24.6	11.6	29.4	5.0

laries: fibres in old active men. The latter group included individuals where the ratio capillaries: fibres was maintained on a satisfactory level very similar to young men. In inactive old men the values were consistently lower (Pařízková et al. 1971a).

In advanced age it was thus not possible to confirm differences in the morphological structure of muscle as revealed between young people engaged and not engaged in sports (Hermansen and Wachtlová 1971). At this advanced age it is not possible to use such an intensive load as in younger subjects because the senile organism cannot cope with these loads and is even less able to adapt to them. If these changes take place earlier in life, most often are not preserved in advanced age (Pařízková 1972i).

6. Indicators of the lipid metabolism in blood in relation to physical activity and body composition

In conjunction with examinations of the ratio of body fat and its possible relationship with the morbidity of the cardiovascular system in groups of active and inactive men *the cholesterol level* (mg), *total lipids* (mg %), *esterified fatty acids* (EFA—mg %) and *lipoprotein index in blood* were investigated in selected men in the seventh decade. *No relationships were found between these indicators and the amount of depot fat in the organism* (Table 58). *A different life-long regime of activity did not affect the levels of these indicators in the blood in a significant way* (Eiselt et al. 1961). Symptoms of cardiovascular disease were not related to the percentage of body fat. It is, however, important to emphasize that our group did not comprise any obese individuals.

7. Long-term investigations (8—10 years) of changes in body composition and somatic characteristics in old men with different activity

The conclusions from comparisons of different indicators in old men with a different life-long physical activity seem to indicate that *adaptation to a different load throughout life exerts a differentiating effect. It is manifested in particular in functional indicators which are specifically developed by this stimulus (aerobic capacity, muscular strength, performance in different disciplines); among morphological indicators it is above all body composition,* i.e. *an increase in LBM,* which is closely related to functional indicators. An analysis of results supports the view that the *above manifestations of adaptation to an increased load are mainly the persisting sequelae of a previous high physical activity,* which are manifest as long as the physical regime is maintained at a certain level. As soon as this level cannot be maintained, most of the differences disappear. It is thus a *delayed manifestation of senile changes as a result of a previously higher level of activity in these subjects* (Pařízková 1972i).

Cross-sectional studies cannot provide a definite answer to a number of questions: the most important shortcoming is that from a single examination and comparison

TABLE 58.
Mean values ($\bar{x} \pm SD$) of blood lipid levels in active, trained (A_7) and control, inactive men (C_7) in the seventh decade of life (Eiselt, Pařízková and Zbuzek 1961)

	A_7 (trained)		C_7 (control)	
n	65		18	
	$\bar{x}$	SD	$\bar{x}$	SD
Cholesterol (mg)	254	54	244	31
Lipoprotein index	2.46	1.17	2.47	1.23
Total lipids (mg %)	835	412	804	179
Esterified fatty acids (EFA, mg %)	177	49	179	32

we do not know the initial level of the assessed indicators, i.e. we cannot rule out a primary difference in constitution and in the level of decisive morphological and functional indicators which lead to a major or minor engagement in physical training. A longitudinal study has the advantage that the trend of these changes during ageing can be evaluated and thus possible differences in their course, rate etc. assessed. This helps to evaluate the influence of training and increased physical activity in old age.

We wanted therefore to resolve the question whether in active subjects investigated longitudinally there is a decline of values of different morphological and functional characteristics similar to that in controls, and whether it is possible in old age to induce at least to a certain extent by systematic training suited for the given age some adaptive changes, similar to those which were observed in subjects who were active throughout life.

In a smaller group of men ($n = 40$) anthropometric indicators and body composition were examined by means of densitometry *after an interval of three years.* The men were divided again into groups of active men and controls ($A_{7,8}$, $C_{7,8}$) as mentioned above. *Measurements after three years failed to confirm a reduction of height,* as described by Büchi (1950—who, however, repeated these measurements after nine years) and others. *Body weight and body composition were also unaltered.* There was a significant *reduction in the arm span, width of the chest and the circumference of the right and left forearm;* the *bitrochanteric and biiliocristal diameters,* on the other hand, *increased significantly along with the chest circumference at rest, during inspiration and expiration.* These changes were *not influenced by physical activity* i.e. in groups $A_{7,8}$ and $C_{7,8}$ the changes were practically the same (Pařízková and Eiselt 1968).

Along with the above men a *longitudinal investigation* was made in a *special group of men in the seventh decade who started with physical training at an average age of 64.5 years and proceeded with it for the course of three years* (physical training once a week for 1.5 hours). The intensity of the training and its type were selected to suit this age group and were conducted throughout the experimental period. The initial values of anthropometric indicators and body composition were the same as in the controls, C_7. The trend of senile changes was again similar to the above mentioned two groups investigated after three years, i.e. $A_{7,8}$ and $C_{7,8}$ (Pařízková and Eiselt 1968). *Physical training commenced at this age did not affect the trend of senile changes in body composition and somatic indicators.*—From the aspect of functional indicators certain changes were apparent—there was a significant increase in the work performed in watt, the caloric expenditure declined and the efficiency of work on a bicycle ergometer increased (Eiselt and Pařízková 1971, 1975).

Examination of somatic and functional characteristics was again *repeated eight—ten years after the initial tests*. It was possible to do so only in 55 men (group I), active and inactive men from the original group of 170 men (i.e. 32.3%).—56 men (i.e. 32.9%; group II) died during the experimental period from various diseases. Another 59 surviving men (34.7%) were unable or unwilling to attend the examination.

31 from the original number of active men belonged to group A_7 and A_8 (i.e. 38.7%). 25 men from the original number (27.7%) were in the group of inactive controls.—The most frequent cause of death was cardiovascular disease (myocardial infarction, hypertension, cerebrovascular attacks, etc.: further selected subgroup III, n = 24). In group A these diseases accounted for 48.7% of deaths, in group C for 56%. Cancer of different organs accounted for 19.6% of deaths. Pneumonia, accidents, and intoxications were very rare causes of death (Pařízková and Eiselt 1971).

The above group of 55 men (group I) is thus a *very selected group of surviving and relatively healthy, fit men* (who were able and willing to be examined in our laboratory), and was divided, as previously into active and inactive men in the seventh and eighth decade ($A_{7,8}$, $C_{7,8}$). *The height, sitting height, and arm span declined significantly during the experimental period of 8–10 years. The biiliocristal diameter,* i.e. *pelvic breadth increased significantly.* Differences according to physical activity were in this group of old men quite rare (Table 59). The *chest circumference also increased significantly; in group A there was a tendency towards lower values. The same applied to the circumference of the trunk at the umbilical level. The circumference of the forearm declined,* the decline being significant *only in group A.* The individuals values of body weight and body composition varied, but in the mean remained the same. In this case however the initial and final values of LBM and fat were calculated from ten skinfolds (*see* Table 9 and Fig. 10a) (Pařízková and Eiselt 1962, 1966), because in the old men during the final examinations it was not possible to apply in all instances the densitometric method. There was no decline in some other lengths and circumferences and widths after eight—ten years which are not mentioned here (Pařízková and Eiselt 1971). The changes in general are in agreement with those recorded after three years only (Pařízková and Eiselt 1968) with the exception of reduced height where the decline after 8–10 years was significant.

When evaluating these results it must, however, be kept in mind that this was a specially selected group of men in relatively good health and functional status. For the reasons given above it was not possible to evaluate the changes in men

TABLE 59.
Mean values ($\bar{x} \pm SD$) of anthropometric measurements and body composition in active, trained ($A_{7,8}$) and control, inactive men ($C_{7,8}$) measured repeatedly after 8—10 year intervals (I — first, initial measurement, II — second measurement) (Pařízková and Eiselt 1971)

		A_7 (Trained)		C_7 (Untrained) control		A_8 (Trained)		C_8 (Untrained) control	
n		14		21		11		10	
		$\bar{x}$	SD	$\bar{x}$	SD	$\bar{x}$	SD	$\bar{x}$	SD
Age (years)	I	61.83	2.01	62.92	1.69	70.36	4.29	69.96	4.28
	II	71.18	1.90	70.46	1.76	79.17	1.18	78.12	4.37
Height (cm)	I	168.9	4.5	168.9	5.35	171.0	6.1	166.4	2.1
	II	167.7	4.2	167.6	5.5	169.5	5.6	164.8	2.7
Weight (kg)	I	68.98	4.48	70.70	8.53	71.69	3.22	70.88	8.83
	II	68.80	5.82	72.50	8.55	71.61	4.87	68.52	8.97
Spread of the arms (cm)	I	174.2	5.7	174.7	6.4	175.7	6.8	173.1	4.1
	II	171.3	5.6	172.7	6.6	171.5	6.9	169.6	4.5
Biiliocristal diameter (cm)	I	27.5	1.3	28.5	1.9	28.2	1.9	28.1	1.8
	II	30.2	0.8	30.7	1.2	30.9	1.6	30.5	1.9
Chest circumference (rest)	I	89.8	3.7	93.5	6.4	93.9	2.9	95.4	5.4
(cm)	II	92.4	6.8	96.1	6.5	97.1	4.2	96.0	5.2
Abdomen circumference	I	80.1	4.0	86.1	7.1	85.9	7.2	88.0	9.0
(cm)	II	86.9	7.5	91.6	8.5	91.6	7.9	92.1	11.8
Fat (%)	I	19.3	5.4	20.3	6.3	20.3	4.2	19.3	7.8
	II	18.9	3.3	20.4	3.1	19.8	2.9	18.9	4.4
Lean body mass (kg)	I	55.3	4.0	56.3	5.7	56.9	4.1	56.7	4.3
	II	55.6	3.4	57.6	5.6	57.4	2.8	55.1	4.3

who were not willing to undergo the examination. In view of different pathological conditions, we may assume certain changes; these however would have to be analyzed with regard to different pathological conditions.

A constant body weight and unaltered body composition seem to be thus marked characteristics of men who survived in a relatively satisfactory health status (Pařízková and Eiselt 1971). The other changes mentioned are an indispensible attribute of ageing: reduced height as a result of contracting intercalar discs etc., increased chest circumference due to senile emphysema (Eiselt 1968). Increase of the waist measurement is probably due to the reduced tonus of abdominal muscles, as total fat and subcutaneous fat on the abdomen did not change significantly (Pařízková and Eiselt 1971). Another explanation would be a shift of fat from the body surface, mainly from the extremities, into the abdominal cavity. The increase in the biiliocristal diameter of the pelvis cannot also be explained by increased deposition of fat. To test these changes of pelvis measurements repeated X-ray examinations would be necessary. It is, however, also possible that the position of pelvic bones can be influenced by the activity of muscles with insertions on these bones along with altered biomechanics of movements in old age (we have in mind in particular gait on a broader base). This assumption too would have to be tested in long-term comprehensive investigations.

8. Body composition and somatic indicators with regard to the perspective of longevity

Another problem which emerged from our investigations was the possibility of certain differences in body composition and other somatic indicators resp. in men who died during the experimental period from various diseases as compared with those who survived in a relatively satisfactory health and functional status. *We compared therefore ex post the initial values of all characteristics during the first measurement of 55 men of group 1 and 56 men in group II.* With the exception of rare unsystematic differences (weight, biiliocristal and bitrochanteric diameters, chest circumference) which were observed episodically between sub-groups of different age and physical activity ($A_{7,8}$ and $C_{7,8}$ who survived—I or died—II) *no marked differences were found.*

The same was evaluated in the other group of 24 men who died of cardiovascular diseases (group III—*see* p. 219). There it did not prove possible to detect marked differences in body build and composition (Table 60). Active and inactive men had to be combined in one group in view of the small number of cases (this was possible due to the absence of differences in relation to physical activity).

From the somatic aspect during the initial examination old men with a favourable health perspective etc. did not differ from those who did not survive the experimental period. The absence of marked differences between groups, i.e. practically the same values of somatic indicators, LBM and fat indicate that as regards morbidity and

TABLE 60.
Mean values ($\bar{x} \pm SD$) of initial anthropometric measurements and body composition in groups of men who died during experimental period (8—10 years) of cardiovascular diseases (n —24, III; combined $A_7 + C_7$, n — 8, $A_8 + C_8$, n — 16) (Pařízková and Eiselt 1971)

	$A_7 + C_7$		$A_8 + C_8$	
n	8		16	
	$\bar{x}$	SD	$\bar{x}$	SD
Weight (kg)	73.5	7.7	74.2	9.6
Fat (%)	20.4	6.3	22.0	5.8
Lean body mass (kg)	58.5	4.9	57.8	5.9
Chest circumference (cm)	95.1	7.7	95.7	6.3
Abdomen circumference (cm)	87.6	10.0	90.4	9.9

mortality these indicators do not play a major role in advanced age. It must, however, be kept in mind that our groups did not comprise extreme individuals, i.e. obese or asthenic ones. It cannot be ruled out either that in these homogeneous groups of men who died earlier, certain differences may have developed after our measurements when these men were not available for further examination (Pařízková and Eiselt 1971).

The investigation of morbidity from cardiovascular diseases revealed a somewhat smaller number of men who died during the 8 – 10 years of the experimental period in the active group $A_{7,8}$; the differences are, however, due to the small size of the group as compared with inactive controls, not conclusive (48 and 56.0 %). Some experience indicates that the relatively most advanced age is reached by those who are engaged in sports on a recreational basis. Those engaged in contests and inactive subjects reach approximately the same age. In our groups the mortality was somewhat higher in group A (38.7 %) than in group C (27.7 %). These *results do not seem to suggest that life-long engagement in physical activity affected the morbidity or mortality in our group of men* (Pařízková and Eiselt 1971).

9. Relationship of body composition and changes in performance and aerobic capacity of old men after 8—10 years

From the group of old men mentioned the functional capacity and physical fitness could be examined only in 39 men. These men (who form part of the above group I) were tested on a bicycle ergometer using the method described above (*see* p. 53). Their total performance, the maximal oxygen consumption and maximal oxygen pulse in confrontation with the somatic indicators and LBM were evaluated (Eiselt and Pařízková 1971, 1975).

From the functional examination of the selected group of old men the conclusion was drawn that *the laboratory performance in the seventh and eighth decade did not change substantially after eight-ten years of experimental period.* The majority of the investigated indicators which characterize fitness had a *slightly declining trend* which *only in rare instances was statistically significant.* Only in those men who were throughout life engaged in physical training and in their younger years participated in contests i.e. in selected nine men ex-champion athletes of group A the maximal oxygen consumption declined significantly. The mean initial value in these nine men was 1727 ml/min, the final one 1435 ml/min. In remaining men who were engaged in physical training only on a recreational basis the inital values were insignificantly lower, and their decline after experimental period was not significant. *In active men as a whole (group $A_{7,8}$) and when divided further into ex-champion athletes and those engaged only in recreational sports, no significant changes developed in the maximal oxygen consumption, body weight, LBM and other somatic indicators.*

In inactive controls the initial value of maximal oxygen consumption was 1448 ml/min, the final one 1314 ml/min. This *decrease was not significant either.*— The maximal oxygen pulse did not change significantly, not even in the group of nine selected men who were engaged in sports contests in the past (Eiselt and Pařízková 1971, 1975). On the same basis as the assessment of LBM, we may conclude from the results of functional tests that *in the surviving men with a satisfactory health status constant body weight and body composition during this period,* i.e. *during the seventh and eighth decade, no marked changes in aerobic capacity occur, provided the health status is maintained on a satisfactory level.* The *functional capacity is, as compared with younger and middle aged men, reduced but during this period it no longer changes in a marked way.* The decline of aerobic capacity has already occurred sooner (*see* Fig. 20) and at this advanced age it remains relatively stable. A significant decline is found only in those in whom the original level of aerobic capacity was markedly raised compared with the normal population due to intensive training when younger (Eiselt and Pařízková 1971, 1975). These conclusions agree with the above findings of cross-sectional measurements pertaining to LBM as well as muscular strength and sports performance (Kuta et al. 1964, 1970).

When evaluating the sum of assembled results in old men with a different activity it was revealed that an *intense regime of physical activity throughout life, i.e. adaptation to a load, lead to a larger LBM and better results of functional tests (aerobic capacity, muscular strength, sports performance etc.) which is manifested up to a certain age* (roughly to the *middle of the seventh decade*). The *subsequent decline of values of these indicators in active men has a similar trend as in inactive old men. Due to higher initial values the senile changes are manifested later,* in particular in those selected indicators, which are closely related to physical activity and muscular work.

In selected men followed up for prolonged periods *who survived and were in a relatively satisfactory health status in the seventh — eighth decade, the body weigh and body composition became relatively stabilized along with indicators of aerobic capacity.* Physical training started at an advanced age was not manifested in morphological or the majority of functional indicators. In these groups of men of advanced age it was *not possible to demonstrate the effect of the regime of physical exercise on total body fat and indicators of lipid metabolism in the blood nor on the morbidity and mortality from different diseases,* incl. those of the *cardiovascular system.*

As already mentioned, this could be due to the absence of more marked differences in the ratio of body fat. E.g. in a longitudinal study in the small town of Framingham (Kannel et al. 1967), comprising some 5000 subjects in the course of ten years it was found that in subjects more than 30% overweight (i.e. with a large amount of body fat which was not found in our old men) angina pectoris is five times more frequent as well as sudden deaths due to myocardial infarction than in the remainder of the group with a lower body weight. In our male population aged 52—57 years it was formerly demonstrated (Samek et al. 1971) that during a work load on a bicycle ergometer subjects with the highest ratio of body fat displayed most frequently signs of coronary insufficiency after a load which was in agreement with the findings of Blackburn (1969) and others. Sanders (1959) found higher amounts of subcutaneous fat in subjects after a recent myocardial infarction than in healthy controls. Also Reiniš et al. (1972) found an increasing incidence of latent and manifest ischaemic heart disease in persons with a high body weight; greatest differences were found when comparing extremely different groups i.e. overweight and underweight subjects. Obesity ranked according to these data as the fourth risk factor after systolic hypertension, positive family history, diastolic hypertension. Ošancová et al. (1972), Ošancová and Hejda (1974) confirmed a higher incidence of ischaemic heart disease in overweight subjects who were furthermore characterized by greater daily caloric intake with increased proportion of fats.—There exist, however, some studies which did not demonstrate clearly the influence of increased weight and fat ratio together with hypokinesia on these diseases as summarized e.g. by Keys et al. (1966), Pyorälä et al. (1967), Mann (1974) etc. Nevertheless, overweight and physical inactivity are still, according to WHO, included among most serious risk factors e.g. in ischaemic heart disease and atherosclerosis (Fejfar 1972). There is an evidence from an epidemiological study in 16882 males that regular dynamic exercise can decrease this risk (Morris et al. 1973).

XII. Relationship between body composition and physical activity and the development of experimental cardiac necrosis in male rats of different age

Changes of morphological characteristics and the functional capacity during ageing are associated with various other degenerative changes. Involution of internal organs (brain, liver, spleen, stomach, etc.) takes place mainly as a result of the reduced density of the capillary network. The permeability of capillaries declines, and so does the body water content; more calcium, lipofuscin and other substances are deposited in tissues along with the reduction of LBM. The general adaptability of the organism to the action of various factors is reduced (Shock 1972) and the aged organism is also more sensitive to various noxious agents. These changes have a considerable individual variability and their course, rate and time at which they commence and develop during ontogenesis depend on many circumstances such as e.g. genetic factors, the past and present health and nutritional status etc. The role of many factors which influence the course of ageing has not so far been elucidated; lack of physical activity is considered as one of the important supporting factors in the onset of senile changes from the functional and morphological aspect (Shock 1972) and also in the development of atherothrombosis (Wright 1972) and other pathological processes (Arinchin 1972, Sirotinin 1972, Chebotarev 1972).

The data presented on old men revealed that in those who were engaged throughout life in intensive and systematic physical training some manifestations of ageing are up to certain age somewhat delayed. On the other hand, the incidence of respiratory, cardiovascular and other diseases was not markedly affected by different amounts of physical activity (Eiselt 1968, Pařízková and Eiselt 1971).

Ischaemic heart disease has been studied in recent years by many clinical and experimental departments. In view of the rising incidence and mortality from cardiovascular diseases the effect of all possible factors is studied which may play a part in their pathogenesis (Kagan 1960, Kannel et al. 1967, Keys et al. 1966). One of these factors is the level of physical activity together with the body fat ratio (Frank et al. 1966, Montoye 1975 etc.). This problem has also been investigated from a certain aspect in old men with varying physical activity (*see* Chapter XI). The small number of experimental subjects, differences in possible interference of various not sufficiently defined factors (including both genetic and environmental ones), the narrow variation of some investigated signs (e.g. lack of difference in the body fat ratio etc.) did not make a satisfactory contribution to this question possible.

One of the methodological approaches is the use of an experimental model with laboratory animals where ischaemia of the heart is induced by administration of different substances including isoprenaline (related to adrenalin—Rona et al. 1959, Chappel et al. 1959 etc.) which among other leads to a sudden increase of oxygen requirement by the heart muscle which the organism is as a rule unable to meet. This is considered one of the most important causes of the development of necrosis. In this connection a number of aspects was investigated, e.g. the effect of the administration of different hormones or the development of necrosis during the long-term administration of certain diets (Rona et al. 1959, Balasz et al. 1962) which cause also body weight changes and alter the body composition.

1. Effect of age, body weight and body composition on the development of experimental myocardial necrosis in male rats

Rona et al. (1959) observed a more marked isoprenaline necrosis in older animals with a higher body weight. This increased sensitivity of aged animals to noxious substances (Selye and Bajusz 1959) was ascribed along with other factors to the adverse development of the relative weight of the heart to the total body weight (Rona et al. 1959). In view of these conclusions we were concerned with the relationship of the body fat ratio and the degree of myocardial necrosis and the mortality after the administration of isoprenaline in animals of different age.

To rats 60 to 102 days old we administered by the s.c. route two doses of isoprenaline (80 mg/kg body weight after an interval of 24 hours). 24 hours after the second dose the surviving male rats were killed by decapitation and the degree of myocardial necrosis was determined using Ronas's (1959) scale: score 0 — no changes, 1 — diffuse pale areas at tip of ventricle, 2 — limited necrosis at tip of ventricle, 3 — necrosis involving one-third of the left ventricle, 4 — necrosis of more than half of the left ventricle, 5 — spontaneous death of the experimental animal during the 48-hour experimental period. The macroscopic evaluation of the necrosis was checked by microscopic examination of the heart muscle — Faltová et al. 1973).

Comparison of male rats of different age shows *an increase in body weight associated with a marked increase in body fat* which corresponds to previous investigations (*see* Fig. 2). This was *paralleled by the degree of cardiac damage and number of spontaneous deaths of the experimental animals* (Fig. 89) which is *highest in the oldest, heaviest animals with the highest body fat content.* To elucidate the effect of the body fat content another aspect was analyzed (Fig. 90); it was shown that older and heavier animals which had a lower body fat ratio had also less severe damage of the heart muscle. Animals with a high body fat content and high body weight always died spontaneously during the experiment (score 5). Thus the highest mortality was

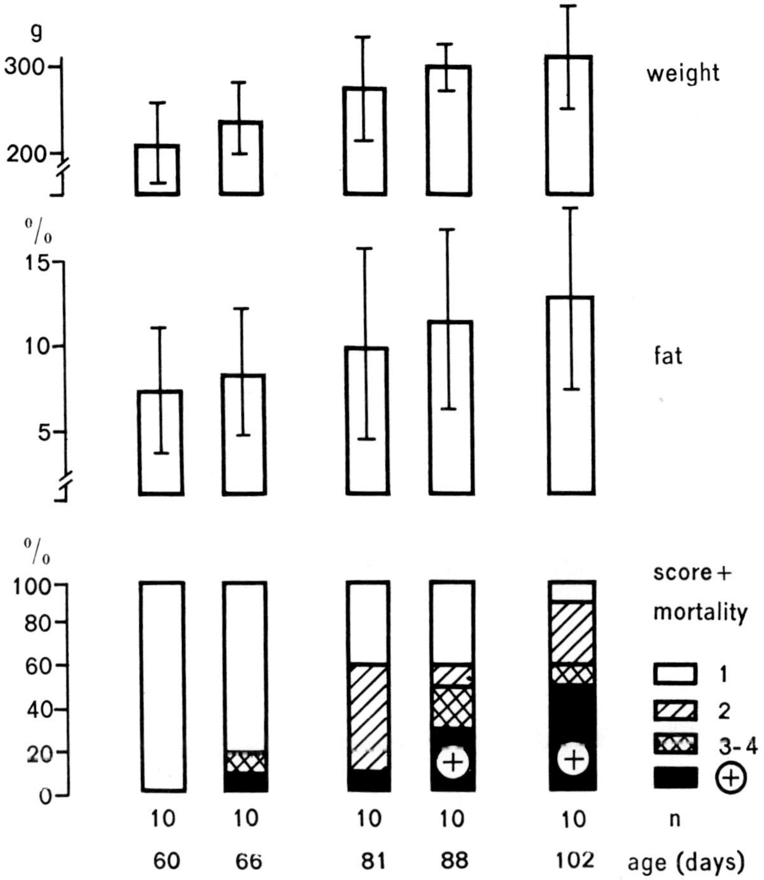

Fig. 89. Comparison of weight (g), depot fat (%) and the degree of experimental cardiac necrosis after administration of isoprenaline (score 1–4; 5 — spontaneous death; according to Rona et al. 1959 — expressed in per cent) in groups of male rats of varying age (*see* bottom: 60–102 days) (Faltová and Pařízková 1970).

recorded in animals with a high body weight who had at the same time a high body fat content (Pařízková and Faltová 1969, 1970, Faltová and Pařízková 1970).

When the body fat ratio in animals of similar age was influenced also by other factors than age the results were similar. In this connection we investigated the *effect of early nutrition,* i.e. the *number of littermates per nest.* Male *rats reared 3 per nest* (n = 24) had, when full grown, a *higher body fat ratio as well as higher body weight.* After administration of isoprenaline these animals displayed on average *greater damage of the heart muscle* and during the 48 hours of the experiment *the number of spontaneous deaths was higher* (Fig. 91). Where *14 animals were reared in one nest* (n = 24) their *body weight,* when full grown, was significantly *lower and so was the*

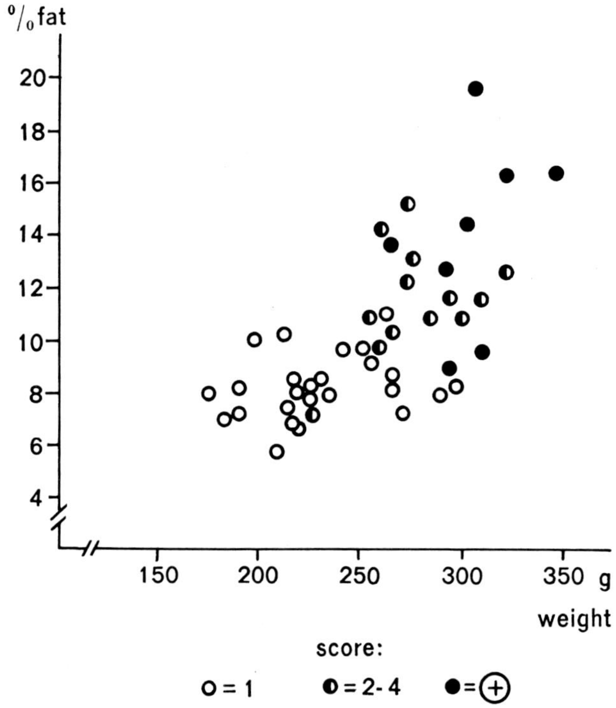

Fig. 90. Relationship of total body weight, depot fat and the degree of experimental cardiac necrosis (score 1–5, for explanation *see* Fig. 89) after administration of isoprenaline in male rats of different age (Pařízková and Faltová 1969, 1970).

body fat content, cardiac necrosis and *the number of spontaneous deaths.* The results of investigations in animals where there were eight per nest were intermediate (Faltová and Pařízková 1970, Pařízková and Faltová 1969, 1970).

It seems thus that a *substantial part in the number of deaths and in the greater damage of the cardiac muscle by isoprenaline in heavy animals is played by the percentage of body fat,* while *factors which cause the difference in body weight and percentage of body fat do not play a primary role.* Similar results were obtained by Balasz et al. (1962) who demonstrated that animals fed a high-fat diet for prolonged periods reached when full grown a higher body weight and had a higher percentage of body fat as compared with animals fed a normal diet; the latter had moreover a lower body weight and lower ratio of body fat.

The *role of the ratio of body fat* was also investigated in the subsequent *experiment with animals weaned after different periods of time.* Male rats weaned on the 18th – 21st day ($n = 10$) did not differ, when full grown, in their body weight and ratio of body fat (385.2 ± 39.8 g, $11.4 \pm 3.0\%$) from controls weaned on the 35th day ($n = 10$) (367.9 ± 30.4 g, $12.0 \pm 3.0\%$). The spontaneous death rate was somewhat higher

Fig. 91. Weight (g), per cent fat (%) and the degree of experimental cardiac necrosis after administration of isoprenaline (score 1–5; for explanation *see* Fig. 89) in male rats 9 weeks old with different nutrition in early period of growth, i.e. weaned in nests of varying litter size 1–3, 8 and 14 (Faltová and Pařízková 1970).

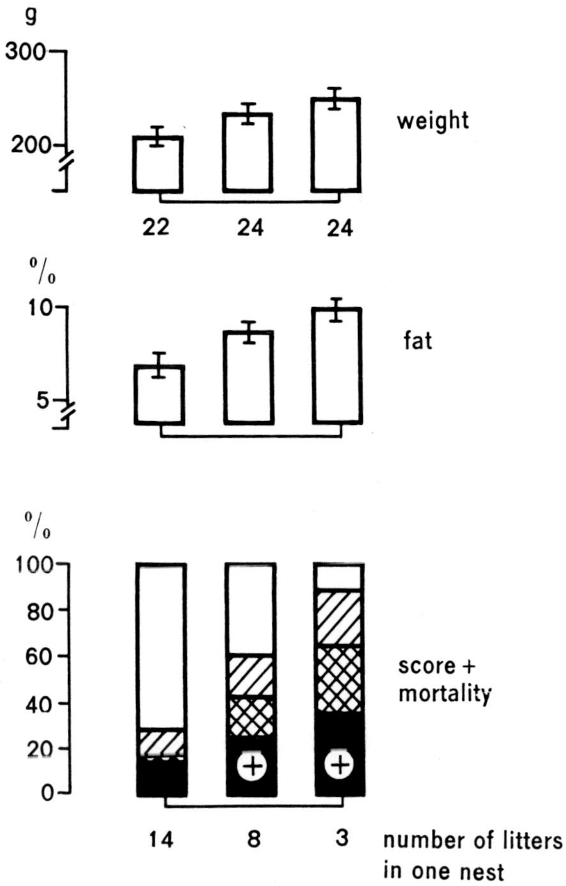

in animals weaned earlier (62 %) than in controls (44 %), in the same way as the mean degree of cardiac necrosis (score 3.3 and 2.5 resp.). All animals which died spontaneously again had a significantly higher body weight (393.0 ± 31.6 g) and higher body fat ratio (13.4 ± 3.1 %) than animals surviving with the lowest score of cardiac damage (score 1, weight 357.0 ± 30.8 g, body fat 10.5 ± 2.3 %).

The results indicate the *important relationship between the size of the organism and ratio of body fat and the development of necrosis of the myocardium after the administration of isoprenaline.* As apparent, *in the foreground is the raised body weight which due to age and diet is to a great extent accounted for by body fat.* A *raised body weight associated with* a *high fat ratio* is thus in our experimental animals, *without interference of other stimuli an important risk factor in association with noxious agents which cause experimental necrosis of the heart muscle in rats.* Similar situation is difficult to interprete in human subjects where too many other factors intervene simultaneously.

2. Effect of adaptation to increased or reduced physical activity

As stated in the previous chapters, animals adapted to an increased physical activity resembled in many respects younger animals, incl. the lower body fat ratio and lower body weight resp. which seemed to be a protective and favourable property during the induction of experimental myocardial necrosis by isoprenaline. From various clinical and experimental investigations it is assumed that reduced physical activity and lack of muscular work may act as an aggravating factor in the genesis, development and mortality from cardiovascular diseases incl. ischaemic heart disease (Morris et al. 1953, 1973, Kagan 1960, Brunner and Kanelis 1960, Montoye 1967, 1975, Kannel et al. 1967, Bruce et al. 1968 etc.). The part played by activity is usually associated with the general effect on the metabolic stereotype, concerning especially lipids, then aerobic capacity of the organism and morphological changes resp. such as the density of capilaries in the heart muscle, etc.

In subsequent experiments we investigated in separate series the relationship between the grade of necrosis of the heart muscle and the intensity of the regime of physical activity to body composition in animals of different age, as well as changes in the capillary density in the heart (and skeletal muscle under the same experimental conditions i.e. the same regime of physical activity without isoprenaline). The effect of activity was evaluated in a series of experiments where body weight and body fat ratio did not change significantly and in long-term experiments where body composition and body weight were influenced in a marked way. This set-up was to differentiate between the effect of exercise alone and the effect of body fat.

It is important to consider *the role of excess fat in thermoregulation of the* organism under these circumstances. *After isoprenaline* the *body temperature rises. Excessive temperature and the inability to loss the excess heat rapidly may in very fat animals play an important role in the final overloading of the circulation resulting in cardiac failure.*

In one of the series of experiments we investigated on a long-term basis a total of 180 male rats divided by age (110, 135, 205 days) and degree of physical activity (exercised animals with daily run on a treadmill; hypokinetic animals where movement was restricted by placing them in a small cage; controls). Changes of the regime of physical activity persisted for varying periods (45, 100, 185 days).
In the youngest group (110 days) training on the treadmill started at the age of 55 days. In the 135-day-old group it started at the age of 32 days (i.e. immediately after weaning) and finally in the oldest group (205 days) already at the age of 18 days. Treadmill exercise was gradually increased up to 90 min/day at a speed of 20 m/min. Isoprenaline was administered in an amount producing in methodological experiments roughly 30 % spontaneous mortality, i.e. it had to be graded by age. The youngest group was given 40 (1st dose) and 20 (2nd dose), the second group 80 and 40 and the oldest group 20 and 5 mg per kg body weight in time intervals mentioned previously. After administration of isoprenaline the rectal temperature was measured by means of a thermocouple in the last group of 205-day-old animals.

Only in the group with the longest training, started before weaning, could we show a weight reduction compared with controls at the age of 205 days; the body weight was, however, also reduced in animals with restricted activity (Fig. 92).

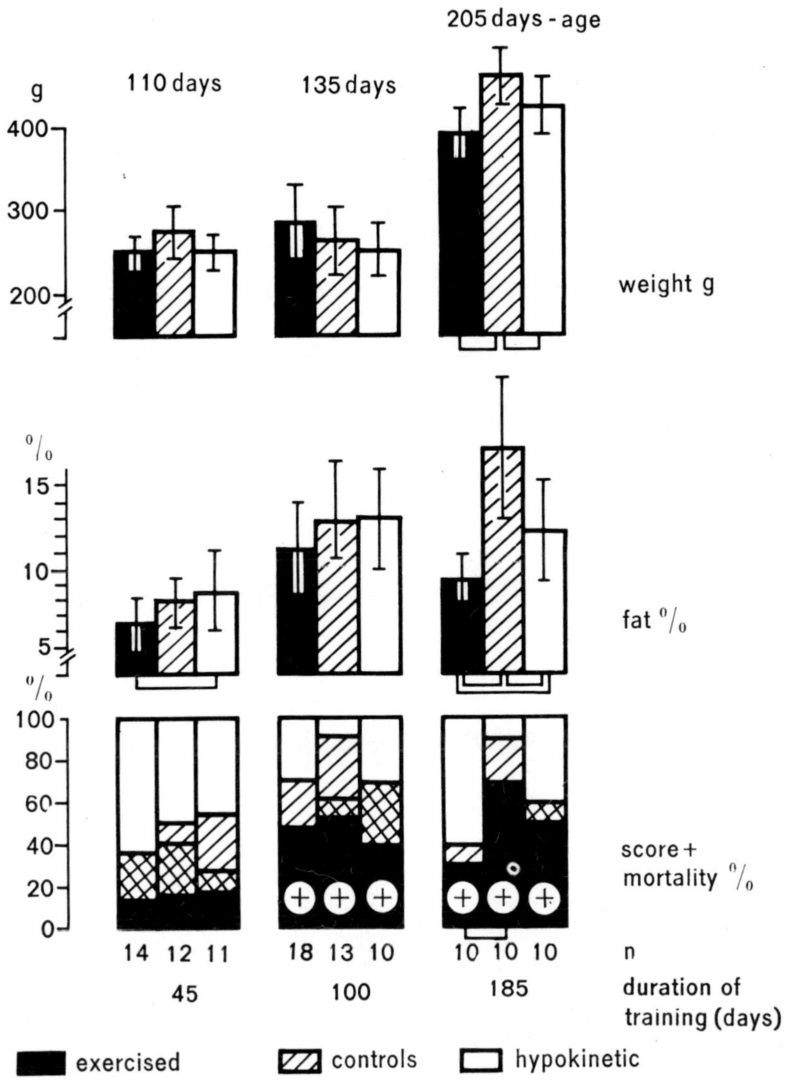

Fig. 92. Comparison of weight (g), per cent fat (%) and the degree of experimental cardiac necrosis (score 1–5, *see* Fig. 89) in male rats of various ages (110, 135 and 205 days) and adapted to different motor activity regime (daily running on a motor-driven treadmill 3 hours supplemented by 3 hours of static work load — black; controls — hatched; hypokinetic — white columns. Score, mortality — for explanation *see* Fig. 89) (Pařízková 1969, Pařízková and Faltová 1969, 1970).

The heart and soleus muscle were significantly heavier in running 110- and 135-day-old animals. We did not find significant differences in the weight of the adrenals and tibialis muscle in relation to physical activity. The body fat ratio was significantly reduced in the youngest running animals (110 days) and in the oldest ones (205 days) (Fig. 92).

The number of spontaneous deaths was slightly lower in the running animals as compared with controls aged 110 and 135 days. The same applies to the average score, i.e. the degree of necrosis of the heart muscle. The overall damage of the heart rose in these younger animals along with the percentage of fat (Fig. 92) (Pařízková 1969, Pařízková and Faltová 1970).

In the oldest group which had the longest period of adaptation to the load on the treadmill (205 days) we also found the most marked differentiation as regards body weight and percentage of body fat, spontaneous mortality and degree of myocardial damage (Fig. 92). *The animals adapted to physical activity had the lowest body weight, the lowest body fat ratio and lowest mean score and mortality*. This could lead to the assumption that adaptation to increased activity influenced in this experimental model in a significant way the sensitivity of the heart muscle to the action of isoprenaline.

Further comparisons did not confirm this assumption: *the animals with restricted activity characterized by the relatively lowest caloric input which according to body weight and body fat ratio were intermediate between the animals adapted to physical activity and controls are also intermediate as regards the mean score expressing the degree of experimental necrosis and the number of spontaneous deaths. The order of cardiac damage did not follow the order of intensity of physical activity but the order of the ratio of body fat and body weight.* The primary role in the sensitivity of the heart muscle to the action of isoprenaline thus does not seem to be played by adaptation to the load alone but rather seems to be related to by body composition, i.e. fat ratio and body weight. Therefore the spontaneous mortality and degree of cardiac damage was highest in controls which were heaviest and had the highest ratio of body fat.

Next we compared our results pertaining to cardiac damage with the ratio of body fat, regardless of physical activity, i.e. animals with the lowest degree of cardiac damage (score 1) after the administration of isoprenaline and animals who died spontaneously during the 48 hours of the experiment (score 5). *The mean body weights and body fat ratios were significantly higher in the animals which died spontaneously* (Pařízková and Faltová 1969, 1970).

The effect of the increased body fat ratio and body weight on the sensitivity of the heart muscle to isoprenaline are obviously very complex. *One of the obvious causal relationships may be the different ability to regulate body temperature in the organism with a high and low body ratio.* Isoprenaline has a direct effect on the metabolism (increased oxygen consumption) and also on the function of the heart muscle and circulation (Rosenblum et al. 1965). The removal of excess heat which is the result of the calorigenic effect of isoprenaline (Strubelt 1964) involves a further load for the circulation and heart muscle. It was proved that a rise of the environmental temperature significantly increases the spontaneous mortality after the administration of isoprenaline. *Shaving* of the experimental animals also *reduced* in a significant way the *mortality and degree of cardiac necrosis* after the same dose of isoprenaline at the same environmental temperature (Faltová 1969). An increased body fat ratio renders heat radiation and thus also the removal of excess heat significantly more difficult. Quaade (1963), Jéquier et al. (1974) demonstrated that obese subjects lose heat substantially more slowly than thin individuals. The same applies to rats (Pullar and Webster 1974). As was demonstrated in the experiment described by individual measurements, the rectal temperature after administration of isoprenaline in dying animals with a high body fat ratio was raised to 42 °C.

In the mechanism of the final heart failure moreover a certain part may be played by the size of the heart, as pointed out by Rona et al. (1959) when comparing young and older animals. In spontaneously dying animals with the highest body weight and highest body fat ratio the relative size of the heart in relation to body weight was actually lowest. Thus at the age of 205 days the surviving rats with the lowest score (1) had a relative weight of the heart 299.4 mg/100 g body weight, while spontaneously dying rats (score 5) only 252.2 mg/100 g body weight. A similar ratio was found when comparing the relative weight of the heart in relation to fat-free, lean body mass (LBM). *A relatively small heart in a fatter and thus more overheated organism with a limited ability to get rid of the excess heat is more heavily loaded. Thus final insufficiency may develop more readily.* Nevertheless we must take into account the difficulty of evaluating the weight of the heart due to oedema which develops after the administration of isoprenaline. This applies, however, to all rats to whom isoprenaline was administered. A relatively larger heart in exercised animals with a lower fat ratio and higher ratio of LBM was, however, demonstrated in other series of experiments (Pařízková et al. 1966b).

3. Density of the capillary network in the heart muscle in male rats after a different load during postnatal ontogenesis

Another aspect which was considered in conjunction with long-term adaptation to an increased load was the possible change in the density of the capillary network of the heart muscle. As was mentioned before, the administration of isoprenaline increases the oxygen consumption in the heart muscle which as a rule cannot be ensured by the organism. An increased density of the capillary network should provide a higher oxygen supply in a critical situation such as the administration of isoprenaline. Several authors examined in experimental animals subjected to different loads of physical work (swimming, running, etc.) the amount of capillaries in the heart using the injection method and demonstrated an increase in animals exposed to a load (e.g. Tepperman and Pearlman 1961, Tomanek 1970). With regard to these results we investigated in the subsequent series of experiments also the density of the capillaries in the heart muscle. We used again several groups of male rats with a different degree of adaptation to a load to differentiate also the effect of age and training of different length. Previous results did not provide evidence of the role of adaptation alone to an increased regime of physical activity without concurrent changes in body composition. We selected therefore in one of the experiments a relatively intense and prolonged load. We respected again the *principle of applying such a load to which all animals included in the experimental groups at a very young age from the onset to the end of the experiment, can be subjected.* As was mentioned on p. 62-5, an *excessive load eliminates sooner or later some animals from daily training* and thus the *factor of selection of the fittest and most readily adapted animals is introduced;* thus we do not know whether or not these animals differ primarily from the rest.

Male rats were adapted to a load from the 18th day of life. The daily run on the treadmill was supplemented by an equally long static load hanging on vertical ladders. We compared the effect of the intensity of the load in two groups: group one aged 65 days where the animals ran eventually as much as two hours a day at a rate of 18—20 m/min. Hanging on the ladder also lasted two hours. The second group followed up to the age of 285 days had originally a similar load as the younger group. At the age of cca 150 days it was necessary to reduce the load, i.e. the speed of the treadmill was decreased to 10—12 m/min, however, the period of running and hanging on the ladder was prolonged to three hours. The distance covered at a more advanced age was thus practically the same, the static load was increased by one third. This prevented the elimination of experimental animals.
Body weight, heart weight, and the characteristics of the microstructure of the heart were evaluated. Density of capillaries and muscle fibres were determined histochemically by the PAS reaction (Hecht 1958). Tissue specimens were taken from the same part (approximately in the middle of the longitudinal axis of the left ventricle) and fixed with 10 % formol during 3—4 weeks. The number of capillaries and muscle fibres was counted in transverse sections only from 5—25 fields (40,000 sq μ) from each heart using a microscope with a vertical camera (Zeiss). From these measurements two other parameters were derived, i.e. the capillary: fibre ratio and the diffusion distance (D/2) according to Krogh (1929) which is the average half-distance between two capillaries on the cross-section (Pařízková et al. 1972c).

The results obtained in animals adapted to the load were again compared with controls and with values obtained in animals with restricted activity. The differences in caloric intake were in this instance very marked, as in previous experiments. The body weight and body fat ratio in animals subjected to daily exercise were lower, as in the last group of animals (205-day-old) which received isoprenaline (*see* p. 230 and Fig. 92) where, however, the load was smaller and shorter. *Despite the more intense and more prolonged exercise we did not find marked differences in the capillarization of the heart muscle* (Table 61) nor of skeletal muscles (m. soleus, m. tibialis). The only significant difference found was in the soleus muscle in animals followed up for only 65 days where at this age the load could be more intensive, as regards speed of the treadmill (the total work performed expressed as the distance covered per day was, however, the same). The results are difficult to interpret: in groups of different age it is not possible to apply the same intensity and the same duration of load as the older organism cannot tolerate such a load for a prolonged period. If we consider the *effect of an exercise tolerable and feasible for all (i.e. without the effect of selection of the fittest) we reach* the *conclusion that the capillary density in the heart as a result of adaptation to such a load was not affected* (Pařízková et al.

TABLE 61.
Mean values ($\bar{x} \pm$ SD) of the characteristics of heart microstructure in groups of male rats of different age and different physical activity regime (A — active, exercised, C — controls) (Pařízková et al. 1972c)

Group (age)	I (65 days)				II (285 days)			
	A (n = 14)		C (n = 14)		A (n = 10)		C (n = 5)	
	$\bar{x}$	SD	$\bar{x}$	SD	$\bar{x}$	SD	$\bar{x}$	SD
Capillaries per mm^2	3672	36	3562	164	2937	114	3198	471
Fibres per mm^2	2997	179	2795	102	2403	173	2770	473
Capillary: fibre ratio	0.82	0.07	0.79	0.06	0.81	0.04	0.87	0.03
D/2	8.2	0.7	8.4	0.7	9.2	0.1	8.9	0.8

1971, 1972c, 1974b). This is why we assume that this factor was not involved in the sensitivity of the heart muscle to isoprenaline.

In experiments with a different regime of physical activity an important role may be played primarily by a different ability of the organism to tolerate a load and to adapt to it. In view of the great variability of different investigated signs (spontaneous physical activity, density of the capillary network, etc.) it may be assumed that the ability to adapt to a load might be related in a significant way to these signs. In several laboratories, which are concerned with the effect of an exercise on the organism, animals which tolerate loads readily are selected for experiments and animals not willing to run etc. are eliminated. Thus it may happen that at the very onset different groups contain experimental animals which differ primarily in signs where the effect exerted by a load is the object of investigation.

Different conclusions reached from our investigations of capillary density after a load as compared with other authors (Tepperman and Pearlman 1961, Tomanek 1970) may also be due to the application of a *different technique*: the *injection method* used by all these authors may lead in some instances due to the different functional state of the vascular system to the capillaries not becoming filled (e.g. in inactive controls) and cannot be detected. On the other hand, *when using the PAS staining method all existing capillaries in the tissue can be detected, whatever their filling.*

Long-term adaptation to a load during ontogenesis which is tolerable for every normal organism acts only on certain selected characteristics and obviously does not affect others in a significant way. The density of the capillary network differs e.g. markedly in wild living animal species. *When comparing the laboratory and wild rat* (*Rattus norvegicus, see* Table 14) *a significantly greater density of the capillaries in the wild rat was found,* the latter being adapted to different types of loads for generations; moreover there is the factor of selection (survival of the fittest). The difference is also marked in the number of capillaries in their skeletal muscle (Wachtlová and Pařízková 1972). The body composition of the wild rat was also different (lower body fat ratio, *see* Table 14), as in the laboratory rat adapted to an increased load. Adaptation to long-term muscular work during ontogenesis as described above is manifested in all these comparisons only at the level of body composition, the capillaries in the heart muscle are not influenced by this stimulus.

Similar conclusions are reached e.g. by *comparison of cell migration from tissue fragments in vitro,* which *characterizes biological age.* From the tissue of wild rats it is significantly higher than from tissue of the laboratory rat. Comparison of this indicator in controls and animals adapted to physical activity at the age of 285 days revealed *no differences,* although in these groups there were concurrent marked differences in the caloric intake, body weight and body composition (Pařízková et al. 1972c).

When interpreting the different results pertaining to the sensitivity of the heart muscle to isoprenaline in animals with different adaptation to physical activity we rather favour the view that the increased mortality of heavy, fat animals with low activity depends above all on the ratio of body fat which is the common factor of increased sensitivity in all the experiments described above. The adverse effect of increased fat content *inter alia,* is related to the thermoregulating abilities of the organism which fail under critical conditions imposing increased demands on the circulation.

The important role of the body fat ratio in conjunction with experimental necrosis of the heart muscle is further supported by findings on the *difference in the affection of the heart muscle after the administration of isoprenaline in two strains of rats which differ genetically in their ratio of body fat.* Male rats of *Wistar strain* with an *increased body weight* (cca 500 g) and *body fat ratio* (cca 26%) have a much *more severe myocardial necrosis* than animals of the *Lewis strain* which at the same age have relatively *low body fat ratios* (cca 8%, usually found in Wistar strain only in the young growing animals). In these animals the *degree of cardiac necrosis is very low* (most often score 1) (Faltová et al. 1973).

The role of body composition comes to the foreground not only from the aspect of thermoregulation but also in other associations: *a certain body composition also involves a certain metabolic stereotype;* this was partly recorded e.g. by following the *caloric intake in relation to physical activity,* or by investigating e.g. the *activity of lipid metabolism* which is decreased in old or inactive animals (*see* Fig. 2, 3, 25, 37, 38, 44 and Tables 19, 20, 21, 25, 26) (Pařízková 1969) and *also manifested typically under risk conditions affecting the cardiovascular system.* The relation of lipid metabolism to the development of isoprenaline-induced cardiac necrosis in rats of different age was also found by Stuchlíková et al. (1974). Deeper insight into all pertinent mechanisms and relations represented by a certain type of body composition, depending on various factors from the earliest stages of ontogenesis will, however, call for further research.

4. The impact of work load during prenatal ontogenesis on the subsequent development of the offspring

The above results pertaining to different indicators in man as well as in experimental animals revealed that *one of the most important circumstances which leads to marked adaptive consequences to* a muscular load is the *early onset* of the stimulus. When using the load of running on a treadmill it is only possible to start at a certain age, i.e. in rats on the 18th – 20st day of life. When using swimming we can begin much sooner; e.g. Oscai et al. (1974) trained male rats as early as the 5th day of life. Although training lasted only up to the age of 28 weeks, during the subsequent 34 weeks, i.e. at the age of 62 weeks significant changes were observed e.g. in the body weight and body fat content which was much lower in animals where training started early. These results demonstrate that exercise in early life is effective in significantly reducing the rate of accumulation of fat cells in epididymal fat pads of rats leading to a significant reduction of body fat later in life.

A load can, however, exert its action even earlier in particular during prenatal ontogenesis, i.e. during pregnancy of the mother. Under these conditions we must consider the consequences immediately after birth and in particular later during postnatal ontogenesis. Arshavski (1967) found a greater weight of the heart in the offspring of rabbit mothers swimming daily during the last third of pregnancy. The question therefore arose of further possible changes in body weight, heart development and depot fat of the offspring from exercise of the mother manifested later during their life.

Young female rats were selected and mated with males (always 4 females with 2 males in one cage) at the age of approximately 120 days. The mean weight of females at the beginning of the experiment was 230 g, that of males 420 g. Half of the females were exercised during the whole period of pregnancy on a treadmill for 1 hour per day at a speed of 14—16 m/min (i.e. mild exercise of an aerobic character). The body weight at the end of pregnancy increased to 295—305 g and did not differ in exercised and control mothers. 9—12 littermates were born to mothers in both experimental groups, but only 8 were left in one nest during the weaning period, which lasted up to 30th day of life. Mothers and later their offspring were fed a standard Larsen diet. No further change in the motor activity regime was induced in the offspring. In the first series of experiments 21 male offspring from 8 mothers exercised during pregnancy and 25 male offspring from 10 control inactive mothers were studied at the age of 50 days. In the second series of experiments 23 male offspring from 7 exercised mothers and 20 male offspring from 10 control mothers were selected and sacrificed at the age of 100 days. The microstructure of the heart was investigated, as previously described, and the epididymal fat pads were weighed.

The *total body weight* of the male offspring in the two experiments *did not differ after birth or later. The same applied to absolute and relative weights of epididymal fat pads.* The heart weight was the same in 50-day-old males both from exercised and control mothers and was significantly higher in 100-day-old male offspring from exercised mothers, compared with the offspring from control inactive mothers (Table 62). Depot fat did not differ.

TABLE 62.
Mean values ($\bar{x} \pm SD$) of the weight of the body and of the heart, and of the heart microstructure in groups of male rat offspring of mothers exercised during pregnancy, and those of control inactive mothers, with no other change in physical activity regime during postnatal life (followed at the age of 50 and 100 days) (Pařízková 1975b).

Male offspring of mothers:			Body weight	Heart weight	Fibres per mm^2	Capillaries per mm^2	Capillary: fibre ratio	D/2
I (50 days)	Exercised	$\bar{x}$	193.9	632.7	2963	2770	0.94	9.5
		SD	18.6	31.8	303	217	0.07	0.3
	Control	$\bar{x}$	192.3	630.8	2065	1796	0.87	12.1
		SD	22.7	75.2	216	259	0.03	1.4
II (100 days)	Exercised	$\bar{x}$	375.5	1182.5	3237	3050	0.97	9.1
		SD	41.5	151.8	364	364	0.08	0.5
	Control	$\bar{x}$	353.4	1077.9	2801	2565	0.92	9.9
		SD	43.3	95.4	177	220	0.08	0.4

The microstructure of the heart muscle differed significantly in both age groups: the *number of muscle fibres and capillaries per mm^2 was always higher in the heart of the offspring from exercised mothers. The capillary: fibre ratio in the heart was always significantly higher and the diffusion distance significantly shorter in the offspring of exercised mothers* (Table 62) (Pařízková 1975b).

The impact of mild exercise of an aerobic character during the prenatal period, as manifested in the offspring of mothers exercised during pregnancy, has obviously a greater impact on the development of the heart than exercise later during postnatal ontogenesis. With this type of work-load, which is tolerable for all animals without selection during prolonged periods of their life, no changes in the heart microstructure developed as shown in previous experiments with 65- and 285-day-old animals in spite of the very early commencement (18th day of life) and much longer duration of exercise (3 hours daily). However, even shorter exercise to which the mothers were subjected during pregnancy had a significant positive effect on the development of the heart of the male offspring even much later in their postnatal life.

Of other members of the litters from the first series of experiments surviving until the 100th day of life and then *injected with isoprenaline, those from the exercised mothers tended to have a lower spontaneous mortality and lower degree of experimental heart necrosis* (Pařízková et al. 1974b). The same was observed in the offspring from the second experiment who were also injected with isoprenaline at the age of 100 days; again those from exercised mothers tended to have better results, but in this case the difference between groups was very small.

As regards mechanisms underlying the changes mentioned in the development of the heart several factors could be considered. Increased vascularization of the heart *could be e.g. due to increased cardiac output during pregnancy with the increased placental blood flow, oxygen transport and nutrient supply to the foetus of the mother exercised during pregnancy.* This change can be assumed but there is very little experimental evidence for it. *Metabolic changes in the blood of the exercised mother* resulting from *increased glycolysis, lipolysis* etc. could also cause later modifications in the cardiac microstructure of the offspring. An *increased release of catecholamines* could also be responsible for triggering the development of an increased number of heart fibres, capillaries, etc. But this situation in the organism cannot be imitated accurately as the injected adrenalin is immediately broken down. Experimental data concerning the problems mentioned are not yet available. Random measurements in the offspring have not shown in following experiments any changes in the level of spontaneous physical activity according to the regime of the mothers. The analysis of possible causes of increased cardiac vascularization, which are no doubt multiple is now being studied not only in males but also in females. Obviously during the prenatal period the developing heart is more susceptible to various stimuli, including exercise and resulting metabolic etc. changes than later during postnatal growth.

As is apparent, there are many other possible factors of work load which can act by various mechanisms via the maternal organism (Harris and Cummings 1973, Eisenberg de Smoler et al. 1974) on the development of the foetus not only as regards immediate consequences, but in particular as regards changes which are manifested during later life of the offspring. It confirms the experience that the mother should have sufficient adequate exercise (i.e. of aerobic character etc.) during pregnancy which is useful for her as well as for her offspring. Little is known so far in this field; most information concerns e.g. nutritional deficiences during pregnancy—the impact of undernutrition of the mother on learning, behaviour, brain development of the offspring etc. (Scrimshaw and Gordon 1968, Zamenhof et al. 1973, Rider and Simmonson 1973, 1974, Smart 1974 etc.).

Generally it is possible that selected properties which are ascribed to hereditary inborn factors may be rather sometimes the result of favourable or adverse influences of different character during prenatal ontogenesis (Arshavski 1967). The same applies also to the effect of muscular work of the mother during pregnancy. This provides a further possibility of using this stimulus, again taking into account individual properties, to influence in a favourable way the development of the organism as regards fitness and the prognosis of the health status incl. cardiovascular health.

XIII. Summary

Body composition, i.e. the relative and absolute amount of lean body mass (LBM) and depot fat is *one of the most variable morphological characteristics of the organism.* It is *differentiated according to sex from the earliest periods of ontogeny,* and undergoes *changes throughout life not only in relation to growth, development and ageing,* but above all *in relation to caloric balance and energy turnover in the organism per unit of time.* This depends mainly on nutrition and physical activity (i.e. muscle work). The growing organism has a relatively high calorie input in relation to body weight, and also a high basal and total energy output, which is, inter alia, mainly due to increased spontaneous physical activity in this period. The reverse applies to the ageing and old organism.

During growth and development *LBM forms a higher proportion of the weight at the expense of depot fat than during later periods of life. During ageing LBM decreases both relatively and absolutely* in human subjects as well as in experimental animals (even when e.g. in human subjects the relative weight does not change, i.e. there is no increase in total body weight). In experimental animals (male rats—*Rattus norvegicus laboratorius*) it was shown that during growth and development heart, liver, spleen, adrenals were relatively greater not only as related to total body weight, but also as related to lean, fat-free body mass than later in adult life and old age. *Adipose tissue also differs during the growth period*—it has a higher content of deoxyribonucleic acid (DNA) indicative of its *greater cellularity,* and is *metabolically more active.* This is manifested e.g. by a *greater ability to release free fatty acids (FFA) from adipose tissue in vitro* into the medium both spontaneously and after addition of adrenalin (which is released in greater quantities e.g. during a work-load) compared with adipose tissue of adult and aged animals. In this connection, a *higher activity of lipoprotein lipase (LPL), an indirect indicator of the increased fatty acid utilization in the heart and skeletal muscle of the growing animals was found.* These findings were also confirmed by the experimental data of other authors.

In full-term newborn infants with normal length and weight, approximately the same range of variability in the amount of subcutaneous fat (measured as skinfold thickness with a caliper) was found as in later periods of life. Together with findings of a greater amount of subcutaneous fat in children of hyperglycaemic mothers (with metabolically decompensated diabetes mellitus) and other indirect data reported in the literature the results mentioned seem to show that the *present and later development of adipose tissue is influenced not only by nutritional factors during the earliest period of life* (i.e. by a temporary high-fat diet during the period around weaning which, in the laboratory animals, influenced the spontaneous food intake, the growth curve, lean, fat-free body mass and proportion of fat in adult life) but *even earlier*, i.e. *by various factors acting during the late period of pregnancy* (i.e. the shift in blood glucose levels stimulating possibly insulin and growth hormone levels in the foetus, which could further influence adipose tissue cellularity, and thus change subsequent potential development of body fatness).

In *newborn infants* there is already a *tendency towards higher values of skinfold thickness in girls, especially over the hips (suprailiac skinfold)*. These *sexual differences both in subcutaneous and total body fat* (ascertained by means of densitometry, i.e. hydrostatic weighing with simultaneous measurement of the air in the lungs and respiratory passages by the nitrogen dilution method) *become more apparent during childhood, are relatively most marked during the period of adolescence and sexual maturation and are preserved in aged subjects* even in the absence of changes in body weight. *Ageing* manifests itself by *reduction of LBM and increase in adipose tissue together with a changed distribution of subcutaneous fat. Regressive changes already start to appear during the third decade of life.* Together with *reduction of LBM* there is a *decrease in its metabolic activity expressed* e.g. by a decrease of both basal and *maximal O_2 uptake in relation to LBM* which is *paralelled by an increase in body fat*. Maximal O_2 uptake as related to LBM is highest at the end of puberty (approximately at the age of 15 years) and then decreases constantly. At the same time the *microstructure of skeletal muscles* as the greatest component of LBM, examined by means of biopsies, also changes significantly. *Muscle fibres in old age have a smaller diameter and their blood supply is poorer compared with that in young subjects*, i.e. the *capillary: fibre ratio is lower in old age*, which means that the oxygen supply and nutrition of the muscle fibres is poorer. In young men a positive correlation was shown between the max O_2/kg body weight and the max O_2 pulse on the one hand and the capillary: fibre ratio on the other. This provides evidence of a relationship between the microstructure of skeletal muscle and the aerobic capacity of the organism.

There exist *significant relationships between subcutaneous and total body fat* which render it possible to *calculate both relative and absolute values of depot fat* (and indirectly also that of LBM) *on the basis of skinfold thickness data* measured by modified Best's and Harpenden calipers only, using regression equations. The *regressions are different according to sex and age;* it is therefore necessary to use the regression appropriate for different population categories, and also special types of calipers. The reliability of prediction differs also—the relatively smallest error of the estimate was found in adults of both sexes, and the relatively greatest in adolescent girls and old men.

The close relationship between changes in body composition and changes in the level of energy turnover during ontogeny brings up the question of what would happen when the level of physical activity alters longitudinally both in a positive (increased work load) and a negative sense (physical inactivity—hypokinesia) which either corresponds, or does not correspond with actual ontogenetical tendencies of spontaneous physical activity.

Adaptation to increased physical activity (daily run on a motor-driven tread mill for 1 – 3 hours per day with a speed up to 20 m/min which is a mild to medium aerobic load tolerable for all animals included in the experiment without any selection) *significantly increased the caloric input* (g Larsen diet/100 g body-weight/1 day). Growth curves during the mentioned optimal gradually increased work-load did not change compared with control or hypokinetic animals (adapted to be kept in a small space 8 × 12 × 20 cm) until the age of 85 – 360 days. Only *after a very intensive work-load* (3 hours running on a treadmill and by 3 hours hanging on a vertical ladder, i.e. 6 hours of work load per day up to 285th day of life) *did the body weight fail to increase after the period of exponential growth in the same manner as in the control animals. Animals adapted to hypokinesia* did not always put on weight as might have been expected in view of the reduced energy expenditure; the *values were somewhat lower or higher than in controls.* This was obviously *due to a spontaneous reduction of the caloric intake* in relation to body weight which was apparent throughout life in the hypokinetic animals. The *development of fat-free body mass was somewhat retarded during growth* (lower values were recorded e.g. in 90-day old rats); in adult life fat-free body mass did not differ significantly in relation to physical activity though there was a considerable interindividual variability.

In the animals adapted to increased physical activity there appeared a *tendency to preserve a more favourable* (i.e. *higher*) *weight ratio of liver, adrenals and in some cases of heart muscle also in relation to both total and lean, fat-free body mass:* this together with the lower proportion of fat made these animals more similar to young, growing individuals.

The same conclusions resulted from observations on the composition and metabolic activity of adipose tissue. *In the animals adapted to increased physical activity the adipose tissue contained a greater proportion of DNA, it contained less palmitoleic acid* (which is always released after the action of adrenalin in relatively larger amounts than other fatty acids), and *released in vitro both spontaneously and after adrenalin significantly higher amounts of FFA* into the medium similar to that from animals during their growth period.

Catecholamines are one of the most important factors which participate in the regulation of the lipid metabolism also during a work load. Investigations of the simple *weight of the adrenals* revealed *somewhat elevated values* (absolute or at least relative) *in animals adapted to a load, compared with controls and in particular com-*

pared with animals adapted to hypokinesia where the adrenals were also smallest. The *corticosterone plasma level at rest was highest in animals adapted to a load. Biosynthesis of catecholamines* in the *adrenal medulla* was also *elevated in these animals as revealed by the activity of catecholamine synthetizing enzymes*, i.e. *tyrosine hydroxylase, dopamine-β-hydroxylase and phenylethanolamine-N-methyl transferase* (measured 24 hours after last work-load). Hypokinesia did not alter the activity of these enzymes. On the contrary, the *activity of catecholamine-degrading enzymes (caecholamine-O-methyl transferase* and *monoamine oxidase) was reduced in the animals exposed to a load*, as was found in the liver and heart. A lower activity of monoamine oxidase in the above organs (liver and heart) of exercised animals again recalls the position encountered as a rule in younger organism. *Long-term adaptation to an increased load caused the organism to have a larger amount of catecholamines than the organism of control or hypokinetic animals.*

The response of adipose tissue to the action of catecholamines *in vitro* differs, depending on the level of the regime of physical activity, the *release of FFA from the epididymal adipose tissue of animals adapted to a load being significantly higher.* In connection with this phenomenon in animals adapted to a load even during rest the *inflow rate of fatty acids to adipose tissue is significantly lower than to muscle* (i.e. the soleus muscle) and *heart* assessed by means of injected palmitate-^{14}C. Also the *LPL activity in heart muscle* and *skeletal muscle was, in animals adapted to exercise, significantly higher.* All these indicators were assessed 24 hours after the last run on a treadmill which indicates within a certain time interval a *relatively constant character for these changes of the lipid metabolism and their independence on acute muscular work.* The mentioned differences suggesting an *increased turnover and utilization of lipid metabolites leading to a lower body fat ratio were more marked the earlier* the increased intensity of the regime of exercise started and *the longer it persisted.*

The reverse happened in *hypokinetic animals. The FFA blood level which was the same at rest in animals adapted to activity and in controls* was *reduced after adaptation to hypokinesia.* The *outflow rate of injected palmitate-*^{14}C from *the plasma was reduced in hypokinetic animals.* The *inflow rate of palmitate-*^{14}C *to the soleus muscle was always lower than to adipose tissue* as previously mentioned while in exercised animals the position was reversed. The *inflow rate of injected palmitate-*^{14}C *to* the *soleus muscle and heart of hypokinetic animals was significantly lower than in animals adapted to exercise,* the *opposite was true for adipose tissue.* Although the rate of palmitate-^{14}C to adipose tissue in hypokinetic animals is significantly lower than in controls, the percentage of body fat in their organism was rather higher, particularly in older animals. The *release of FFA from adipose tissue of hypokinetic animals in vitro was significantly the lowest* which suggests a *reduced metabolic activity of adipose tissue after adaptation to restricted activity* which leads to the *greatest accumulation of body fat despite the significantly lowest caloric intake.* The *regulation of energy intake obviously cannot compensate for lack of physical activity. Adequate exercise thus plays an important irreplaceable positive role in lipid metabolism.*

Similar conclusions were also reached by investigation of $^{14}CO_2$ in the expired air collected by means of a special hood during 30 min infusion into the femoral vein under pentobarbital anaesthesia of rat serum (diluted with Krebs-Ringer phosphate buffer with 5% albumin and FFA obtained by hydrolysis of rat adipose tissue labelled with palmitate-^{14}C). Assesssment of ^{14}C *activity in the expired air revealed a higher ratio in animals adapted to a load* than in controls and hypokinetic animals. This difference also indicates that the *fatty acid utilization remains at a higher level even during rest* and *anaesthesia*. As apparent *modifications of the lipid metabolism* which are the result of adaptation to a different regime of exercise *are not manifested only during exercise but also without a work-load*. Even if animals adapted to exercise ingest more calories, they have as a result of the higher rate of lipid metabolism a lower body fat ratio. The higher aerobic capacity previously described, e.g. in human subjects adapted to work-load, to this also contributes by promoting a higher P_{O_2} in tissues incl. adipose tissue and this obviously is enough to prevent a major shift of NADH/NAD. Increased formation of NADH as well as dihydroxyacetone phosphate resulting from an inadequate oxygen supply (e.g. in hypokinetic or older subjects) produces a greater amount of alpha-glycerophosphate to match the catecholamine-induced triglyceride hydrolysis and FFA release during the load; thus reesterification can predominate and the fatty acid turnover declines.—Assessment of the O_2 *consumption/24 hours revealed again even during rest much higher values in animals adapted to exercise* (similar to younger animals), compared with controls and hypokinetic animals. During the above everyday load the daily oxygen consumption increases further (cca by 10–20%).

In the above groups the cholesterol formation *in vitro* was also assessed, measuring the incorporation of acetate-^{14}C into total cholesterol in liver slices. The *highest cholesterogenesis was found in rats adapted to exercise, and the lowest in hypokinetic animals;* however, the *cholesterol serum level and its concentration in the liver were lowest in animals adapted to exercise,* while they were *highest in the hypokinetic animals.* Long-term increase in activity thus leads even when the cholesterol formation is raised to a lower serum cholesterol level which again reminds us of the conditions encountered in growing animals with a higher rate of lipogenesis and lower body fat ratio. In some indicators of the lipid metabolism, as well as others (oxygen consumption, morphological parameters) this adaptation to increased activity induces a state commonly found in younger age groups.

The results of adaptation to different regimes of physical activity were dependent on the stage of ontogeny, and thus on the actual level of spontaneous physical activity. *In adult life the changes of adaptation to increased physical activity were more apparent;* on the other hand *during growth and development adaptation to hypokinesia manifested itself more markedly.*

The metabolic and morphological differences mentioned were always *related to the actual level of physical activity,* i.e. *after a certain period of its discontinuation* (2–4 weeks) *these characteristics approached the values for control animals.* But *this return to expected normal values took a very characteristic individual course.*

After discontinuation of daily running some experimental animals significantly increased their weight and proportion of fat, while this was not the case in the others. This obviously *resulted from primordial constitutional characteristics* especially concerning the *level of excitability of central nervous system (CNS)* which is closely related to the level of spontaneous physical activity.

Study of the relationship between body composition and CNS excitability (evaluated by means of the habituation test) showed, that *adaptation to increased physical activity resulted in a significantly decrease of CNS excitability.* This could imply results of an opposite character in relation to ontogeny as compared with the conclusions based on morphological and metabolic data: a decreased CNS excitability is characteristic for older animals (but it is possible to interpret it as a greater "economy" of the reactions under the test conditions). The *highest CNS excitability was found in hypokinetic animals.* The analysis of the degree of CNS excitability after a certain period of latency following a period of different regimes of physical activity showed similar but much less apparent results. As with body composition, individual animals reacted to the discontinuation of a certain type of physical activity regime in a very different way—in some the level of CNS excitability increased, but others showed no change.

In human subjects the influence of adaptation to an intensive regime of physical activity is also manifested clearly in the development of morphological, functional, metabolic, motor and other parameters incl. *changes in body fat ratio* which can be found *from youth to old age.* At preschool age there are already marked differences not only between boys and girls but also differences depending on oecological conditions, participation in systematic physical exercise, kindergarten attendance, etc. As shown in a representative sample of children just before entering the first class of the primary school, *children from large towns,* in particular the capital of Prague *were taller and heavier but their posture and performance were poorer than in children from smaller towns and villages.* Only the level of sensomotor development tended to be higher in Prague children. As is apparent, *accelerated somatic development in preschool age did not imply better performance,* despite a higher level of sensomotor development. A preliminary analysis of causes revealed among various oecological conditions in particular the influence of inadequate motor stimulation and exercise which is the reason that in Prague children the motor abilities and performance do not develop to the same level as in the more slender and smaller children from other Bohemian and Moravian regions. Further analysis of the above material revealed not only significant *sexual differences (i.e. greater body dimensions, better performance, a somewhat lower level of sensomotor development and a tendency of poorer posture in boys)* but also *differences* as *regards the economic standard of the family, family background, parity of the child,* etc. (i.e. larger bodily dimensions, but not always better performance etc. in children from families with a higher per capita income, from orderly families, or first born children etc.).

Examination of this representative sample of preschool children from Bohemia and Moravia revealed that only *10% of boys and 18% girls participated in regular physical education classes before they entered school;* these children displayed *not only accelerated somatic development, but also better posture, improved performance and higher level of sensomotor development.*—Also further *children who attended special physical education classes for parents and children* (2–5 years old) had even when their *height and weight were equal a lower amount of subcutaneous fat along with a good level of motor performance.*

In a selected sample of Prague children aged 3–6 years we were moreover able to test in more detail developmental changes as well as sexual differences and the influence of some of the above mentioned factors on somatic development, body fat, functional development and performance incl. sensomotor development. Cross-sectional and longitudinal measurements revealed, as compared with other somatic indicators, the highest variability in body weight and body fat. *The skinfold thickness was the only indicator which did not change markedly between 3–6 years* and this was in agreement with previous measurements. This finding suggested that *during this period in particular LBM increases.*—The results of the *modified step-test* showed that *at rest, during a load and during recovery the values of the pulse rate declined gradually with increasing age;* the values of the *step-test index increased significantly.* This conclusion is characteristic for the *improved work economy of the cardiovascular system* which at this age had a tendency to improve particularly in children with a tendency to an accelerated somatic development. Furthermore *sexual differences were confirmed,* e.g. in *greater muscle strength and better performance in some disciplines in boys, a tendency to better posture in girls, and finally improvement of the motor development with age in both sexes.*

Longitudinal studies of different groups of children and adolescents during four to eight years made a more detailed analysis of somatic development and changes of body composition during different periods of physical activity possible. The role of exercise can be evaluated more accurately than in cross-sectional studies which cannot eliminate even marked primordial constitutional etc. differences between children who decide to take exercise regularly and persevere, and inactive children.

Longitudinal measurements of boys from 10.7 to 14.7, or 17.7 years respectively revealed a *more marked development of LBM at the expense of fat* together with a *typical body build (relatively narrow pelvis, i.e. biiliocristal diameter in relation to height or biacromial, shoulder breadth) and a higher aerobic capacity in boys training in track and field athletics and basket-ball* (at least six hours per week). The reverse applied to relatively inactive boys who developed a significantly greater proportion of fat, relatively broader pelvis, lower aerobic capacity, etc.

The development of LBM displayed according to the results of correlation analysis between values obtained in different boys in different years *a characteristic stability* (as with height) *which was higher than that of total body weight.* The *maximal yearly increment in height, weight and lean body mass of individual subjects coincided in the same year;* the respective mean values for that year of peak height velocity were 9.4 cm, 8.1 and 7.5 kg. Throughout the growth spurt, the contribution of fat to increase in body weight was very small. *Individual skinfolds had also a relatively constant developmental trend, contrary to the total percent of body fat which varied considerably.*

Somatotypes evaluated by *Carter-Heath method* were, however, *variable during adolescence: every boy had changes of at least one unit in one or more components between 10.7–17.7 years. Exercise did not influence somatotypes.*

The development of LBM correlated significantly with bone age (X-ray of the wrist), *heart volume, height, aerobic capacity* etc. This *steady development* of the above indicators incl. the *size of LBM and distribution of body fat* indicates the *important role of genetic, constitutional factors in their development.* These factors imply at the same time better or less favourable prerequisites for sports activity which develop further positively during adaptation to an increased work-load.

Body composition of girls developed in a similar manner as in boys during *long-term adaptation to increased exercise (four-five years of gymnastic or swimming training): the deposition of fat declined,* and there was a *more marked development of LBM. The analysis of weight increments during periods of exercise of different intensity,* rendered possible by densitometric measurements, showed a *great variability as regards their composition.* The proportion of LBM and fat in weight increments differed both depending on the period of growth and the intensity of actual training. E.g. in boys and girls followed longitudinally the *increments of LBM during certain period of intensive training were often greater than the total increase in body weight due to simultaneous reduction of body fat.* During growth and development a reduction of LBM usually does not occur under physiological conditions.

Body composition in human subjects changes, similar to that in experimental animals, due only to the actual intensity level of physical activity. *After discontinuation of training the body weight increases rapidly from enhanced deposition of fat. Quantitative and qualitative studies of caloric input showed during various periods of training* (i.e. different energy output) *corresponding changes in the regulation of the caloric input,* i.e. an increase in calories during most intensive training, and a significant decrease after its interruption. These results indicate that the *enhanced deposition of fat after discontinued training was not caused by failure in the regulation of caloric input,* but was obviously due to *more profound adaptive changes of fat metabolism concerning the mobilization and utilization of fat metabolites* in a way *indicated above by experiments on laboratory animals adapted to various levels of physical activity. In human subjects* also the *decrease of caloric input could not compensate the lack of physical activity which resulted in an accumulation of superfluous fat.*

These problems were further elucidated by means of clinical studies performed in *obese children* during *reducing therapy using intensive systematic physical exercise in special therapeutic summer camps* lasting seven weeks. These children were obese due to hyperalimentation; all children with endocrinological disturbances were eliminated in our measurements. Obese children characterised as a rule by a *lower spontaneous physical activity* have not only a *higher body weight and depot fat* (*distributed in a manner reminiscent of adult women even in boys*) and *relatively broader pelvis* (higher absolute values of biiliocristal diameter even in boys) but also a *higher absolute amount of LBM*. Intensive exercise proved a suitable physiological means for normalization in these children.

Longitudinal studies of selected indicators of lipid metabolism in the blood during and after a work load on a treadmill before and after reduction showed *significant changes not only in the quantity*, but also in the *metabolic characteristics of the adipose tissue*. The changes in the blood level of FFA during the maximal work load after the period of adaptation to increased physical activity and exercise seemed to indicate *an increased ability to mobilize and obviously to utilize FFA* as a source of energy during the muscle work with resulting fat reduction. After the stay in the summer camp and weight reduction the FFA and *cholesterol blood level at rest decreased significantly*, the latter *only in boys*. Blood levels of esterified fatty acids and glucose did not change either at rest or after work load.

After reduction of weight and fat due to adaptation to increased physical activity the economy of work and overall physical fitness also improved significantly. The same or even a greater work-load was performed with a lower oxygen uptake and lower pulse rate, i.e. the *energy cost of work under the same conditions was lowered after reduction.—The results of the step test correlated significantly with the proportion of depot fat:* the greater the relative amount of fat, the poorer the results of the step test, and vice versa.

Aerobic capacity expressed as maximal O_2 *uptake was the same in the obese boys and boys with normal body weight: the same level of maximal oxygen consumption, however, was achieved in the obese at a lower speed of the treadmill. Maximal* O_2 *uptake as related to total body weight and LBM was significantly lower in the obese.* After reduction of weight and fat the value of maximal O_2 uptake did not change markedly (provided LBM also remained equal), but was *achieved as in normal boys after a longer run on a treadmill with greater speed per minute, than before the reduction*. This result indicates a *more favourable situation after reduction of superfluous fat:* it is possible to utilize a greater proportion of energy for an actual practical performance (i.e. cover a certain distance at a certain speed), and a smaller proportion of the energy is used for the transport of one's own body weight—especially fat (i.e. unprofitable work). These conclusions were also tested by comparing the performance and energy cost of other children with different body weight and body fat proportion; *significant differences in performance and economy of work appeared not only when obese and subjects with normal weight were compared, but even in the range of so-called normal body weight and body composition.*

These observations led to reflections on the *relationships between body dimensions, weight and LBM in relation to the functional capacity of the organism*. Experimental elucidation of selected questions was made possible by a *field study performed in children from a developing country (Tunisia)* where the *range of socio-economic conditions* (which have an important impact on somatic etc. development of children) *is markedly greater than in industrially developed countries*. This study including the evaluation of *body build and composition* together with *functional measurements* (*cardiorespiratory efficiency, muscle strength and sport performance*) showed that *children from poorer families with lower height, weight and even LBM*, who on the basis of usual growth grids based on data from industrially developed countries *seem to be retarded* in their development, display *the highest level of physical fitness and optimal economy of work performance.*

In the adults the *relatively greatest changes in body composition were found after adaptation to increased physical activity*, this ensues from the possibility of *most intensive training* in this life period (i.e. mostly third decade). *In athletes of Olympic teams an increased proportion of LBM at the expense of fat* can be found, especially in *participants of dynamic, cyclic sport disciplines* (runners, track and field athletes, but also gymnasts) where it is necessary to carry one's own weight. *In athletes adapted to* predominantly *static work* a *large absolute amount of LBM was found, but the proportion of depot fat reached relatively high values* (e.g. weight-lifters). In top Olympic sport the *body build and constitution differed in various disciplines* (e.g. relatively short lower extremities and relatively broad shoulders in gymnasts or weight-lifters who both were of low height, or markedly linear type with high values for height and narrow trunk and shoulders in runners etc.), which is obviously *mostly due to a primary selection of special constitutional types favoured for a particular sport. The changes in body composition* can be *explained predominatly by adaptation to increased physical activity and muscle work as well as the increase in the capacity of the transporting system for O_2. The development of LBM at the expense of fat runs parallel with the increase of aerobic capacity especially in protagonists of dynamic sport disciplines* (runners etc.). *In sports of predominantly static character a relatively low aerobic capacity is accompanied by a higher deposition of fat* (e.g. weight-lifters). In top sports there occurs a marked and typical morphological and functional differentiation in individual sport disciplines.

In top athletes significant variations in body composition occur regularly in relation to the actual level of training intensity, e.g. during various stages of olympic training, and after Olympic games when decrease of training intensity occurs. These changes are relatively less apparent than in untrained or obese subjects due to high initial level of these characteristics. The trend of changes is the same as in other groups mentioned; only *after sudden and complete discontinuation of intensive top training* it is possible in adult life *to demonstrate a decrease of LBM* as *a manifestation of functional involution*. The decrements of LBM are mostly marked in *overtrained athletes*, or *after an illness*.

In advanced age it is also possible to show *an increased relative and absolute amount of LBM in men adapted during their whole life to increased physical activity and exercise;* this is *associated also with an increased aerobic capacity* in absolute and relative values (i.e. maximal oxygen consumption as related to body weight and LBM). This is *mostly apparent up to the middle of the 7th decade*, when it is still possible to *maintain a significantly higher level of physical activity* and exercise. During the 8th decade these differences in LBM are no longer significant. This applies also to some functional characteristics (muscle strength, performance in different sport disciplines). At this more advanced age it is also not possible to find significant differences in the microstructure of the muscle, i.e. in the size and number of muscle fibres in relation to their capillary supply. *Systematic exercise started during the 7th decade* selected to suit this age period *had no significant impact* on somatic characteristics, body composition and aerobic capacity.

A life-long intensive physical activity regime causes a delay in senile involutionary changes in the organism, especially *of those systems which are related to the muscular work—LBM and aerobic capacity, muscle strength and sport performance, but only up to a certain age range.* This delay in senile involution is, however, mostly *due to a higher level of all these indicators, attained in earlier periods of life.*

Longitudinal studies performed in men in the 7th and 8th decades of life *showed in a selected sample of surviving and relatively healthy and fit subjects a significant decrease of body height, increase in chest and abdominal circumference, and biiliocristal diameter after 8–10 years. Weight and body composition in this group remained constant:* this was typical for this selected group of old men (who represented only one third of men examined initially at the beginning of experimental period). Another third of the men died during the experiment, and the remaining third could not participate in our laboratory examinations for different reasons (mainly illness). Changes in these groups therefore could not be ascertained.

The comparison of initial values ascertained in this *sample of healthy and fit old men with the initial data recorded in men who died during the experimental period showed no marked differences in somatic characteristics and body composition. The same applies to the comparison of initial data* of *men who died due to cardiovascular disease only.*

In this longitudinal study of aged men it was not possible to demonstrate differences in body fat proportions or selected indicators of lipid metabolism in the blood in relation to physical activity. Also the mortality—both overall and due to cardiovascular diseases in the groups of active, exercising and non exercising men did not differ significantly in this age range. The latter could be, however, related to the above mentioned lack of any differences in per cent fat, cholesterol, etc.

The role of physical activity or inactivity together with changes in body composition in an induced pathological situation concerning the cardiovascular system was therefore studied separately in our experimental model with laboratory animals adapted to daily work load and/or hypokinesia in whom it is easier to exclude the interference of genetic, constitutional, environmental etc. factors than in humans. *Isoprenaline causing experimental cardiac necrosis was administered* to these animals. *The degree of heart damage after administration of this substance was always smaller in younger, lighter and leaner animals with a low proportion of depot fat than in old, heavy and fat animals. If adaptation to increased physical activity caused a decrease in body fat and total body weight, experimental cardiac necrosis was also smaller and the mortality of experimental animals was lower.* In the absence of body composition changes, however, activity itself did not affect experimental cardiac necrosis. Hypokinetic animals which due to a lower caloric intake had in some cases lower total body weight and fat had also correspondingly less cardiac necrosis after isoprenaline compared with control rats. As follows, it is therefore *not possible to explain the lower degree of experimental cardiac necrosis in animals adapted to increased physical activity primarily by the influence of a daily work load, but rather by changes of body composition and weight, and by some more profound changes in the metabolic pattern concerning also lipids and manifesting itself also by a relative increase of lean, fat-free body mass at the expense of depot fat.*

Similar results, i.e. *smaller extent of experimental cardiac necrosis* after isoprenaline could also be *achieved by different nutrition in the very early periods of life* (i.e. weaning in large or small groups) *causing the lowering of fat proportion in the adult life* or by *genetic factors* (differences in fat proportion in different genetic strains of laboratory rats—e.g. Wistar or Lewis strain).

Adaptation to a different work load as described in our experiments *did not change the density of capillaries in the heart* and skeletal muscle in male rats adapted to increased physical activity or hypokinesia, which otherwise differed in caloric intake, body composition and weight. In these relationships a *different proportion of body fat appears, when excluding other intervening circumstances, as a risk or protective factor resp., which can be significantly modified during ontogeny by means of caloric balance and energy turnover using an adequate and differentiated regime of physical activity.* This is also borne out by some clinical observations.

It is important to emphasize *the importance of optimal caloric balance and energy turnover in* the organism resulting from dietary intake and the intensity of physical activity and muscular work *from the beginning of life.* Further experiments showed that the *above mentioned mild aerobic load had a marked effect on the microstructure of the heart muscle even during prenatal ontogenesis,* i.e. in the offspring (male rats) of mothers who throughout pregnancy were exercised on a treadmill for one hour per day some positive changes were found. At the age of 50 and 100 days *the offspring of exercised mothers* (kept during postnatal ontogenesis without further changes of the regime of physical activity) *had a more favourable development of the heart,* i.e. *a higher heart weight, greater density of fibres and capillaries per sq mm, a higher capillary fibre ratio* and *lower diffusion distance (D/2) than offspring of control mothers.* In one of the experiments with the offspring of exercised mothers aged 100 days a *trend towards a lower mortality and slighter damage of the heart muscle after isoprenaline* was also found. Total body weight and weight of the epididymal fat pads (which correlate with per cent fat in the organism) did not differ.—Finally the most recent experiments revealed that *increased loading of pregnant mothers can produce e.g. changes in the lipid and fatty acid concentration in the liver which is elevated in female offspring while the lipid and fatty acid formation is reduced;* in males these differences were not found. It seems thus that a certain regime of physical activity of the mothers and the resulting metabolic and other changes of their internal environment along with an increased placental blood flow may have an important effect on the development of the heart muscle or lipid metabolism of the offspring *in utero* and influence late sequelae during postnatal life.

XIV. General conclusions and perspectives

A summary of the above results focused on the sphere of metabolic consequences of adaptation to different physical activity provides certain prerequisites for deriving some more general conclusions, analyses of further relationships and for attention to some new, ensuing problems. In the first place we should like to emphasize the *ontogenetic aspect* which leads under contemporary oecological conditions to a *very different impact of increased physical activity in different stages of life.* This is suggested by data obtained in experimental animals as well as men.—Increased physical activity results in the *relatively greatest differences* in body composition but also in other indicators in the period when the trend of spontaneous activity is already declining (i.e. an increase in physical is a relatively great change) but when the adaptive abilities of the organism are still at a high level and when the organism has also a great resistance, i.e. in *early adult life* (Pařízková 1963a, 1968a). These manifestations, however, obviously *depend largely in the entire previous period of life incl. childhood* and on the regime of physical activity and adaptation to an increased load in those developmental stages when the organism is formed and is more sensitive to external stimuli which influence immediate as well as late sequelae.

In the normal healthy child *opportunity for exercise and intensive physical activity* is *a basic need* the implementation of which is the *prerequisite for optimal development;* moreover it is *one of the formative factors* by means of which it is possible to influence, taking into account the sensitivity and peculiarities at this age, the organism in a natural way (Berdychová 1972, Seefeldt 1975). It was e.g. shown that the motor stimulation in earliest childhood (1st year) not only promotes the motor and somatic, but also psychic development of the child (Koch 1969). From the aspect of other functions (in particular metabolic adaptations) the sequelae of motor stimulation in this early period were not investigated in detail. Experiments in laboratory animals showed e.g. a positive impact of exercise during earliest ontogenesis on adipose tissue development. Based on the evaluation of adaptive sequelae induced during a later stage of growth it is, however, justifiable to assume that by means of favourable directed influence on the motor regime of the child during the earliest stage of ontogenesis it should be possible to achive optimal results from this aspect too. By this we mean first of all a *good opportunity for spontaneous physical activity and games of children in preschool age* (which is not at all a self-evident nowadays, especially in large towns), and then a *sensitive individualised motor education aimed for acquiring optimal motor habits from which the child can profit in subsequent years* (when he has, inter alia, no more so much free time) and which are suitable for this age period. *Unnaturally high demands* at this period (even if they sometimes lead to succesfull championship in later years) *do not seem acceptable* for *health, psychological and further reasons when considering an optimal overall development and health of the child as well as his prognosis for future life.*

In view of the acceleration of somatic development due to the secular trend in particular in advanced industrial countries (Tanner 1962, Prokopec 1961, Suchý 1971, Vlastovskij 1963, etc.) *this period could be used to a greater extent and more intensively* to give an *optimum orientation not only to the contemporary but also the later development of the child until adult and advanced age.* It is a period about which relatively little is known, which gives rise to a certain reserve in planning directed action in the sphere of pedagogic, health, metabolic and other aspects.

In this connection we must also emphasize the great importance of *factors which influence the organism even during prenatal ontogenesis via the action of various factors on the mother.* This applies also to an *adequate dynamic exercise of an aerobic character of the pregnant mother.* Sequelae on the circulation, metabolism and endocrine glands etc. are obviously transmitted to the foetus, and due to mechanisms which are so far not well understood, they influence e.g. the development of some indicators of the lipid metabolism and development of cardiac muscle during postnatal life (Pařízková 1975b, Pařízková and Petrásek 1976). Again, such a physical activity regime of the pregnant mother must not mean physical overburdening, but an *optimal motor activity,* always recommended by physicians already in the past; however, often neglected even today by quite healthy and fit women.—Also *in the earliest stages of postnatal ontogenesis it is possible to influence the "programming" of the subsequent development* of some properties of the organism. As regards body composition—in particular changes in the development of adipose tissue (e.g. by a certain type of diet—Knittle and Hirsch 1968, which alters self-selection of foods and thus body weight and body composition in later periods of life—Pařízková 1961b, or physical activity—swimming from the 5th day—Oscai et al. 1974) are manifested more markedly only after a prolonged latent period. *These factors obviously can contribute in a substantial way to the great variability of various indicators,* which characterize the organism (and which *may often be ascribed to genetic and constitutional factors because they act at the very onset of development*) from the normal and pathological point of view.

Another aspect to which little attention has been paid so far are the *sequelae of prolonged hypokinesia.* Under contemporary oecological conditions and with the present living and working pattern permanent restriction of physical activity is found and moreover this limited load of muscular work is very unbalanced. The adverse effect of hypokinesia (Krasnykh 1969, Åstrand and Rodahl 1970, Pařízková et al. 1972c, etc.), is also due to its long-lasting duration. *Minor sequelae add up during a prolonged period* and *eventually lead to pathological manifestations* (e.g. obesity or orthopaedic defects, etc.). In view of developmental trends as regards spontaneous physical activity this is a negative feature, in particular during childhood and early adolescence. Examples of the action of hypokinesia on youth, mentioned in the chapter on preschool or obese children, have revealed clearly the negative sequelae of an incorrect energy balance (Pařízková 1970a, 1972c,f) and low level of energy turnover in early childhood as well as the marked effect produced by a more favourable motor regime (Pařízková 1975a,c, Pařízková et al. 1962, 1971b). *Lack of physical activity cannot be compensated by a reduced caloric intake,* as was demonstrated in man as well as experimental animals (Pařízková and Poupa 1963), Pařízková and Poledne 1974a,b, etc.). It leads usually (even *when the body weight is not particularly elevated*) to a *considerable accumulation of body fat* which can be characterized as *"hidden obesity"*—Pařízková 1962a, 1963a, 1968b,g, etc.) and which is very frequent in subjects living in developed industrial countries (Mašek et al. 1970, Ošancová and Hejda 1974). *Subjects adapted to hypokinesia resemble in some respect older individuals—their caloric intake is low, they deposit more body fat,* the *activity of the lipid metabolism is reduced,* etc. (Pařízková 1974c).

Occasionally views may be encountered that contemporary life does not call for physical fitness with all its morphological and functional attributes; aesthetic demands are rather in the foreground. It is however worth mentioning that a *higher level of fitness and aerobic capacity of the organism* as a result of adaptation to increased physical loads also *means in contemporary everyday life—through lacking special physical demands—the use and mobilization of a much smaller proportion of bodily reserves* (Åstrand and Rodahl 1970). This leads to a lower fatiguability, a feeling of well-being and eventually it might *prevent the development of various pathogenic situations* which in conjunction with other factors *create conditions for the development of various diseases, and in particular those of the cardiovascular system.*

Contemporary man is exposed to the influence of mental and emotional stress in particular and under its influence the alarm reaction develops in the organism. Man is the victim of emotional anachronisms and internal stimuli which were essential for survival in the primitive past but are undesirable in a civilized world. *Old fixed phylogenetic mechanisms are involved which under contemporary conditions lead to an inexpedient response,* the liberation of catecholamines, a more rapid pulse rate, increase of the *cardiac output*, rise of the blood pressure, enhanced fatty acid mobilization (Mallow and Witt 1961) etc. which are the *preparation for fight or flight, i.e. muscular work.* And *because this muscular work is not implemented, various disharmonious conditions develop* in the organism which are assumed to be the *basis of so-called "diseases of civilization"* (Leytes and Chon-Su 1963, Charvát 1970). But e.g. the level of free fatty acids (FFA) increases not only in liminal situations (injury, fear, anxiety etc.) but also under more trivial conditions, e.g. in students during examinations (when the cholesterol level also rises—Wertlake et al. 1958) or during discussions of exciting subjects or in the morning before an experiment in the laboratory (Bogdanoff 1960, Bogdanoff et al. 1959) etc. Some authors assume that these lipid metabolites not used for muscular work may be deposited e.g. in the vascular wall and this may lead in association with the mobilized lipoproteins to the onset of arteriosclerosis (e.g. Charvát 1970). In immobilized fixed rats (restraint stress) along with a rise of FFA a gradual decline of the lipolytic activity of the heart and aortal wall was also demonstrated (Leytes and Chon-Su 1963).

In this connection the changes described in the organism induced by adaptation to increased physical activity (which applies to dynamic activity of an aerobic character) may appear as a factor facilitating compensation of some metabolic sequelae of stress situations. It would be perhaps premature also to present in this connection results gathered so far only in experimental animals in the sphere of the CNS (Pařízková and Lát 1973); after adaptation to a load experimental animals display a lower level of excitability, while animals adapted to hypokinesia had a higher level of excitability. Without further confirmation so far conclusions for the human organism cannot be drawn although empirical findings seem to support this hypothesis.

Let us mention rather some facts pertaining to metabolic sequelae of stress. For instance a raised level of FFA liberated from adipose tissue exerts a toxic effect on the heart of the dog under conditions of ischaemia and glucose deficiency, and also causes changes of the action potential of the isolated hypoxic heart cell (arrhythmia, fibrillation—Oliver and Yates 1971–2, Mjös and Kjekshus 1971). According to clinical experience there exists a relationship between the FFA level and arrhythmia in patients. The organism adapted to increased physical activity is, among other things, characterized even at an advanced age by high aerobic capacity (Åstrand and Rodahl 1970, Shephard 1969 etc.) ensuring the maintenance of a high pO_2 in tissues, which is one of the prerequisites of an increased ability to utilize FFA as an energy source. This ability could *promote a more rapid elimination of some metabolic sequelae of stress including the impact of an increased FFA level on the heart metabolism* (Shug and Shrago 1973) manifested e.g. by increased moycardial oxygen consumption (Mjös and Akre 1971, Mjös and Kjekshus 1971, etc.) which could be critical in certain situations (infarction).—There is some evidence that physically fit individuals survive more often especially the first myocardial infarction, and recover sooner than those with a very low level of physical fitness; but no scientific prove has been assembled in a representative number of subjects until now (Fejfar 1972). Animal experiments seem to indicate that the *facility of increased fatty acid utilization is manifested e.g. in animals adapted to dynamic exercise not only during muscular work* (Issekutz et al. 1965) *but also at rest or even during anaesthesia* (Poledne and Pařízková 1974b, 1975) which could be helpful in the context mentioned previously.

Last but not least, under special pathological situations the mere effect of *reduced body fat ratio may play a part;* e.g. clinical observations or some epidemiological studies (Sanders 1959, Kannel et al. 1967 etc.) suggest a more frequent incidence of fatal myocardial infarctions in very obese subjects. The experimental model of myocardial necrosis, using the administration of isoprenaline in laboratory rats revealed (Pařízková and Faltová 1969, 1970) that the *body fat ratio* acted (but provided all interfering factors were excluded, which has been hardly possible until now in epidemiological studies with human subjects) *as a significant pathogenic factor in proportion to its amount in the body already within a range below the borderline of obesity.* Any factor incl. an *intensive regime of physical activity which contributes to a reduction of the fat ratio in the organism thus implies also a reduction of this hazard* (Tremolières 1971a,b). *The same implies e.g. to lowered cholesterolaemia of trained subjects* (Campbell 1965, Hoffmann et al. 1967, Ahrens and Broxton 1970 etc.). In this we can see certain positive role of adequate individualized physical activity regime.

The young organism with a low body weight: fat ratio and greater ability to utilize lipid metabolites as an energy substrate during stress is thus exposed to a smaller danger as regards its pathological consequences. The organism adapted to increased physical activity which is one of the attributes of the young organism has some typical features which may provide it with some advantages during stress and the elimination of its consequences as in a younger organism. In this context the *state of adaptation to a higher level of dynamic physical activity may appear, to certain extent, as one of the natural preventive means against the negative features of contemporary civilization* (Kasch and Boyer 1969, Costill et al. 1974). *Static exercise does not seem to have this effect.*—There are obviously more mechanisms so far not well understood which are involved than those mentioned here: if we consider, however, the *effect of adaptation to exercise which can be implemented by any organism without exception* (i.e. without selection of the primarily fittest and most efficient individuals) *within a time also feasible for the normal subject,* the sequelae of adaptation to dynamic exercise pertaining to the lipid metabolism and body composition, manifested in every instance, will be in the foreground of interest.

The state of adaptation to an increased load is thus obviously a more natural situation in the human organism from the aspect of the hitherto completed morphological and functional development during phylogenesis, and is associated with certain properties which might reduce selected hazards ensuing from oecological living conditions in industrialized society. The reverse applies to the organism living under conditions of hypokinesia (Krasnykh 1969 etc.). Nevertheless, how and when, in what range or under what special set-up such mechanisms can be of use is still not fully understood or experimentally proved.

In this connection it is, however, essential to emphasize the *necessity of a permanent balanced optimum regime of physical activity which plays its part in many respects only when maintained during prolonged periods.* In connection with the finding of an increased cholesterol formation in the liver of the organism adapted to increased physical activity (Petrásek and Pařízková 1976, Petrásek et al. 1975) which does not lead to an elevated cholesterol level due only to enhanced catabolic processes as a result of an increased energy expenditure, we must keep in mind *possible adverse sequelae of sudden complete discontinuation of exercise.* In this connection we may even consider the hazard of hypokinesia greater than in an organism adapted to a lower but steady level of activity. This fact could also, at least partly, help to explain the incidence of various cardiovascular diseases e.g. in former sportsmen (in whom without training aerobic capacity, performance etc. decrease, and fat ratio increases) which in this case is often used as an argument against the favourable effect of a higher physical activity on the organism (we are of course omitting cases of obvious overburdening of the organism by sports training on a top level which unfortunately is no rarity).

We must also take into account other circumstances such as e.g. the *incidence of certain latent abnormalities or even malformations* of various types which are *manifested negatively only during extreme loads* (e.g. contests at a top level) or *various dispositions—either of hereditary origin* (Jokl and McClellan 1971) or those *ensuing from factors acting during prenatal and postnatal ontogenesis.* When comparing the morbidity and mortality from cardiovascular diseases in groups of active and inactive individuals it is therefore *not possible to ensure absolute homogeneity of the groups with regard to all other factors which may interfere.* It is therefore very difficult in groups of human subjects (mainly of a more advanced age and with different anamnesis, frequently compared from very different aspects) to interpret solely the effect of physical activity and inactivity and resulting changes in lipid metabolism and body composition, and differentiate them from the concurrent influence of other factors. The *solution of these problems calls for further directed investigation and experiments in large population groups,* and if possible, *longitudinal investigations,* where *these interferences would be eliminated.*

In this connection it is important to recall again the *ontogenetic aspect.* As revealed by some experimental observations, the effect of increased physical activity or hypokinesia produces the most marked results during prolonged or permanent action from early stages of ontogenesis. There exists a certain threshold age for the beginning of exercise which can influence e.g. longevity in male rats (Eddington et al. 1972). In the experimental model of laboratory animals by adaptation to different physical activity the caloric intake, energy turnover and balance, the level of lipid metabolism in adipose and muscular tissue along with changes in body composition, the sensitivity of the heart muscle to isoprenaline when inducing cardiac necrosis was influenced. The *consequences were graded depending on the intensity and duration of the stimulus; this was rendered possible in particular by the fact that the organism became gradually adapted to a given load, starting at a very early age.*—The example of young people engaged in training in different sport disciplines and their somatic development (advanced growth, greater LBM) along with increased aerobic capacity and improved physical fitness, revealed how the average growing organism develops when subjected to optimal physical loads (Pařízková 1968a,d). Positive changes produced by adaptation to increased activity in obese children (reduced body fat ratio due to increased ability to utilize lipid metabolites as an energy source during muscular work, increase of fitness and aerobic capacity per kg body weight with better practical performance at the same level of maximal oxygen consumption etc.) are particularly instructive examples of the consequences of an optimal load during the developmental period, acting as measures focused on improving an abnormal situation. The attainement of a maximal level of adaptation from all aspects (body composition, aerobic capacity, performance) in adult life with the maintenance of a higher, more favourable level of these indicators in advanced age provide evidence of the *beneficial effect of life-long optimal stimulation by activity in the later stages of life.* This implies in general not only an *extension of selected positive abilities of the organism but also their longer maintenance at a level usually found at an earlier age.* Prolongation of human life, common in recent decades in developed countries with favourable hygienic, health and dietary conditions (Mašek 1974), etc. does not imply under conditions of an optimum regime of physical activity prolongation of existence only but of a really active life. An essential prerequisite is, however, the *maintenance of a permanently increased level of physical activity throughout life, differentiated and adapted to individual needs optimally since early childhood. Most beneficial consequences* seem to result from regular *dynamic exercise of aerobic character* (e.g. running,"jogging" etc.) leading to increased aerobic capacity, reduced deposition of fat, higher level of activity of lipid metabolism etc. Static work load does not lead to such changes (see the exemple of weight lifters, sumo-wrestlers etc.) and is not recommended from this point of view. Moreover, sumo-wrestlers or e.g. lumberjacks (in whom static work prevails) display high mortality from cardiovascular diseases.

Investigations of body composition and other parameters in conjunction with physical activity and physical fitness bring up the question of *what parameters should be used when evaluating the child's development and fitness,* taking into account broader concepts and perspective development. One of the conclusions is that evaluation according to the most traditional indicators—*height and body weight*—appear insufficient and attention must be devoted to some further criteria. Based on our experience it is, in particular, *body composition*, i.e. the percentage of lean body mass and depot fat. The latter has an adverse effect on the economy of functions even within a range beneath the borderline of obesity; this applies in particular to indicators of circulatory and respiratory efficiency, and lipid metabolism.

It was revealed that *taller and heavier children with a higher ratio of body fat, but in some instances also a greater amount of LBM, have from this aspects no advantage even if from the aspect of growth standards they appear to be superior to smaller and more slender children.* Comparison of results obtained in a selected group of Tunisian children (Pařízková and Merhautová 1970, 1973) indicates that *children from more modest conditions (including nutrition) with more ample physical activity have from the aspect of functional fitness and economy of functions the best results.* This finding also applies, however, to our conditions (Pařízková 1974c, Vamberová et al. 1971). It leads therefore to the assumption that it is necessary to *re-evaluate criteria for the optimum development of children* (Karsayevskaya 1964) and *supplement it by further indicators which characterize body composition, and by parameters which render it possible to evaluate functional and also metabolic development.*

This leads also to *reflections whether the steady acceleration of somatic development of children in advanced industrial countries* (so far it is not even established that all organs incl. the heart grow proportionately—Kaluzhnaya 1972) *which is not associated with a similarly accelerated functional development implies satisfactory results as regards the perspective for future development and life and the possible predisposition to so-called diseases of civilization during later life and old age.* Here we would like to recall the example of experimental animals which due to a more restricted diet during early stages of ontogenesis did not attain an equally high body weight and body fat ratio in adult life as animals fed more abundantly, but had under equal conditions a lower mortality and less serious damage of the heart muscle after administration of isoprenaline (Faltová and Pařízková 1970). Although the results cannot be directly extrapolated to humans, the results seem to indicate that in this case also "bigger was not better". The living conditions in contemporary society characterized mainly by hypokinesia and relative (and frequently also absolute) overeating from an early age may be a negative factor which has an impact not only on the actual conditions of the child but also his future health prognosis. *"Homo sedentarius" of the 20th century develops in this way almost from the cradle.*

In our previous investigations we demonstrated when *different age groups were compared* in 1959 – 1972 *that in adolescents there was a trend towards greater body fat ratio after only a ten—thirteen year interval* (Pařízková 1973b). This was also shown by Soviet authors (Gladysheva et al. 1974), in particular in girls. Durnin et al. (1974) found when *comparing measurements in 1964 and 1971 an increased body fat content* together *with significant reduction of energy intake* which according to author's opinion could be accounted for by a marked reduction in physical activity. Guminskiy et al. (1972) showed moreover that the *relative aerobic capacity (max. O_2/kg body weight) declines significantly after a longer time interval from 1948 up to 1968 in children of the same age who have now greater height and weight,* which seems to suggest a *decline of physical fitness of the normal untrained organism in the secular trend of growth acceleration. But these phenomena can be completely prevented by regular physical training* (Gladysheva et al. 1974). The reduction of aerobic capacity is also clearly manifested in adult life, as apparent when comparing the max. O_2/kg body weight in men in the third decade of life who were measured e.g. by Robinson (1938) and Shephard (1969), Kozlowski (1975) demonstrated for instance that it is sufficient to transfer a man for six months to a less strenuous occupation for the aerobic capacity of the organism to decline significantly. Fučík (1975) found when investigating university students, not only a significant decline of fitness during their studies (18–23 years) but a gradually increasing proportion of students with a low and very low performance after only an interval of five years (1967 – 1972). These results necessarily lead to the conclusion that *we cannot consider growth acceleration and an increase of bodily dimensions in developed industrial countries,* mainly as a result of an improved diet, *an unequivocally positive phenomenon* (Fomon 1971,

Fomon et al. 1969). It was also demonstrated that very old subjects had a poor diet in childhood (Hejda 1968).

If we consider moreover that *this living pattern from developed industrial countries spreads along with industrialization and technical progress to developing countries also, this implies the transmission of negative associated phenomena of our civilization* (as inadequately increased caloric input, physical inactivity etc.—Fejfar 1972) *to localities where it would be theoretically possible to direct the development of further generations on a scientific basis in a better way than hitherto.* These problems are one of the most important spheres of care of the present contemporary and future development of new generations under the conditions of the scientific and technological revolution. Not in vain are doctors beginning to *seek the roots of cardiovascular disease* (in particular atherosclerosis) *in childhood* and in changes of the lipid metabolism resulting not only from genetic factors, pathological processes and diet (Kannel and Dawber 1972) but also from hypokinesia. In gerontology also in conjunction with the rate of *onset and course of senile changes* and the *pathogenesis of diseases of old age today, reflections extend over the whole range of ontogenesis* starting not only with early postnatal stages (Chebotarev 1972) but also prenatal ontogenesis.

Criteria for the evaluation of optimum development and growth thus should not be the attainment of greater body dimensions (as it is currently the case in particular in the youngest children) but also *an optimal health prognosis not only for present but also for future life incl. old age.* There are already some examination methods which make it possible to evaluate these aspects, but it is clear—for reasons which need not be explained—that it would hardly be possible to use them widely in common practice. Moreover, it must be emphasized that it is necessary to test and elaborate further comprehensive examinations based on most recent scientific findings which will render it possible to meet the above demands when evaluating child development.

Emphasis on an optimal regime for children as regards physical activity which is beyond doubt one of the most important factors which ensure optimal function and health development may quite rightly be considered as a repetition of old and well know facts. ..."*The more the child is employed in something, runs about, is occupied in doing something, the sweeter is its sleep, the more easily it digests, the more richly it grows, becomes vigorous and flourishing both in body and mind; solely, as long as one sees that it is protected from injury. For this purpose a safe place where children may run about and exercise themselves, should be meant for them and found for them; and a harmless way of such exercise should be shown to them...*" *(John Amos Comenius, Informatorium of the school of infancy—Schola infantiae 1632 Mss; ed. in Latin, Amsterdam 1657).* But *not only in this* but also in *other respects contemporary scientific observations and experiments must detect anew and confirm the importance of natural factors which favourably influence child development, factors about which we have known for a long time* (effect of early nutrition and weaning, the effect of emotional deprivation at an early age, etc.). Analysis of the effect of shortcomings in these respect shows not only the need to prevent them consequentially; it provides at the same time a *basis for applying these factors in an optimal manner not only to maintain but more emphatically to expand the positive abilities and improve the human organism.* An optimally differentiated regime of physical activity should from the aspect of its volume, structure and temporal distribution act in such a way as to *promote self-realization of man throughout life in all the varied spheres of his activity.* Physical training and sports adequately directed are one of the most important forms, in particular under conditions common in developed industrial countries. The basis for inducing a desirable optimal regime is to create prerequisites and correct habits of activity in the child from the earliest age which will be the basis for his whole subsequent life.

References

Abell L. L., Levy B. B., Brodie B. B., Kendall E. F.: J. biol. Chem. 195:357, 1951.
Adolph E. F., Hegeness F. W.: Growth 35:55, 1971.
Ahrens R. A., Broxton M. H.: Proc. Soc. exp. Biol. 134:1043, 1970.
Allen T. H., Peng M. T., Chen K. B., Huang T. F., Chang C., Fang H. S.: Metabolism 5:346, 1956.
Allen T. H., Anderson E. C., Langham W. H.: J. Geront. 15:348, 1960.
Altschuler H., Lieberson M., Spitzer J. J.: Experientia 18:91, 1962.
Anderson E. C., Langham W. H.: Science 130:713, 1959.
Anton A. H., Sayre E. D.: J. Pharmacol. exp. Ther. 138:360, 1962.
Arinchin N.: The cardiovascular system and ageing. 9th Internat. Congress Geront., Kiev 1972. Proc. Vol. 1, p. 236.
Arshavski I. A.: In: Advances in psychobiology. Vol. 1. Ed. G. Newton and A. H. Riesen. Wiley-Interscience, J. Wiley and Sons, New York 1972, p. 1.
Arshavski I. A.: Ocherki po vozrastnoy fiziologii. Ed. "Meditsina", Moscow 1967.
Askew E. W., Dohm G. L., Huston R. L., Sneed T. W., Dowdy R. P.: Proc. Soc. exp. Biol. 141:123, 1972.
Åstrand P. O.: Sport and age. Scient. Congress "Sport in the modern world-chances and problems". XXth Olympiade, Munich 1972. Proc., p. 173 (a)
Åstrand P. O.: In: "Nutritional aspects of physical performance". Papendal (Holland) 1971. Mouton & Comp., The Netherlands 1972, p. 1. (b).
Åstrand P. O., Rodahl K.: Textbook of work physiology. McGraw-Hill Book Comp., New York etc. 1970.
Avoye D. R., Swyryd E. A., Gould R. G.: J. Lipid Res. 6:368, 1965.
Axelrod J.: J. biol. Chem. 237:1657, 1962.

Baker N., Rostam H.: J. Lipid Res. 10:83, 1969.
Balasz T., Sahazrabudhe M. R., Grice H. C.: Toxicol. appl. Pharmacol. 4:613, 1962.

Bashkirov P. N.: Soviet. Anthropologiya Vol. 1958, p. 95.
Bass A., Vondra K., Rath R., Vítek V., Teisinger J., Macková E., Šprynarová Š., Malkovská M.: Pflügers Arch. ges. Physiol. 361:169, 1976.
Bayley N., Pinneau S.: J. Pediat. 40:423, 1952.
Beatty G., Bocek R. M.: Amer. J. Physiol. 219:1311, 1970.
Behnke A. R., Jr.: Ann. N.Y. Acad. Sci. 56:1095, 1956.
Behnke A. R., Jr., Feen G. B., Welham W. C.: J. Amer. med. Ass. 118:495, 1942.
Behnke A. R., Jr., Royce J.: J. Sport Med. 6:75, 1966.
Behnke A. R. Jr., Wilmore J. H.: Evaluation and regulation of body build and composition. Prentice Hall, Inc. Englewood Cliffs, N. Jersey, USA 1974.
Benjamin W., Gellhorn A., Wagner M., Kundell H.: Amer. J. Physiol. 201:540, 1961.
Berdychová J.: Teor. Praxe těl. Vých. 20:321, 1972.
Berdychová J., Pařízková J.: Teor. Praxe těl. Vých. 21:398, 1973.
Berglund G., Björntorp P., Sjöström L., Smit U.: Acta med. scand. 195:213, 1974.
Bergstrøm J.: Scand. J. clin. lab. Invest. Suppl. 68, 1962.
Bernet F., Denimal J.: Europ. J. appl. Physiol. 33:57, 1974.
Best W. R.: J. Lab. clin. Med. 43:967, 1954.
Biale Y., Gorin E., Shafrir E.: Israel J. Chem. 3:112, 1956.
Blackburn H. V.: In: "Measurement in exercise electrocardiography". Ch. C. Thomas, Springfield, Ill. 1969.
Blažek F.: Čs. Pediat. 26:265, 1971.
Bogdanoff M. D.: Arch. intern. Med. 105:505, 1960.
Bogdanoff M. D., Estes E. H., jr., Trout D.: Proc. Soc. exp. Biol. 100:503, 1959.
Bottin R., Juchness J., Deroanner R., Pirnay F., Petit J. M.: Int. Z. angew. Physiol. 25:25, 1968.
Boyd E.: Hum. Biol. 5:646, 1923.
Brans Y. W., Summers J. E., Dwyck H. S., Cassady G.: Pediat. Res. 8:215, 1974.
Brody S.: Bioenergetics and growth, with special reference to the efficiency complex in domestic animals. Reinhold, New York 1945.
Brook C. G.: Lancet II:624, 1972.
Brown B. S., Van Huss W.: J. appl. Physiol. 34:664, 1973.
Brožek J., Chen K. P., Carlsson W., Bronczyk F.: Fed. Proc. 12:21, 1953.
Brožek J., Grande F., Anderson J. T., Keys A.: Ann. N.Y. Acad. Sci. 110:113, 1963.
Brožek J., Keys A.: Brit. J. Nutr. 5:194, 1951.
Bruce R. A., Hornstein T. R., Blackmon J. R.: Circulation 38:552, 1968.
Bruch H.: Amer. J. Dis. Child. 60:1982, 1940.
Brunner D., Kannelis M. O.: Lancet 2:1049, 1960.
Büchi E. C.: Anthropol. Forschungen Anthrop. Gesellschaft Wien, F. Berger, Horn-Wien, Heft 1., 1950.
Bunak V. V.: Voprosy Antropologii No. 28, 1968.
Burmeister W., Fromberg G.: Arch. Kinderheilkunde 180:228, 1970.
Buskirk E., Taylor H. L.: J. appl. Physiol. 11:72, 1957.

Campbell D. E.: J. Lipid Res. 6:478, 1965.
Carlsson L. A.: Fed. Proc. 26:1755, 1967.
Carlsson L. A., Ekelund L., Fröberg S. O.: J. clin. Invest. 50:248, 1971.
Carlsson L. A., Mossfeld F.: Acta physiol. scand. 62:51, 1964.
Carter J. E. L.: Hum. Biol. 42:535, 1970.
Carter J. E. L., Heath B.: Kinesiology Rev. 1971, p. 10.
Čermák J.: Cardiologia (Basel) 53:99, 1969.
Čermák J.: Brit. J. Sports Med. 7:241, 1973.
Čermák J., Brousil J., Pařízková J.: Čs. Fyziol. 16:46, 1967.
Čermák J., Kuta I., Pařízková J.: J. Sports Med. 15:243, 1975.
Čermák J., Pařízková J.: (1) Čs. Pediat. 113:1181, 1974. (2) Rev. czech. Med. 21:134, 1975.
Čermák J., Pařízková J., Venclík Z., Mařatková A.: Physiol. bohemoslov. 22:377, 1973.
Čermák J., Tůma Z., Pařízková J.: Z. Kreisl.-Forsch. 62:1, 1970.
Chappel C. I., Rona G., Balasz T., Gaudry E.: Can. J. Biochem. 37:36, 1959.
Charvát J.: Life, adaptation and stress (in Czech). Avicenum, Prague 1970.
Chebotarev D. F.: In: Proc. 9th Int. Congress Geront. Kiev 1972. Proc. Vol. 1. p. 22.
Cheek D. B.: Human growth. Lea & Febiger, Philadelphia 1968.
Cherkes A., Gordon B. S., Jr.: J. Lipid Res. 1:97, 1957.
Chtetsov V. P., Lutovinova N. Y., Utkina M. I.: In: Proc. VIIth Int. Congress Anthrop. Ethnolog. Sci., Moscow 1964. Ed. Nauka, Moscow 1967. Vol. 2, p. 253.
Cohn C.: Ann. N.Y. Acad. Sci. 110:395, 1963.
Collier G.: (1) Comp. Physiol. Psychol. 77:155, 1971. (2) Lecture Inst. Clin. Exp. Med. 1971.
Consolazio F. C., Krzywicki H. J., Nelson R. A.: In: Proc. 7th Int. Congress Nutrition, Hamburg 1966. Ed. Verlag F. Vierweg and Sohn, G.m.b.H. Braunschweig, Vol. 4, p. 1.
Correnti V., Zauli B.: Olimpionici. Marques, Roma, Italy 1964.
Costill D. L., Branam G. E., Moore J. C., Sparks K., Turner C.: Med. Sci. Sports 6:95, 1974.
Cournand A., Darling R. C., Mansfield J. S., Richards D. W., Jr.: J. clin. Invest. 19:599, 1940.
Crass M. F., Meng H. C.: Biochem. biophys. Acta 125:1, 1966.
Crawford M. A.: Lancet I:329, 1968.
Cureton T. K.: Physical fitness of champion athletes. Univ. Illinois Press, Urbana, USA, 1951.

Damon A., Stoudt H. W.: Hum. Factors 5:485, 1963.
Dancis J.: In: Early diabetes in early life. Ed. R. A. Camerini-Davalos and H. S. Cole. Academic Press, New York 1975, p. 233.
Davies C. M. T.: Clin. Sci. 42:1, 1972.
Davies M.: J. cell. comp. Physiol. 57:135, 1961.

Dole V. P.: J. clin. Med. 35:150, 1956.
von Döbeln W.: Acta physiol. scand. 37, Suppl. 126, 1956.
Drummond G. J., Black E. C.: Ann. Rev. Physiol. 22:169, 1960.
Durnin J. V. A. G., Lonergan M. E., Good J., Ewan A.: Brit. J. Nutr. 32 : 169, 1974.
Durnin J. V. A. G., Rahaman M. M.: Brit. J. Nutr. 21:681, 1967.
Durnin J. V. A. G., Womersley J.: Brit. J. Nutr. 32:77, 1974.
Eddington D. W., Cosmas A. C., McCafferty W. B.: J. Geront. 27:341, 1972.
Edwards D. A. W., Hammond W. H., Healy M. J. R., Tanner J. M., Whitehouse R. H.: Brit. J. Nutr. 9:133, 1955.
Eiselt E.: In: Proc. 2nd. Int. Seminar Ergometry, Berlin 1967. Inst. Leistungsmedizin, Berlin 1968, p. 192.
Eiselt E., Pařízková J.: Z. Altersforsch. 24:259, 1971.
Eiselt E., Pařízková J.: Med. sportiva 28:99, 1975.
Eiselt E., Pařízková J., Zbuzek V.: Sportärztl. Prax. Heft 12, p. 210, 1961.
Eisenberg de Smoler P., Armass-Domínguez J., Domínguez-Manguín C., Karchmer S.: Arch. Investigación 5:595, 1974.
Elmajian F., Hope J. M. et al.: Recent Progr. Hormone Res. 14:513, 1958.
Erankö O., Karvonen M. J., Reisanen L.: Acta endocrin. (Khb) 39:285, 1958.
Euler U. S., Lishajko F.: Acta physiol. scand. 51:348, 1961.

Fábry P.: Feeding pattern and nutritional adaptations. Academia, Prague 1969.
Fábry P., Petrásek R., Kujalová V., Holečková E.: Adaptation to changed caloric intake (in Czech). Státní zdravotnické nakladatelství, Prague 1962.
Falkner F.: In: Puberty. Biologic and Psychological components. Ed. S. R. Berenberg. H. E. Stenfert Kroese B. V. Leiden 1975, p. 123.
Faltová E.: Canad. J. Physiol. Pharmacol. 47:295, 1969.
Faltová E., Albrecht I., Pařízková J., Pilný J.: Čs. Fyziol. 22:71, 1973.
Faltová E., Pařízková J.: Physiol. bohemoslov. 19:275, 1970.
Fee B. A., Well W. B.: Ann. N.Y. Acad. Sci. 110:869, 1963.
Fejfar Z.: Acta cardiol. (Brux.) Suppl. XVI, 1972, p. 7.
Felder O.: Klin. Wschr. 37:844, 1959.
Fetter V., Prokopec M., Suchý J., Tittelbachová S.: Anthropologie. Academia, Prague 1967
Fidanza F.: Nutr. et Dieta No. 21. Ed. S. Karger Basel 1975. P. 110.
Fisher R. A.: Statistical methods for research workers. Edinburgh: Oliver and Boyd 1950.
Fischer A., Pařízková J., Roth Z.: Int. Z. angew. Physiol. 21:269, 1965.
Fomon S. J.: Bull. N.Y. Acad. Med. 47:569, 1971.
Fomon S. J., Filer L. J., Thomas L. N., Rogers R. R., Proksch A. M.: J. Nutr. 98:241, 1969.
Forbes G. B.: Pediatrics 31:308, 1964.
Forbes G. B.: In: Puberty. Biologic and Psychosocial Components. Ed. S. R. Berenberg. Stenfert Kroese N. V. Leiden 1975, p. 132.

Forbes G. B., Amirhakimi G. H.: Hum. Biol. 42:401, 1970.
Forbes G. B., Hursh J. B.: Ann. N. Y. Acad. Sci. 110:255, 1963.
Foster B. J., Bloom M. E.: Amer. J. Physiol. 205:453, 1963.
Frank Ch. W., Weinblatt W., Shapiro S., Sager R. V.: Circulation 34:1022, 1966.
Fredericson D. S., Gordon R. S.: J. clin. Invest. 27:1054, 1958.
Freinkel N., Metzger B. E.: In: Early diabetes in early life. Ed. R. A. Camerini-Davalos and H. S. Cole. Academic Press, New York 1975, p. 289.
Friedberg S. J., Harlan W. R., Trout D. L., Estes E. H.: J. clin. Invest. 39:215, 1960.
Frisancho A. R., Sanchez J., Pellardel D., Yanez L.: Amer. J. phys. Anthrop. 39:255, 1973.
Frisch R., Revelle R., Cook S.: Hum. Biol. 45:469, 1973.
Fritz I. B.: Physiol. Rev. 41:52, 1961.
Fröberg S. O.: Metabolism (1) 20:714, 1971; (2) 20:1044, 1971.
Fučík A.: Čs. Hyg. 20:405, 1975.

Gaidash T. V., Savostyanova E. B.: In: Proc. Symp. "Basic laws of child development and its periodization", Odessa 1975, p. 93.
Gapon A. J.: In: Physical activity of man and hypokinesia (in Rusian) Acad. Sci. USSR, Sibirian Dept. Novosibirsk 1972, p. 46.
deGaray A. L., Levine L., Carter J. E. L.: Genetic and anthropological studies of Olympic athletes. Academic Press Inc., New York 1974.
Garn S. M., Greaney G. R., Young R. W.: Hum. Biol. 28:232, 1956.
Gellhorn A., Benjamin W., Wagner M.: J. Lipid. Res. 3:314, 1962.
George J. C., Jyoti D.: J. anim. Morphol. Physiol. 3:37, 1955.
George J. C., Naik R. M.: Nature (Lond.) 181:709, 1958.
George J. C., Vallyathan N. V.: Amer. J. Physiol. 202:268, 1962.
George J. C., Vallyathan N. V.: Canad. J. Physiol. Pharmacol. 42:447, 1964a.
George J. C., Vallyathan N. V.: J. cell. comp. Physiol. 63:381, 1964b.
DiGirolamo M., Esposito J.: Amer. J. Physiol. 229:107, 1975.
Gladysheva A. A., Guminskiy A. A., Shidlovskaya E. I.: In: Proc. Int. Congress "Sport in the modern society". Moscow 1974.
Goldberger A. L.: Amer. J. Physiol. 213:1193, 1967.
Gollnick P. D., Simmons S. W.: Int. Z. angew. Physiol. 23:322, 1967.
Gollnick P. D., Soule R. G., Taylor A. W., Williams C., Ianuzzo C. D.: Amer. J. Physiol. 219:729, 1970.
Gollnick P. D., Taylor A. W.: Int. Z. angew. Physiol. 27:144, 1969.
Gordon R. S. Jr., Cherkes A.: J. clin. Invest. 35:206, 1956.
Greulich W. W., Pyle S. I.: Radiographic atlas of skeletal development of the hand and the wrist. 2nd. Ed. Calif. Univ. Press, Stanford, 1959.
Grimm H.: Grundrisse der Konstitutionsbiologie und Anthropometrie. VEB Verlag Volk und Gesundheit, Berlin 1960.
Guillemin R., Clayton G. W., Lipscomb H. S., Smit D.: J. Lab. clin. Med. 53:830, 1959.

Guminskiy A. A., Elizarova O. S., Zhurkova N. N., Zolotayko G. A., Novozhilova A. D.: Pediatriya 1972, No. 3, p. 6.

Hagenfeldt L., Wahren J.: In: Muscle metabolism during exercise. Ed. B. Pernow and B. Saltin. Plenum Press, New York — London 1971, p. 153.
Hampton M. C., Huenemann R. L., Shapiro L. R., Mitchell R. W., Behnke A. R.: Amer. J. clin. Nutr. 19:422, 1966.
Hannon J. P., Larson A.: Amer. J. Physiol. 203:1055, 1962.
Harris W. H., Cummings J. N.: J. appl. Physiol. 34:584, 1973.
Harris P., Gloster J.: Cardiology 56:43, 1972.
Havel R. J.: In: Muscle metabolism during exercise. Ed. B. Pernow and B. Saltin. Plenum Press, New York — London 1971, p. 315.
Havel R. J., Carlsson L. A.: Life Sci. 9:651, 1963.
Hebbelinck M., Casier H.: Int. Z. angew. Physiol. 22:185, 1966.
Hecht A.: Virchows Arch. path. Anat. 331:26, 1958.
Hejda S.: Z. Altersforsch. 21:159, 1968.
Hejda S., Hátle J.: Čs. Gastroenterol. 14:557, 1960.
Hellander E.: Acta morphol. neerl.-scand. 3:92, 1959.
Hermanssen L., Saltin B.: J. appl. Physiol. 26:31, 1969.
Hermanssen L., Wachtlová M.: J. appl. Physiol. 30:860, 1971.
Hess G. H., Riegle G. D.: J. Geront. 25:354, 1970.
Himms-Hagen J.: Lipids 7:310, 1972.
Hirsch J., Knittle J. L.: Fed. Proc. 29:1516, 1970.
Hoet J. J.: In: Proc. XIIIth Int. Congress Pediatrics. Metabolism, p. 397. Ed. Verlag Wiener Med. Acad., Vienna 1971.
Hoffman A. A., Nelson W. R., Goss F. H.: Amer. J. Cardiol. 20:516, 1967.
Hollander C. F.: Exp. Geront. 5:313, 1970.
Holliday M. A., Potter D., Jarrah A., Bearg S.: Pediat. Res. 1:185, 1967.
Hollman W.: Höchst- und Dauerleistungsfähigkeit des Sportlers. J. Ambrosius Barth, Munich 1963.
Hrdlička A.: Proc. Amer. Phil. Soc. 76:847, 1936.
Hunt E., Heald F. P.: Ann. N.Y. Acad. Sci. 110:532, 1963.

Issekutz B., Jr., Miller H.: Proc. Soc. exp. Biol. 110:237, 1962.
Issekutz B., Jr., Miller H., Paul P., Rodahl K.: J. appl. Physiol. 20:293, 1965.
Issekutz B., Jr., Miller H., Rodahl K.: Fed. Proc. 25:1415, 1966.
Issekutz B., Jr., Spitzer J. J.: Proc. Soc. exp. Biol. 21:105, 1960.

Janda F.: Čs. Hyg. 4:204, 1959
Jelínková M., Myslivečková Z.: Physiol. bohemoslov. 14:146, 1965.
Jéquier E., Cygax P. H., Pittet P., Vanotti A.: J. appl. Physiol. 36:674, 1974.
Johnson P. R., Stern J. S., Greenwood M. R. C., Zucker L. M., Hirsch K.: J. Nutr. 103:738, 1973.

Jokl E.: Nutrition, exercise and body composition. Chc. Thomas, Springfield, III., USA 1964.
Jokl E., McClellan J. T.: Exercise and cardiac death. Medicine and Sport Vol. 5. Univ. Park Press, Baltimore-London-Tokyo 1971.
Juřinová I.: In: Proc. Scient. Comm. ČSTV (Czechoslovak Sport Organization), Prague 1968, p. 19.

Kagan A.: Proc. roy. Soc. Med. (Lond.) 53:8, 1960.
Kagi N. T.: Acta physiol. scand. Suppl. 39, p. 132, 1956.
Kaluzhnaya R. A.: Pediatriya 1972, No. 5, p. 56.
Kannel W. B., Dawber T. R.: J. Pediat. 80:544, 1972.
Kannel W. B., LeBauer E. J., Dawber T. R., McNamara P. M.: Circulation 35:734, 1967.
Kapalín V.: In: Handbook of practical medicine (in Czech), Avicenum, Prague 1967. p. 109.
Kasch F. W., Boyer J. L.: Med. Sci. Sports 1:156, 1969.
Karsayevskaya T. V.: Akhiv Anat. gistol. Embriol. 46:93, 1964.
Kennedy G. C., Mitra J.: J. Physiol. (Lond.) 166:395, 1963.
Kenyon B. S., Torresani R.: Res. Quart. Amer. Ass. Hlth phys. Educ. 34:21, 1963.
Keys A.: Ann. N.Y. Acad. Sci. 134:1046, 1966.
Keys A., Aravanis C., Blackburn H. B. et al.: Acta med. scand. Suppl. 460, 1966, p. 392.
Keys A., Brožek J.: Physiol. Rev. 33:245, 1953.
Keys A., Mickelson O., Anderson A. A., Bethesda B. S.: J. Lab. clin. Med. 53:282, 1959.
Khanina K. P., Chagovets P. V.: Dopovidi Ukrainskoi Akademii Nauk, No. 2, 1954, p. 94.
Kirton A. H., Pearson A. M.: Ann. N.Y. Acad. Sci. 110:221, 1963.
Kitagawa K., Ikuta K., Hara Y., Hiirta K.: J. Phys. Fitness Japan 23:96, 1974.
Kleiber M., Rogers T. A.: Ann. Rev. Physiol. 23:15, 1961.
Knittle J.: In: Puberty. Biologic and Psychosocial Components. Ed. S. R. Berenberg. H. E. Stenfert Kroese B. V. Leiden 1975, p. 158.
Knittle J., Ginsberg-Fellner F.: Diabetes 21:754, 1972.
Knittle J., Hirsch J.: J. clin. Invest. 47:2091, 1968.
Koch J.: In: Bericht 26. Kongress Deutsch. Gesellsch. Psychol. 1969. Ed. Verlag für Psychologie. Dr. Hofrege, Gottingen, p. 413.
Kohout M., Braun T., Pařízková J.: Physiol. bohemoslov. 14:276, 1965.
Kozlowski S.: In: Proc. Int. Symp. "Methods of checking the development of human beings and changes in the population structure in connection with transformations of the environments". Polska Akad. Nauk. Jablonna, Aug. 1975, Poland. In press.
Kozlowski S., Brzezinska Z., Nazar K., Kowalski W.: Bull. Pol. Acad. Sci. 20:897, 1972.

Krasnykh I. G.: In: Problemy kosmicheskoi meditsiny i biologii, Vol. XIII. Ed. Nauka, Moscow 1969, p. 93.
Krogh A.: Physiology of capillaries. Yale Univ. Press, New Haven 1929.
Krzywicki H. J., Vhinn K. S. K.: Amer. J. clin. Nutr. 20:305, 1967.
Kuta I., Pařízková J., Eiselt E.: Teor. Praxe těl. Vých. 12:348, 1964.
Kuta I., Pařízková J., Dýcka J.: J. appl. Physiol. 29:168, 1970.
Kuzuya T., Akanuma Y., Kosaka K.: In: Proc. Xth Int. Congress Nutrition, Kyoto 1975. In press.
Kvetňanský R., Mikulaj L.: Endocrinology 87:738, 1970.
Kvetňanský R., Pařízková J., Mikulaj L., Torda T., Poledne R., Petrásek R.: Physiol. bohemoslov. 24:75, 1975.
Kvetňanský R., Weise W. K., Kopin I. J.: Endocrinology 87:744, 1970.

Lát J.: In: "Pharmacology of conditioning, learning and retention". Proc. 2nd Int. Pharmacol. Meeting, Prague 1963. Pergamon Press 1963, p. 47.
Lát J., Gollová E.: In: Experimental approaches to the study of emotional behavior. Ed. E. Tobach. Ann. N.Y. Acad. Sci. 159:710, 1969.
Ledovskaya N. M.: In. Physical activity of man and hypokinesia (in Russian). Acad. Sci. USSR, Siberian Dept., Novosibirsk 1972, p. 30.
Lee M. M. C., Lasker G. W.: Amer. J. Phys. Anthrop. 16:125, 1958.
Lemonnier D., Suquet J. P., Aubert R., Rosslin G.: Horm. Metab. Res. 5:223, 1973.
Leshkevich L. G.: Ukrainsk. biokhem. Zhurnal 32:692, 1960.
Lesser G. T., Deutsch S., Jarkofsky J.: J. Geront. 25:108, 1970.
Leusink J. A.: In: Proc. Nutricia Symp. "Nutritional aspects of physical performance", Papendal 1971. Mouton & Comp. The Hague, Netherlands 1972, p. 100.
Leytes S. M., Chon-su: Fed. Proc. (Trans. suppl.) 22:244, 1963.
Lincoln J. E.: Amer. J. clin. Nutr. 25:390, 1972.
Link R. P., Pedersoll W. M., Safanie A. H.: Atherosclerosis 15:107, 1972.
Luft U. C.: In: "Physical Fitness". Ed. V. Seliger, Universitas Carolina, Prague 1973, p. 237.
Luštinec K.: Čs. Fysiol. 5:250, 1956.
Lutovinova N. I., Utkina M. I., Chtetsov V. P.: In: Proc. VIIth Int. Congress Anthropol. Ethnograph. Sci. Moscow 1964. Nauka, Moscow 1967. Vol. 2, p. 253.

Macho L., Kolena J.: Endocrinol. exper. 9:93, 1975.
Mack R. M., Kleinhenz M. E.: Hum. Biol. 46:345, 1974.
Macková E.: Physiol. bohemoslov. 17:279, 1968.
Malina R.: In: Exercise and Sports Sci. Rev., Vol. 3, Academic Press Inc., New York 1975, p. 249.
Malina R. M., Harper A. B., Avent H. H., Campbell D. R.: Med. Sci. Sports 3:32, 1971.
Malinow M. R., Perley A., McLoughlin P.: J. appl. Physiol. 27:662, 1969.
Malkovská M.: Anthropologia 9:63, 1971.

Mallow S., Alousi A. A.: Amer. J. Physiol. 216:794, 1969.
Mallow S., Witt P. N.: J. Pharmacol. exp. Ther. 126:132, 1961.
Mann G. V.: New Engl. J. Med. 291:178, 1974.
Mann M. D., Bowie M. D., Hansen J. D. L.: Pediat. Res. 8 : 879, 1974.
Marshall N. B., Engel F. L.: J. Lipid Res. 1:339, 1960.
Mašek J.: In: "Nutrition. Proc. VIIIth Int. Congress, Prague 1969. Ed. J. Mašek, K. Ošancová, D. P. Cuthbertson. Excerpta Med., Amsterdam 1970, p. 358.
Mašek J.: Ecol. Food Nutr. 3:55, 1974
Matiegka J.: Čs. Vlastivěda Vol. II. Sphinx Janda, Prague 1933, p. 193.
Mayer J.: Overweight: Causes, cost and control. Prentice Hall. Inc., Englewood Cliffs, New Jersey, USA 1968, p. 116.
Mayer J.: Nutrition. Proc. VIIIth Int. Congress, Prague 1969. Ed. J. Mašek, K. Ošancová, D. P. Cuthbertson. Excerpta Med. Amsterdam 1970, p. 354.
McCance R. A., Widdowson E. M.: Proc. roy. Soc. (B) London 156:326, 1962.
Merhautová J., Pařízková J.: (1) Physiol. bohemoslov. 20:71, 1971; (2) Anthropologie 11 : 121, 1973a.
Merhautová J., Pařízková J.: Brit. J. Sports Med. 7 : 247, 1973b.
Métivier O.: In: Metabolic adaptations to prolonged exercise. Proc. 2nd. Int. Symp. "Biochemistry of exercise", Magglingen 1973. Ed. H. Howald and J. R. Poortmans. Birkhäuser Verlag, Basel 1975, p. 276.
Mikulaj L., Komadel L., Vigaš M., Kvetňanský R., Starka L., Vencel P.: In: Metabolic adaptations to prolonged exercise. Proc. 2nd Int. Symp. "Biochemistry of exercise". Ed. H. Howald and J. R. Poortmans. Birkhäuser Verlag, Basel 1975, p. 333.
Mikulaj L., Kvetňanský R., Murgaš K., Pařízková J., Vencel P.: In: Proc. Int. Symp. "Catecholamines and stress", Bratislava 1975. Ed. E. Usdin et al. Pergamon Press, Oxford 1976, p. 445.
Milicer H.: Studia i Monogr. AWF, No. 5. Warszawa 1973.
Miller A. T., Blyth C. S.: J. appl. Physiol. 8:139, 1955.
Mitchell S., Blount S. G., Blumenthal S., Jesse M. J., Weidman W. H.: Pediatrics 49:165, 1972.
Mjös O. D., Akre S.: Scand. J. clin. Lab. Invest. 27:221, 1971.
Mjös O. D., Kjekshus J.: Scand. J. clin. Lab. Invest. 28:389, 1971.
Möhr M.: Dtsch. Gesundheitswes. 24:954, 1969.
Molé P. A., Holoszy J. O.: Proc. Soc. exp. Biol. 134:789, 1970.
Molinoff P. B., Weinshilboum R., Axelrod J.: J. Pharmacol. exp. Ther. 178:425, 1971.
Montoye H.: Canad. med. Ass. J. 96 : 813, 1967.
Montoye H.: Physical activity and health: an epidemiologic study of an entire community. Prentice-Hall, Inc. Englewood Cliffs, New Jersey 1975.
Moody D. L., Kolkas J., Buskirk E. R.: Med. Sci. Sports 1:75, 1969.
Morant G. M.: Proc. roy. Soc. (B) 137:443, 1950.
Morris J. N., Heady J. A., Raffle F. A. B., Roberts C. G., Parks J. N.: Lancet II:1053, 1111, 1953.

Morris J. N., Chave S. P. W., Adam C., Sirey C., Epstein L., Sheehan D. J.: Lancet I:333, 1973.
Moser P. D., Berdanier C. D.: J. Nutr. 104:687, 1974.
Mosinger M., Wenkeová J.: Proc. 5th Nat. Congress Physiol. Sci. Karlovy Vary 1961. Academia, Prague 1963, p. 86.
Motyčka J.: Teor. Praxe těl. Vých. 14:40, 1966.
Moulton C. R.: J. biol. Chem. 57:79, 1923.
Musshoff K., Reindell H.: Dtsch. med. Wchschr. 81:1001, 1956.

Nagamine S., Yamakawa K., Tsuji K.: Ann. Report Nat. Inst. Nutr. Tokyo, Japan No. 23, 1974, p. 29.
Nagatsu T., Levitt M., Udenfried S.: Analyt. Biochem. 9:122, 1964.
Navrátil M., Křeček V., Cvachová L.: Čas. Lék. čes. 97:782, 1958.
Nikityuk B. A.: In: Proc. 9th Int. Congress Geront. Kiev 1972, Vol. 1, p. 289.
Nikkilä E. A., Konttinen A.: Lancet II:1151, 1962.
Nikkilä E. A., Torsti P., Pentillä O.: Metabolism 12:863, 1963.
Novak L. P.: Ann. N.Y. Acad. Sci. 110:545, 1963.
Novak L. P.: J. Amer. med. Ass. 197:891, 1966.
Novak L. P.: J. Geront. 27:438, 1972.
Novak L. P.: J. nucl. Med. 14:550, 1973.
Novak L. P., Hamamoto K., Orvis A. L., Burke E. C.: Amer. J. Dis. Child. 119:419, 1970.
Novak L. P., Hyatt R. E., Alexander J. F.: J. Amer. med. Ass. 205:764, 1968.
Novotný V.: Teor. Praxe těl. Vých. 10:127, 1962.

Oliver M. F., Yates P. A.: Cardiology 56:359, 1971/2.
Oliverau J. M.: Z. vergl. Physiol. 72:435, 1971.
Ošancová K., Hejda S.: Problems of obesity in the population (in Czech). Avicenum Prague 1974.
Ošancová K., Zvolánková K., Hejda S.: Nutrition (Lond.) 26:162, 1972.
Oscai L. B., Babirak S. P., McGarr J. A., Spirakis C. N.: Fed. Proc. 33:1956, 1974.
Oscai L. B., Molé P. A., Holloszy J. O.: Amer. Physiol. 220:1944, 1971.
Ostman I., Sjöstrand N. D.: Acta physiol. scand. 82:202, 1971.

Palmer W. K., Tipton C. M.: Fed. Proc. 33:1964, 1974.
Pařízková J.: Čs. Pediat. 12:310, 1957.
Pařízková J.: Physiol. bohemoslov. 8:112, 1959a.
Pařízková J.: (1) Čs. Fyziol. 8:426, 1959b; (2) Ph. D. thesis, Czechosl. Acad. Sci. Prague 1956—9.
Pařízková J.: Physiol. bohemoslov. 9:516, 1960a.
Pařízková J.: Čs. Fyziol. 9:253, 1960b.
Pařízková J.: In: Actes VIe Congrès Int. Sciences Anthropol. Ethnologiques Paris 1960. Vol. 1, p. 349 (1960c).

Pařízková J.: J. appl. Physiol. 16:173, 1961a.
Pařízková J.: Nutr. et Dieta 3:236, 1961b
Pařízková J.: Metabolism 10:794, 1961c.
Pařízková J.: The development of lean body mass and fat in children and adolescents (in Czech). Ed. Státní zdravotnické nakladatelství, Prague 1962a.
Pařízková J.: Teoriya i Praktika fizitcheskoy kultury i sporta 25:37, 1962b.
Pařízková J.: Ann. N.Y. Acad. Sci. 110:661, 1963a.
Pařízková J.: Current Anthropol. 4:26, 1963b.
Pařízková J.: *In:* "L'obésité." Proc. Symp. Int. Paris 1963. Problèmes actuels d'endocrinologie et de nutrition, Série No. 7. Ed. Expansion Scientifique Française, Paris 1963. P. 271 (1963c).
Pařízková J. In: "Body composition." Proc. Conf. SSHB, London 1963. Ed. J. Brožek. Pergamon Press, Oxford 1965, p. 161.
Pařízková J.: *In:* (1) Proc. Int. Seminar on Ergometry, Berlin 1965. Inst. Leistungsmedizin, Berlin 1966, p. 62; (2) *In:* Ergebnisse der Ergometrie. Ed. H. Mellerowicz, E. Jokl, G. Hansen. Perimed, Germany 1975, p. 37.
Pařízková J.: Proc. Nutr. Soc. 25:93, 1966.
Pařízková J.: *In:* Proc. Int. Congress Anthropol. Ethnolog. Sci. Moscow 1964. Nauka, Moscow 1967. Vol. 2, p. 164.
Pařízková J.: (1) Hum. Biol. 40:212, 1968; (2) Teor. Praxe těl. Vých. (Suppl.) 16:31, 1968a.
Pařízková J.: Current Anthropol. 9:273, 1968b.
Pařízková J.: *In:* "Human body composition" (in Dutch). Ed. A. Haak et al. Van Gorcum & Comp. N. V. Assen 1968 (1) p. 27 (1968c); (2) p. 142 (1968d); (3) p. 274 (1968e).
Pařízková J.: Nutrition, body fat and physical fitness. Borden's Rev. Nutr. Res. Vol. 29 (Fourth Quarter). 1968f.
Pařízková J.: Compositional growth in relation to metabolic activity. Opening plenary session — XIIth Int. Congress Pediatrics, Mexiko City 1968. Proceedings, Vol. 1, p. 32. (1968g).
Pařízková J.: *In:* "Biochemistry of exercise" — 1st Int. Symp. Bruxelles 1968. Medicine and Sport, Vol. 3. Ed. J. R. Poortmans. S. Karger, Basel 1969, p. 37.
Pařízková J.: Monogr. Soc. Res. Child. Devel. 28:35, 1970a.
Pařízková J.: Glasnik antropol. Drušstvo 7:33, 1970b.
Pařízková J.: Antropologie 8:73, 1970c.
Pařízková J.: Čs. Pediat. 26:14, 1971a.
Pařízková J.: Ärztl. Jugendkunde 62:437, 1971b.
Pařízková J.: Čs. Pediat. 27:443, 1972a.
Pařízková J.: *In:* Nutricia Symp. "Nutritional aspects of physical performance", Papendal 1971. Ed. Nutricia, Mouton & Comp. The Hague, Netherlands, 1972 (1) p. 89 (1972b); (2) p. 146 (1972c).
Pařízková J.: Kinanthropologie 4:95, 1972d.
Pařízková J.: Teor. Praxe těl. Vých. 20:430, 1972e.

Pařízková J.: In: "Alimentation et travail", 1er Symp. Int. Vitell 1971. Ed. G. Débry and L. Blayer. Masson, Paris, 1972, p. 85 (1972f).

Pařízková J.: Body composition and exercise during growth and development. Chap. 5. *In:* "Physical activity: human growth and development". Ed. G. L. Rarick. Academic Press Inc. New York 1972, p. 97. (1972g).

Pařízková J.: Anthropologie 10:3, 1972h.

Pařízková J.: In: Proc. 9th Int. Congress Geront., Kiev 1972. Vol. 3, p. 243 (1972i).

Pařízková J.: Teor. Praxe těl. Vých. (1) 21:301, 1973; (2) ibidem 21:352 (1973a).

Pařízková J.: Proc. Nutr. Soc. 32:181, 1973b.

Pařízková J.: Body composition, nutrition and exercise. Opening adress, 3° Convegno Internazionale "Nutrizione, dietetica e sport", Roma 1973. Med. sportiva 27:2, 1974a.

Pařízková J.: Acta paediat. belg. Suppl. 23, 1974, p. 28 (1974b).

Pařízková J.: Interrelationships between nutritional status, body size and body composition. *In:* "Nutrition and Malnutrition", ed. A. Roche and F. Falkner. Advances in experimental medicine and physiology, vol. 49. Plenum Press, New York 1974, p. 119 (1974c).

Pařízková J.: In: Recent advances in obesity research. Proc. 1st Int. Symp. Obesity, London 1974. Ed. A. Howard. Newman Publ., Ltd. London 1975, p. 293 (1975a).

Pařízková J.: Europ. J. appl. Physiol. 34:331, 1975b.

Pařízková J.: In: Puberty. Biologic and psychosocial components. Ed. S. R. Berenberg. Stenfert Kroese B. V. Leiden 1975, p. 198 (1975c).

Pařízková J.: In: Proc. Int. Symp. "Criteria for determination of biological age in man". Leningrad, Oct. 1974. In press.

Pařízková J.: The impact of physical activity and nutrition during prenatal and postnatal ontogeny on body composition, lipid metabolism and fitness. *In:* Proc. Xth Int. Congress Nutrition, Kyoto Aug. 1975. In press. (d).

Pařízková J.: Pediat. Res. 10:647, 1976.

Pařízková J., Berdychová J.: (1) *In:* Proc. Conf. Int. FIEPS "Éducation physique avant la puberté", Gdansk 1974. Éd. Scient. Pol., Varsovie 1976, p. 506. (2) Metod. Bull. ČSTV (Czechoslovak Sport Org.), Prague 1976.

Pařízková J., Bůžková P.: Hum. Biol. 16:43, 1971.

Pařízková J., Carter J. E. L.: Amer. J. Phys. Anthropol. 44:327, 1976.

Pařízková J., Čermák J.: In: Proc. Symp. Int. "Physiologie de l'effort chez l'enfant", Trois Rivières, Québec, Canada 1975. In press.

Pařízková J., Čermák J., Horná J.: In: Proc. 2ème Symp. Int. "Alimentation et travail", Vitell 1974. Ed. G. Débry et R. Blayer, p. 37 (1974a).

Pařízková J., Eiselt E.: Čs. Hyg. 7:295, 1962.

Pařízková J., Eiselt E.: Hum. Biol. 38:351, 1966.

Pařízková J., Eiselt E.: Hum. Biol. 40:331, 1968.

Pařízková J., Eiselt E.: Hum. Biol. 43:318, 1971.

Pařízková J., Eiselt E., Šprynarová Š., Wachtlová M.: J. appl. Physiol. 31:323, 1971a.

Pařízková J., Faltová E.: (1) Physiol. bohemoslov. 18:503, 1969, (2) Brit. J. Nutr. 3:24, 1970.
Pařízková J., Faltová E., Wachtlová M.: Int. Symp. "Adaptability of cardiac muscle", Prague 1974.
Pařízková J., Goldstein H.: Hum. Biol. 40:436, 1970.
Pařízková J., Kaldovský O., Pípal M.: Čs. Hyg. 7:405, 1960.
Pařízková J., Koutecký Z.: Physiol. bohemoslov. 17:177, 1968.
Pařízková J., Koutecký Z., Staňková L.: Physiol. bohemoslov. 15:237, 1966a.
Pařízková J., Kreipl J.: Čs. Hyg. 16:123, 1971.
Pařízková J., Lát J.: In: Physical fitness. Ed. V. Seliger, Universitas Carolina, Prague 1973, p. 304. (1973a).
Pařízková J., Lát J.: Physiol. bohemoslov. 22:422, 1973b.
Pařízková J., Merhautová J.: (1) Hum. Biol. 42:391, 1970; (2) Physiol. bohemoslov. 20:76, 1971; (3) Anthropologie 11:115, 1973.
Pařízková J., Merhautová J., Mazzorra R., Radojevič R.: Voprosy antropologii No. 47, p. 124, 1974c.
Pařízková J., Merhautová J., Prokopec M.: Rev. Biometrie hum. 7:1, 1972a.
Pařízková J., Petrásek R.: Int. Symp. "Nutrition, Dietetics and Sport", Bordighera 1976.
Pařízková J., Poledne R.: Physiol. bohemoslov. 23:165, 1974a.
Pařízková J., Poledne R.: Europ. J. appl. Physiol. 33:1, 1974b.
Pařízková J., Poledne R.: Physiol. bohemoslov. 24:75, 1975a.
Pařízková J., Poledne R.: In: Proc. "Int. Symp. on athlete's nutrition", Leningrad 1975. In press. (b).
Pařízková J., Poupa O.: Brit. J. Nutr. 17:341, 1963.
Pařízková J., Roth Z.: Hum. Biol. 44:613, 1972.
Pařízková J., Šprynarová Š.: In: (1) Proc. Int. Seminar Ergometry, Berlin 1967. Inst. Leistungsmedizin, Berlin 1968; p. 115; (2) Ergebnisse der Ergometrie. Ed. H. Mellerowicz et al. Perimed 1975, p. 47.
Pařízková J., Šprynarová Š.: In: "Nutrition". Proc. VIIIth Int. Congress, Prague 1969. Ed. J. Mašek et al. Excerpta Medica, Amsterdam 1970, p. 316.
Pařízková J., Šprynarová Š.: In: Proc. Sci. Congress "Sport in the modern world-chances and problems". XXth Olympiade, Munich 1972 (summ.) Springer Verlag, Berlin etc. 1973, p. 504.
Pařízková J., Šprynarová Š., Macková E., Eiselt E.: Physiol. bohemoslov. 22:425, 1972 (1972b).
Pařízková J., Staňková L.: Brit. J. Nutr. 18:325, 1964a.
Pařízková J., Staňková L.: (1) J. Physiol. (Paris) 56:625, 1964b; (2) Nutr. et Dieta 9:43, 1967.
Pařízková J., Staňková L., Fábry P., Koutecký Z.: Physiol. bohemoslov. 15:31, 1966b.
Pařízková J., Staňková L., Šprynarová Š., Vamberová M.: Nutr. et Dieta 7:21, 1965.
Pařízková J., Vamberová M.: Devel. Med. Child. Neurol. 9:202, 1967.

Pařízková J., Vamberová M., Oppelt J., Vaněčková M.: In: Proc. 5th Nat. Congress Physiol. Sci. Karlovy Vary 1961. Academia, Prague 1963, p. 66.
Pařízková J., Vaněčková M., Šprynarová Š., Vamberová M.: Acta paediat. scand. Suppl. 217, p. 80 (1971b).
Pařízková J., Vaněčková M., Vamberová M.: Physiol. bohemoslov. 11:351, 1962.
Pařízková J., Wachtlová M., Soukupová M.: (1) Physiol. bohemoslov. 20:397, 1971; (2) Int. Z. angew. Physiol. 30:207, 1972c.
Paul P.: In: Metabolic adaptation to prolonged physical exercise. Proc. 2nd. Int. Symp. "Biochemistry of exercise", Magglingen 1973. Ed. H. Howell and J. R. Poortmans. Birkhäuser Verlag, Basel 1975, p. 156.
Paul P., Issekutz B., Jr.: J. appl. Physiol. 22:615, 1967.
Peterson R. D., Gaudin D., Bocer R. M., Beatty C. H.: Amer. J. Physiol. 206:599. 1964.
Petrásek R., Pařízková J., Poledne R.: Physiol. bohemoslov. 24:77, 1975.
Petrásek R., Pařízková J.: Physiol. bohemoslov. in press.
Petrásek R., Rath R., Mašek J.: Rev. czech. Med. 11:267, 1965.
Petrásek R., Reiniš K., Loubová J., Misíková J., Rath R.: Amer. J. phys. Anthrop. 1976. In press.
Pett L. B., Ogilvie G. F.: In: Body measurement and human nutrition. Ed. J. Brožek. Wayne Univ. Press 1956, p. 67.
Pette D.: In: Proc. Symp. "Progressive Muskeldystrophie". Springer Verlag, Berlin 1966, p. 492.
Piechaczek H.: Materialy i Pracy Antropol. No. 85, 1975, p. 3.
Pike R., Brown M.: Nutrition: an integrated approach. 2nd ed. J. Wiley and Sons, Inc. New York etc. 1975.
Pokrovsky A. A.: In: Proc. "Int. Symp. on athlete's nutrition", LNIIFK, Leningrad 1975. In press.
Poledne R., Pařízková J.: In: "Metabolic adaptation to prolonged physical exercise", 2nd Int. Symp. "Biochemistry of exercise", Magglingen 1973. Ed. H. Howald and J. R. Poortmans. Birkhäuser Verlag, Basel 1975, p. 201 (1975a).
Poledne R., Pařízková J.: Int. Symp. "Adaptability of cardiac muscle", Prague 1974.
Poledne R., Pařízková J.: Physiol. bohemoslov. 24:75, 1975b.
Poledne R., Pařízková J.: In: Proc. "Int. Symp. on athlete's nutrition". LNIIFK, Leningrad 1975. In press.
Přibylová H., Znamenáček K.: In: Proc. XIIIth Int. Congress Pediatrics, Vienna 1972. Metabolism, p. 456. Verlag Wiener Med. Akad. Wissensch., Vienna 1971.
Prokopec M.: Acta Fac. Rer. Natur. Univ. Comen. 6:81, 1961.
Pullar J. D., Webster A. J. F.: Brit. J. Nutr. 31:377, 1974.
Puzanová L., Pařízková J.: Sborn. lék. 78:85, 1976.
Pyorälä K., Karvonen M. J. et al.: Amer. J. Cardiol. 20:191, 1967.

Quaade F.: Lancet II:429, 1963.

Raben M. S., Hollenberg C. H.: J. clin. Invest. 39:435, 1960.

Rath R.: In: "Nutrition." Proc. VIIIth Int. Congress, Prague 1969. Ed. J. Mašek et al. Excerpta Medica, Amsterdam 1970, p. 366.
Rath R.: Čas. Lék. čes. 110:391, 1971.
Rath R., Slabochová Z.: Nutr. et Dieta 6:273, 1964
Rehs H. J., Berndt I., Rutenfranz J., Burmeister W.: Z. Kinderheilk. 120:121, 1975.
Reiniš Z., Pokorný J., Bazika V., Hejda S. et al.: Vnitřní Lék. 18:9, 1972.
Reitman J., Baldwin K. M., Holloszy J. O.: Proc. Soc. exp. Biol. 142:628, 1973.
Restrepo C., Tracy R. E.: Atherosclerosis 21:179, 1975.
Reynolds E. L.: Monogr. Soc. Res. Child. Devel. 15:189, 1950.
Richet C.: La chaleur animal. Bibl. Scient. Int. Felix Alcan, Paris 1889.
Rider A. A., Simonson M.: Nutr. Rep. Int. (1) 7:361, 1973; (2) Ibidem 10:19, 1974.
Robinson S.: Arbeitsphysiologie 10:251, 1938.
Robinson D. S.: J. Lipid Res. 1:332, 1960.
Robinson D. S.: Fed. Proc. 34:103, 1975.
Rogozkin V. A.: In: Proc. "Int. Symp. on athlete's nutrition", LNIIFK, Leningrad 1975. In press.
Rona G., Chappel C. I., Balasz T., Gaudry R.: J. Geront. 14:169, 1959.
Rose H. E., Mayer J.: Pediatrics 41:18, 1968.
Rosenblum I., Wohl A., Stein A. A.: Toxicol. appl. Pharmacol. 7:344, 1965.
Ross W. D., Day J. A. P.: J. Sport Med. 12:30, 1972.
Roux W.: Die Entwicklungsmechanik. Leipzig 1905.
Rowell L. B.: Med. Sci. Sports 1:15, 1969.
Rowell L. B.: Physiol. Rev. 54:75, 1974.
Rubner M. (quot. Krogh A.): The respiratory exchange of animals and man. Longmans, New York 1916.

Salans L. B., Cushman S. W., Weisman R. E.: J. clin. Invest. 52:929, 1974.
Sámek L., Geizerová H., Novotný V. et al.: In: Proc. Symp. "Weight of the human organism" (in Czech), Prague 1971. Ed. E. Vlček. Nat. Museum, Prague 1971, p. 193.
Sanders K.: Lancet II:432, 1959.
Schmit-Nielsen K.: Fed. Proc. 29:1524, 1970.
Schotz M., Baker N.: J. Lipid Res. 10:1, 1969.
Scrimshaw N. S., Gordon J. E.: Malnutrition, learning and behavior. The MIT Press, Cambridge, Mass. and London, England 1968.
Seefeldt V.: Critical learning periods and program of early intervention. Presented in Nat. Convention, AAHPER, Atlantic City, N. J. 1975.
Seliger V.: Int. Z. angew. Physiol. 25:104, 1968.
Selye H., Bajusz E.: J. Geront. 14:164, 1959.
Shafrir E., Steinberg D.: J. clin. Invest. 39:310, 1960.
Sheldon W. H., Dupertuis C. W., McDermott E.: Atlas of man. Ed. Harper and Bros. New York 1954.
Shephard R. J.: Endurance fitness. University of Toronto 1969.

Shock N. W.: In: Proc. 9th Int. Congress Gerontol., Kiev 1972. Vol. 1, p. 13.
Shug A. L., Shrago E.: J. Lab. clin. Med. 81:214, 1973.
Simko V., Horvathová V.: Physiol. bohemoslov. 17:583, 1968.
Sirotinin N. N.: In: Proc. 9th Int. Congress Gerontol. Kiev 1972. Vol. 1, p. 254,
Sklad M.: Wych. fiz. Sport No. 3, 1972, p. 119.
Slabochová Z., Placer Z.: Die Nahrung 6:525, 1962.
Sloan A. W., Shapiro M.: Hum. Biol. 44:29, 1972.
Slonim A. D., Smirnov K. M.: Physical activity of man and hypokinesia (in Russian) Acad. Sci. USSR, Sibirian Dept. Novosibirsk 1972.
Smart J. L.: Devel. Psychol. 7:315, 1974.
Smith L. C., Dugal L. P.: Can. J. Physiol. Pharmacol. 43:852, 1965.
Sokal R. R., Rohlf J.: Biometry. W. H. Freeman Comp., San Francisco 1968, p. 239.
Spitzer J., McElroy W. T.: Amer. J. Physiol. 201:815, 1961.

Šprynarová Š.: In: Proc. IInd Int. Symp. Physical fitness of youth, Prague 1966, p. 374.
Šprynarová Š.: Acta paed. belg. 1974, Suppl. 28, p. 204.
Šprynarová Š., Pařízková J.: Čs. Fysiol. 11:217, 1962.
Šprynarová Š., Pařízková J.: J. appl. Physiol. 20:934, 1965.
Šprynarová Š., Pařízková J.: J. Sport. Med. 9:3, 1969.
Šprynarová Š., Pařízková J.: Int. Z. angew. Physiol. 29:185, 1971.
Šprynarová Š., Pařízková J.: Physiol. bohemoslov. 22:440, 1972.
Šprynarová Š., Pařízková J.: In: Proc. Int. Symp. "Physiologie de l'effort chez l'enfant", Trois Rivières, Québec, Canada 1975. In press.
Šprynarová Š., Pařízková J., Juřinová I.: In: Proc. VIth Int. Symposium Pediat. Working Physiol., Seč 1974. Ed. Scient. Comm. ČSTV, Prague 1975, p. 41.

Stern J. R., Shapiro B.: J. clin. Path. 6:158, 1953.
Stini W. A.: Amer. J. phys. Anthropol. 31:417, 1969.
Stoffel W., Chu F., Ahrens E. H.: Anal. Chem. 31:307, 1959.
Strubelt O.: Biochem. Pharmacol. 13:845, 1964.
Stuchlíková E., Faltová E., Deyl Z., Reiniš Z.: Scand. J. clin. Lab. Invest. 34 (Suppl. 141):83, 1974.
Stupin G. K.: In: Proc. VIIth Int. Congress Anthropol. Ethnolog. Sci. Moscow 1964. "Nauka", Moscow 1967. Vol. 2, p. 262.
Suchý J.: Čas. Lék. čes. 110:935, 1971.
Sukop J.: In: Proc. Scient. Comm. ČSTV (Czechoslovak Sport Org.) Prague 1966, p. 127 (in Czech).
Sulkin N. M.: In: Proc. 9th Int. Congress Gerontol. Kiev 1972. Vol. 1, p. 271.
Suzuki S.: In: Proc. Xth. Int. Congress Nutrition, Kyoto 1975. In press.
Suzuki S., Kuga T., Oshima S. et al.: Jap. J. Nutr. 19 (No. 5):1, 1961.
Szabo A. J., Opperman W., Hanover B., Gugliucci C., Szabo O.: In: Early diabetes in early life. Ed. R. A. Camerini-Davalos and H. S. Cole. Academic Press, New York 1975, p. 167.

Tanner J. M.: Growth at adolescence. 2nd ed. Blackwell Scient. Publ. Oxford 1962.
Tanner J. M.: The physique of olympic athlete. George Allen and Unwin, Ltd., London 1964.
Tanner J. M.: Nature 243:95, 1973.
Tanner J. M., Whitehouse R. H., Takaishi M.: Arch. Dis. Childh. Part I 41:454, 1966. Part II 41:613, 1966.
Tepperman J., Pearlman D.: Circulation Res. 9:576, 1961.
Tipton C. M.: Fed. Proc. 33:1947, 1974.
Tittel K., Wutscherk H.: Sportanthropometrie. Johann Ambrosius Barth, Leipzig 1972.
Tomanek R. J.: Anat. Res. 1:167, 1970.
Tremolières J.: L'obésité. Actualités diététiques. Cahiers 1970, Les Éditeurs ESF, Paris 1971a.
Tremolières J.: Infarctus et hypertension — maladies du savoir vivre. Les Éditions ESF, Paris 1971b.
Trotter M.: In: Body measurement and human nutrition. Ed. J. Brožek, Wayne Univ. Press 1956. P. 36.
Trotter M., Gleser G.: Amer. J. phys. Anthrop. 9:311, 1951.

Ulbrich J.: Med. Sportiva 24:118, 1971.
Ulbrichová M.: In: Proc. Anthrop. Conference, Olomouc 1976, in press.

Vallyathan N. V., Cherian K. M., George J. C.: J. Anim. Morph. Physiol. 12:235, 1966.
Vamberová M.: Prakt. Lék. 41:589, 1961.
Vamberová M., Pařízková J., Tejralová J.: Čs. Pediat. 17:1057, 1964.
Vamberová M., Pařízková J., Vaněčková M.: Physiol. bohemoslov. 20:415, 1971.
Viteri F. E., Alvarado J., Alleyne G. A. O.: Amer. J. clin. Nutr. 24 : 386, 1971.
Vlastovskiy V. G.: Voprosy antropologii 14:50, 1963.

Wachtlová M., Pařízková J.: Physiol. bohemoslov. 21:489, 1972.
Wahren J., Felig P., Ahlborg J., Jorgfeldt L.: Clin. Invest. 50:2715, 1971.
Walker R. N.: Ann. human Biol. 1:149, 1974.
Weiner J. S., Laurie J. A.: Human Biology. International Biological Programme, Handbook No. 9. Blackwell Scient. Publ. Oxford and Edinburgh 1969.
Wells J. B., Pařízková J., Jokl E.: J. Ass. phys. ment. Rehab. (1) 16:34, 1962; (2) 16:55, 1962; (c) 16 : 59, 1962.
Wenke M., Mühlbachová E., Hynie S.: In: Proc. 5th Nat. Congress Physiol. Soc. Karlovy Vary 1961. Ed. Academia, Prague 1963, p. 82.
Wertlake P. T., Wilcox A. A., Haley M. I., Peterson J. E.: Proc. Soc. exp. Biol. 97:163, 1958.
Wetzel N. V.: Growth. *In:* Medical Physics. The Year Book Publ., Chicago 1942, p. 513.

Widdowson E. M.: Proc. Nutr. Soc. 21:121, 1962.
Widdowson E. M., Kennedy G. S.: Proc. roy. Soc. (B) 156:96, 1962.
Widdowson E. M., McCance R. A.: Proc. roy. Soc. (B) 152:188, 1960.
Widdowson E. M., McCance R. A.: Pediat. Res. 9:154, 1975.
Widdowson E. M., Shaw W. T.: Lancet II:905, 1973.
Wilmore J. H., Haskell W. L.: J. appl. Physiol. 33:564, 1972.
Wilmore J. H., McNamara J. J.: Pediatrics 84:527, 1974.
Winkler R., Steele R., Altszuler H., deBodor C.: Amer. J. Physiol. 174:216, 1964.
Wirths W.: In: Proc. Xth Int. Congress Nutrition, Kyoto 1975. In press.
Wolański N.: Hum. Biol. 42:349, 1970.
Wolański N.: Methods of control and norms of development of children and adolescents (in Polish). Państwowy Zakład Wydawnictw lekarskich, Warszawa 1975.
Wolański N., Pařízková J.: Physical fitness and development of man (in Polish). Sport i turystyka, Warszawa 1976.
Wolf J. V., Doležal J., Luxa J.: J. appl. Physiol. 29:51, 1970.
Wright I. S.: In: Proc. 9th Int. Congress Geront. Kiev 1972. Vol. 1, p. 64.
Wurtman R. J., Axelrod J.: Biochem. Pharmacol. 12:1439, 1963.

Yakovlev N. N., Korobkov A. V., Yananis S. V.: Physiological and biochemical basis of sport training (in Czech). Státní tělovýchovné nakladatelství, Prague 1962.
Young Ch., Blondin J., Tensuan R., Fryer J. H.: Ann. N.Y. Acad. Sci. 110:589, 1963.
Young D. R., Price R.: J. appl. Physiol. 16:351, 1961.

Zamenhof S., VanMarthens E., Grauel L.: Nutr. Rep. Int. 7:371, 1973.
Zhdanova A. G., Pařízková J.: Teoriya i praktika fizicheskoy kultury i sporta 9:27, 1962.
Zook D. F.: Amer. J. Dis. Child. 1347, 1938.